Kidney Diseases and Renal Replacement Therapies

Guest Editors

MARK J. ACIERNO, MBA, DVM
MARY ANNA LABATO, DVM

VETERINARY CLINICS OF NORTH AMERICA: SMALL ANIMAL PRACTICE

www.vetsmall.theclinics.com

January 2011 • Volume 41 • Number 1

SAUNDERS an imprint of ELSEVIER, Inc.

W.B. SAUNDERS COMPANY
A Division of Elsevier Inc.

1600 John F. Kennedy Blvd. ● Suite 1800 ● Philadelphia, PA 19103-2899
http://www.vetsmall.theclinics.com

VETERINARY CLINICS OF NORTH AMERICA: SMALL ANIMAL PRACTICE Volume 41, Number 1
January 2011 ISSN 0195-5616, ISBN-13: 978-1-4557-0524-5

Editor: John Vassallo; j.vassallo@elsevier.com
Developmental Editor: Donald Mumford

Veterinary Clinics of North America: Small Animal Practice (ISSN 0195-5616) is published bimonthly (For Post Office use only: volume 41 issue 1 of 6) by Elsevier Inc., 360 Park Avenue South, New York, NY 10010-1710. Months of issue are January, March, May, July, September, and November. Business and Editorial Offices: 1600 John F. Kennedy Blvd., Ste. 1800, Philadelphia, PA 19103-2899. Customer Service Office: 3251 Riverport Lane, Maryland Heights, MO 63043. Periodicals postage paid at New York, NY and additional mailing offices. Subscription prices are $262.00 per year (domestic individuals), $427.00 per year (domestic institutions), $128.00 per year (domestic students/residents), $347.00 per year (Canadian individuals), $525.00 per year (Canadian institutions), $385.00 per year (international individuals), $525.00 per year (international institutions), and $186.00 per year (international and Canadian students/residents). To receive student/resident rate, orders must be accompanied by name of affiliated institution, date of term, and the *signature* of program/residency coordinator on institution letterhead. Orders will be billed at individual rate until proof of status is received. Foreign air speed delivery is included in all *Clinics* subscription prices. All prices are subject to change without notice. **POSTMASTER:** Send address changes to *Veterinary Clinics of North America: Small Animal Practice*, Elsevier Health Sciences Division, Subscription Customer Service, 3251 Riverport Lane, Maryland Heights, MO 63043. Customer Service (orders, claims, on-line, change of address): Elsevier Periodicals Customer Service, Elsevier Health Sciences Division Subscription Customer Service 3251 Riverport Lane Maryland Heights, MO 63043. Tel: 1-800-654-2452 (U.S. and Canada); 314-447-8871 (outside U.S. and Canada). Fax: 314-447-8029. E-mail: journalscustomerservice-usa@elsevier.com (for print support); journalsonlinesupport-usa@elsevier.com (for online support).

Reprints. For copies of 100 or more of articles in this publication, please contact the Commercial Reprints Department, Elsevier Inc., 360 Park Avenue South, New York, NY 10010-1710. Tel.: 212-633-3812; Fax: 212-462-1935; E-mail: reprints@elsevier.com.

Veterinary Clinics of North America: Small Animal Practice is also published in Japanese by Inter Zoo Publishing Co., Ltd., Aoyama Crystal-Bldg 5F, 3-5-12 Kitaaoyama, Minato-ku, Tokyo 107-0061, Japan.

Veterinary Clinics of North America: Small Animal Practice is covered in *Current Contents/Agriculture, Biology and Environmental Sciences, Science Citation Index, ASCA, MEDLINE/PubMed (Index Medicus), Excerpta Medica,* and *BIOSIS.*

Printed in the United States of America.

Contributors

GUEST EDITORS

MARK J. ACIERNO, MBA, DVM
Diplomate, American College of Veterinary Internal Medicine; Associate Professor/Dialysis Service Coordinator, Companion Animal Center, School of Veterinary Medicine, Louisiana State University, Baton Rouge, Louisiana

MARY ANNA LABATO, DVM
Diplomate, American College of Veterinary Internal Medicine (Small Animal Internal Medicine); Clinical Professor, Department of Clinical Sciences, Cummings School of Veterinary Medicine, Tufts University, North Grafton, Massachusetts

AUTHORS

MARK J. ACIERNO, MBA, DVM
Diplomate, American College of Veterinary Internal Medicine; Associate Professor/Dialysis Service Coordinator, Companion Animal Center, School of Veterinary Medicine, Louisiana State University, Baton Rouge, Louisiana

CARLY ANNE BLOOM, DVM
Head, Small Animal Internal Medicine, University of Queensland School of Veterinary Science, Small Animal Hospital, St Lucia, Queensland, Australia

SERGE CHALHOUB, DVM
Renal Medicine Service, The Animal Medical Center, New York, New York

RACHEL L. COOPER, DVM
Internal Medicine Resident, Department of Clinical Sciences, Matthew J. Ryan Veterinary Hospital, University of Pennsylvania, Philadelphia, Pennsylvania

LARRY D. COWGILL, DVM, PhD
Diplomate, American College of Veterinary Internal Medicine; Professor, Department of Medicine and Epidemiology, and Associate Dean for Southern California Clinical Programs, School of Veterinary Medicine, University of California-Davis, Davis, California

DENISE A. ELLIOTT, BVSc, PhD
Diplomate, American College of Veterinary Internal Medicine; Diplomate, American College of Veterinary Nutrition; Director of Health and Nutritional Sciences: The Americas, Research and Development, Royal Canin SAS, Aimargues, France

MARY ANNA LABATO, DVM
Diplomate, American College of Veterinary Internal Medicine (Small Animal Internal Medicine); Clinical Professor, Department of Clinical Sciences, Cummings School of Veterinary Medicine, Tufts University, North Grafton, Massachusetts

CATHY E. LANGSTON, DVM
Diplomate, American College of Veterinary Internal Medicine; Renal Medicine Service, The Animal Medical Center, New York, New York

MERYL P. LITTMAN, VMD
Diplomate, American College of Veterinary Internal Medicine; Associate Professor of Medicine, Clinical Studies-Philadelphia, University of Pennsylvania School of Veterinary Medicine, Philadelphia, Pennsylvania

KELLY N. MONAGHAN, DVM
Resident, Department of Small Animal Internal Medicine, Cummings School of Veterinary Medicine, Tufts University, North Grafton, Massachusetts

KAREN POEPPEL, LVT
Renal Medicine Service, The Animal Medical Center, New York, New York

DAVID J. POLZIN, DVM, PhD
Diplomate, American College of Veterinary Internal Medicine; Professor and Chief, Department of Veterinary Clinical Sciences, Veterinary Internal Medicine, College of Veterinary Medicine, University of Minnesota, St Paul, Minnesota

LINDA ROSS, DVM, MS
Diplomate, American College of Veterinary Internal Medicine (Small Animal Internal Medicine); Associate Professor, Department of Clinical Sciences, Cummings School of Veterinary Medicine, Tufts University, North Grafton, Massachusetts

SHERI ROSS, DVM, PhD
Diplomate, American College of Veterinary Internal Medicine; Coordinator, Nephrology, Urology, Hemodialysis, University of California Veterinary Medical Center–San Diego, San Diego, California

HARRIET SYME, BVetMed, PhD, FHEA, MRCVS
Diplomate, American College of Veterinary Internal Medicine; Diplomate, European College of Veterinary Internal Medicine (Companion Animal); Senior Lecturer in Small Animal Internal Medicine, Department of Veterinary Clinical Sciences, Royal Veterinary College, North Mymms, Hatfield, Hertfordshire, United Kingdom

Contents

smooth and efficient patient management, whereas a poorly functioning catheter frustrates the technician, doctor, and patient. These catheters are fairly quick to place but require meticulous care for optimal function. The most common complications are thrombosis and infection. Monitoring catheter performance should be a routine part of dialysis patient care.

Several methods to prevent extracorporeal circuit clotting during hemodialysis have been used in human medicine. Unfractionated (UF) heparin remains the mainstay of anticoagulant therapy in both human and veterinary intermittent hemodialysis. Different UF heparin regimes may be used depending on the bleeding risk of the patient. In patients with active bleeding or with a recent history of surgery or hemorrhagic episodes, hemodialysis may be performed without any anticoagulation or with regional anticoagulation.

Hemodialysis is a highly technical procedure that requires specialized equipment that is not used in other areas of veterinary medicine. Certain hemodialysis-specific monitoring equipment is also employed.

Hemodialysis improves survival for animals with acute kidney injury beyond what would be expected with conventional management of the same animals. Clinical evidence and experience in human patients suggest a role for earlier intervention with renal replacement to avoid the morbidity of uremia and to promote better metabolic stability and recovery. For a large population of animal patients, it is the advanced standard for the management of acute and chronic uremia, life-threatening poisoning, and fluid overload for which there is no alternative therapy.

Renal replacement therapies (RRT) are increasingly used for the treatment of acute and chronic kidney diseases as well as intoxications and accidental drug overdoses. These therapies offer a mechanism for the removal of toxic substances from the patient's blood and supplement the standard detoxification protocols. If instituted early, RRT can have a significant effect on the course of the toxicity; however, this process is not selective for the removal of only harmful products and can also result in the clearance of medications intended for therapeutic use.

Nutritional therapy has a key role in the conservative management of renal disease. This role is even more vital with the advent of advanced renal replacement therapies to support patients with life threatening severe oliguric or anuric acute uremia or the International Renal Interest Society stage IV chronic kidney disease. Nutritional assessment and institution of nutritional support is crucial because dialysis only partially alleviates uremic anorexia. Dialytic patients have a higher risk of protein calorie, iron, zinc, vitamin B6, vitamin C, folic acid, 1,25-dihydroxycholecalciferol, and carnitine malnutritions.

THE CLINICS ARE NOW AVAILABLE ONLINE!

Access your subscription at:
www.theclinics.com

Preface

Kidney Diseases and Renal Replacement Therapies

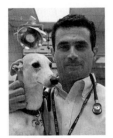 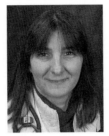

Mark J. Acierno, MBA, DVM   Mary Anna Labato, DVM
Guest Editors

We are both very excited to have had the opportunity to edit this issue of *Veterinary Clinics of North America: Small Animal Practice*. In the summer of 2009, we had a vision to enlist experts who were working on various aspects of kidney disease in order to develop a concise and up-to-date reference that would be suitable for both the general practitioner as well as those working in more specialized areas of nephrology. One and a half years later, this issue is the realization of that vision. The initial articles present the latest information in the pathogenesis, diagnosis and treatment of acute kidney injury, chronic kidney injury, proteinuria, and hypertension. Later articles cover increasingly advanced aspects of renal replacement therapy.

Perhaps the most humbling aspect of working on this issue was realizing how far we have come in the treatment of kidney disease; however, at the same time, we understand that there is so much more to learn. When we started out in veterinary medicine, understanding and treatment of kidney disease were relatively limited. There was fluid therapy, dietary management, and very little else in the way to alleviate the clinical signs or slow the progression of disease. Since that time, increasing advanced treatment modalities, including renal replacement therapies, have become available. Even the names of the diseases have changed as our understanding of the processes has become more sophisticated with acute renal failure becoming acute kidney injury and chronic renal failure becoming chronic kidney disease. At the same time, there is still much work to be done before we fully understand the physiology of kidney disease and how to arrest or even reverse its damaging effects.

We would like to thank those who have contributed to this issue, to whom we owe a debt of gratitude. It is an honor to have colleagues such as these and it is their hard work that has produced a reference that is suitable for readers interested in providing

Vet Clin Small Anim 41 (2011) xi–xii
doi:10.1016/j.cvsm.2010.12.003
0195-5616/11/$ – see front matter © 2011 Elsevier Inc. All rights reserved.

vetsmall.theclinics.com

their clinical cases the best possible care as well as those interested in the more advanced aspects of veterinary nephrology. We would also like to acknowledge the staff at Elsevier, especially John Vassallo, for all their assistance.

Mark J. Acierno, MBA, DVM
School of Veterinary Medicine
The Louisiana State University
Skip Bertman Drive
Baton Rouge, LA 70803, USA

Mary Anna Labato, DVM
Small Animal Medicine
Department of Clinical Sciences
Cummings School of Veterinary Medicine
Tufts University
200 Westboro Road
North Grafton, MA 01536, USA

E-mail addresses:
dialysis@vetmed.lsu.edu (M.J. Acierno)
mary.labato@tufts.edu (M.A. Labato)

Acute Kidney Injury in Dogs and Cats

Linda Ross, DVM, MS

KEYWORDS

• Acute kidney injury • Oliguria • Glomerular filtration rate

Acute kidney injury (AKI) has 4 stages. The first, or initiation phase, occurs during and immediately after the insult to the kidneys when pathologic damage to the kidney is initiated. The second stage is the extension phase, during which ischemia, hypoxia, inflammation, and cellular injury continue, leading to cellular apoptosis, necrosis, or both. Clinical and laboratory abnormalities may not be evident during the first 2 stages. The third stage, or maintenance phase, is characterized by azotemia, uremia, or both and may last for days to weeks. Oliguria (<0.5 mL urine per kg body weight per hour) or anuria (no urine production) may occur during this stage, although urine production is highly variable. The fourth stage is recovery, during which time azotemia improves and renal tubules undergo repair. Marked polyuria may occur during this stage as a result of partial restoration of renal tubular function and of osmotic diuresis of accumulated solutes. Renal function may return to normal, or the animal may be left with residual renal dysfunction. Nonazotemic renal failure can occur and is characterized by abnormalities similar to those seen during the polyuric recovery phase of AKI.[1,2]

There are many potential causes of AKI in dogs and cats (**Box 1**). Because the prognosis and outcome have been shown to be heavily dependent on the cause, every attempt should be made to identify the cause as early as possible in the management of the case.[3,4]

PATHOPHYSIOLOGY

The decrease in renal function that occurs with AKI is multifactorial and includes decreased intrarenal blood flow (RBF) and cellular damage. Ischemia causes a rapid degradation of intracellular adenosine triphosphate (ATP) to adenosine diphosphate and adenosine monophosphate (AMP). AMP may be further degraded to other adenine nucleotides that diffuse out of cells, preventing ATP resynthesis. Decreased intracellular ATP leads to several metabolic and structural changes within renal tubular cells. It causes an increase in intracellular calcium, which may activate proteases and phospholipases, with subsequent cellular damage. It also results in decreased activity of Na^+K^+-ATPase, which can alter the intracellular concentration gradient. This can

Department of Clinical Sciences, Cummings School of Veterinary Medicine, Tufts University, 200 Westboro Road, North Grafton, MA 01536, USA
E-mail address: linda.ross@tufts.edu

Vet Clin Small Anim 41 (2011) 1–14
doi:10.1016/j.cvsm.2010.09.003
0195-5616/11/$ – see front matter © 2011 Elsevier Inc. All rights reserved.

Box 1
Common causes of AKI in the dog and cat

Ischemia

Infarction

Toxins

    Ethylene glycol

    Heavy metals

    Organic compounds

    Grapes or raisins[a]

    Hemoglobinuria/myoglobinuria

    Lily plant[b]

    Envenomation (eg, snake, bee, wasp, bull ants)

    Melamine/cyanuric acid

Infectious diseases

    Pyelonephritis

    Leptospirosis[a]

Drugs

    Aminoglycoside antibiotics

    Amphotericin B

    Cisplatin

    Nonsteroidal anti-inflammatory drugs

    Radiographic contrast agents

Hypercalcemia

    Calciferol-containing rodenticides

    Human dermatologic preparations containing vitamin D analogues

Hyperviscosity

    Hyperglobulinemia

    Polycythemia

Multiple organ dysfunction syndrome

Sepsis

Acute pancreatitis

[a] Reported only in dogs.
[b] Reported only in cats.

---

result in movement of water into the cell and cell swelling, which may contribute to tubular obstruction.[2,5] The breakdown of other substances may result in the generation of hydrogen peroxide and superoxide. Ischemia induces nitric oxide synthase in renal tubular cells. Nitric oxide can react with superoxide to form peroxynitrite, which in turn can directly oxidize molecules, such as lipids and sulfhydryls. Also, peroxynitrite can inhibit renal tubular cell-matrix attachment, delaying recovery of tubular epithelial regeneration.[6,7]

The renal tubular cellular cytoskeleton undergoes significant changes with ischemia. Microvillar actin cores disassemble, resulting in loss of apical microvilli. Cells lose their polarity, resulting in altered solute trafficking. Na^+K^+-ATPase dissociates from its normal location on the basolateral plasma membrane (where it is anchored by the actin cytoskeleton) and is redistributed to the apical cell membrane. This alters proximal tubular sodium handling and results in an increased fraction of filtered sodium reaching the macula densa. The resulting afferent arteriolar constriction as the result of tubuloglomerular feedback leads to decreased glomerular filtration rate (GFR). Tight junction integrity is lost, affecting the "gate" and "fence" functions of this structure; this may contribute to the "backleak" phenomenon in AKI. Integrins are heterodimeric glycoproteins that mediate cell-cell adhesion. With ischemia, they redistribute from the basal to the apical tubular cell membrane. This results in loss of anchorage of tubular cells to the basement membrane and cell desquamation. Expression of integrin receptors may result in clumping of desquamated cells and adherence to the apical cell membrane of intact tubular cells, contributing to tubular obstruction.[2,6,8]

The inflammatory response is now believed to play a major role in AKI. Neutrophil activation, resulting in the release of inflammatory mediators, plays an important role in renal ischemia/reperfusion injury. Neutrophils adhere to endothelial cells, mediated, at least in part, by adhesion molecules P-selectin and intracellular adhesion molecule I. They migrate into the interstitium, resulting in changes in vascular permeability and endothelial and renal tubular cell integrity. Capillary plugging may be caused by neutrophil accumulation along with platelets and red blood cells. Neutrophils also release proteases and cytokines, exaggerating the inflammatory response.[6,9–11]

In humans, the mortality rate from AKI remains high (50%–60%), despite the availability of dialysis.[8] Death in these patients is frequently the result of distant organ damage secondary to AKI and/or uremia. Acute lung injury (ALI) in patients with AKI is common, and mortality of people with both AKI and ALI increases to 80%.[8] The mechanism of ALI is not well understood and is an area of current research. Studies have shown an increase in circulating cytokines in animals with AKI, including the proinflammatory cytokines interleukin-6 and interleukin-1β.[12,13] Others have demonstrated upregulation of certain lung genes that involve proinflammatory and proapoptotic pathways in rodents with AKI.[14,15] Neurologic dysfunction, including abnormal mentation, obtundation, and seizures are seen in people with AKI. Experimental studies in rodents have found increased neuronal pyknosis and microgliosis and elevated levels of proinflammatory cytokines (keratinocyte-derived chemoattractant and granulocyte colony-stimulating factor (G-CSF) in the brain.[16] Other possible mechanisms of neurologic dysfunction include AKI-induced changes in the blood-brain barrier, allowing passage of cytokines and uremic toxins, such as guanidine compounds and indoxyl sulfate.[17,18]

Necrosis is the process by which cells die acutely and is characterized by rapid metabolic collapse, cell swelling, and loss of plasma membrane integrity. Cell rupture results in release of proteolytic enzymes, which then incite inflammation. Apoptosis, or programmed cell death, is an active, energy-dependent process in which affected cells detach and nuclear chromatin becomes condensed while the plasma membrane remains intact. Eventually, the cell disintegrates into membrane-bound vesicles containing cell debris, including condensed chromatin, called apoptotic bodies. Phagocytic cells can recognize and ingest apoptotic bodies or even entire apoptotic cells Apoptosis usually occurs without inciting tissue injury or inflammation. In AKI, tubular necrosis is known to occur as a result of ischemia and toxic injury. However, apoptosis of renal tubular cells also occurs. It seems that less severe insults may result in apoptosis, whereas those that are more severe cause necrosis. Different types of renal insults may produce necrosis or apoptosis or may cause either to occur in different portions of the renal tubule. For example, apoptosis can occur as the result of some endotoxins, gentamicin, and cyclosporine. Lower doses of cisplatin cause apoptosis, whereas higher doses result in necrosis. A *second wave* of tubular cell apoptosis seems to occur during the recovery phase of acute renal failure, which may play a part in the tubule remodeling process by limiting proliferation of regenerating cells.[8,19]

DIAGNOSIS

Although AKI is defined as the rapid loss of nephron function, exact criteria defining the decrease in renal function and the duration of loss have not been well defined in animals. In humans, a recent classification scheme has been proposed to address this issue (RIFLE: risk, injury, failure, loss, end-stage renal disease; **Table 1**).[20] Unfortunately, it is difficult to apply to veterinary patients, because pre-AKI information about serum creatinine concentration and urine output are rarely available. A scoring system using various laboratory and clinical parameters for outcome prediction in dogs with AKI that underwent hemodialysis has recently been described.[4] Further studies are needed to validate this system in other settings.

Examination of the animal with AKI should include a clinical estimate of hydration, assessment of cardiovascular status, evaluation of renal or abdominal pain, and measurement of arterial blood pressure. Diagnostic imaging is indicated for the assessment of renal size and shape and the presence of uroliths. Abdominal radiographs allow evaluation of renal size (normal length as measured on the ventrodorsal view is 2.5 to 3.5 times the length of the second lumber vertebra in dogs and 2 to 3 times, in cats); identification of radio-opaque uroliths (especially feline ureteroliths); and assessment of the amount of urine in the bladder. Ultrasonography may be performed in addition to or instead of radiography, yielding more precise measurements of renal size, determination of the echogenicity of the renal parenchyma, and identification of cysts or masses in the kidneys. Pyelectasia (dilation of the renal pelvis) may

Table 1		
RIFLE classification scheme for AKI		
	GFR Criteria	**Urine Output Criteria**
Risk	Increased SCreat × 1.5 or GFR decrease >25%	<0.5 mL/kg/h × 6 h
Injury	Increased SCreat × 2 or GFR decrease >50%	<0.5 mL/kg/h × 12 h
Failure	Increased SCreat × 3 or GFR decrease >75% or SCreat ≥4 mg/dL or Acute increase in SCreat ≥0.5 mg/dL	<0.3 mL/kg/h × 24 h or anuria × 12 h
Loss	Persistent acute renal failure; complete loss of kidney function >4 wk	
End-Stage Renal Disease	End-stage renal disease >3 mo	

Abbreviation: SCreat, serum creatinine concentration.

be seen with pyelonephritis and diffuse thickening of the cortex, with lymphosarcoma; an echogenic "rim" at the corticomedullary junction may be seen with ethylene glycol toxicity; abnormal subcapsular fluid accumulation can be seen with inflammation, infection, toxicity (ethylene glycol, lily), or neoplasia (feline lymphoma). Intravenous urography (IVU) is usually not beneficial in identifying causes of AKI, with the exception of ureteral obstruction by uroliths in cats. Animals with a serum creatinine concentration greater than 4 mg/dL should not have a diagnostic IVU, because they lack sufficient renal function to excrete and concentrate the contrast medium; also, iodinated contrast media are potentially nephrotoxic. Computerized tomography and magnetic resonance imaging do not usually provide more information than ultrasonography and have the disadvantage of requiring general anesthesia.

Initial laboratory evaluation should include a complete blood count, serum biochemistry profile, assessment of acid-base status, urinalysis, and urine culture. Additional serum and urine should be saved in case further tests are necessary. Leukocytosis may indicate an infectious cause of AKI. Blood urea nitrogen (BUN) and creatinine may be elevated, but AKI should not be ruled out if azotemia is not present. Sodium concentration may be low, normal, or high depending on the disease process, degree of vomiting and/or diarrhea, and any prior therapy. Hyperkalemia occurs primarily in animals that are in the oliguric or anuric phase of AKI. Other causes of azotemia and hyperkalemia, such as hypoadrenocorticism (Addison's disease) and postrenal azotemia, must be differentiated from AKI. Serum calcium levels are usually normal in the absence of hypercalcemia-induced AKI; hypocalcemia may occur in animals with ethylene glycol toxicity. Serum phosphorus levels are often elevated; however, the degree of elevation may reflect the degree of reduced GFR rather than the duration of disease. Metabolic acidosis is often present. Urinalysis shows isosthenuria with AKI, whereas a prerenal cause of the azotemia may be suspected with an increased urine specific gravity. Measurement of urinary electrolytes and/or creatinine can help distinguish prerenal from primary renal azotemia. Animals with prerenal azotemia but normal renal function retain sodium and chloride while excreting creatinine; those with AKI have increased urinary levels of sodium and chloride while retaining creatinine (**Table 2**).[21] Mild-to-moderate glucosuria may be seen with acute tubular damage, and microscopic hematuria can occur with glomerular or tubular damage. Urine pH level is usually acidic, although it may be alkaline in the presence of some bacterial urinary tract infections. The urine sediment should be carefully examined for the presence of casts, white blood cells, bacteria, and crystals.[1]

Tests to identify specific causes of AKI should be performed as appropriate to the animal. Serum ethylene glycol levels can be measured with a rapid in-house test (EGT Test Kit, PRN Pharmacal, Pensacola, FL, USA). This kit detects intact ethylene glycol molecules, and negative results may occur with low blood levels or if sufficient time has passed since ingestion such that all of the intact ethylene glycol has been metabolized. False-positive results can occur if the animal has received drugs containing

Table 2 Selected urinary parameters in prerenal azotemia and AKI		
Test	**Prerenal**	**AKI**
Urine sodium	<20 mEq/L	>40 mEq/L
Urine chloride	<20 mEq/L	>40 mEq/L
Urine creatinine/plasma creatinine	>40	<20
Fractional excretion of sodium	<1%	>2%

propylene glycol, such as some activated charcoal products, injectable diazepam, and etomidate, or ingested nontoxic antifreeze containing propylene glycol instead of ethylene glycol.[2,22] Serum levels of intact ethylene glycol or its metabolites can be measured by some medical laboratories. In the absence of blood levels, metabolic acidosis with an elevated anion gap supports a diagnosis of ethylene glycol toxicity. Animals with hypercalcemia suspected to be due to ingestion of rodenticides or vitamin D supplements should have serum cholecalciferol levels measured. All dogs with AKI living in endemic areas should initially be suspected of having leptospirosis.[1,23] Microscopic agglutination titers for the most common infecting serovars should be submitted. Vaccination can produce a low titer, and there is some cross-reactivity between serovars; however, a single titer of 1:800 or greater in conjunction with appropriate clinical signs has been considered diagnostic.[24] Titer results may be negative early in the course of disease, and in the absence of other causes, leptospirosis should not be ruled out until convalescent titers performed 2 to 4 weeks later also have negative results. A recent study found that dogs most often had positive titer results, defined as 1:1600 or greater, to serovars Autumnalis, Grippotyphosa, Pomona, and Brastislava; although titers to Autumnalis may indicate cross-reactivity with other serovars rather than actual infection.[23] Fluorescent antibody testing for leptospires can be performed on blood, urine, or tissue. More recently, polymerase chain reaction (PCR) testing has become available for early diagnosis. However, the sensitivity and specificity of PCR testing is not yet known, and false negatives can occur if the dog has received antibiotics before testing.[25] Serologic screening can be performed if other infectious diseases are suspected.

Histopathologic examination of renal tissue yields the most definitive information about the chronicity of the disease process but does not necessarily identify a specific cause. Because much of the therapy for AKI is the same regardless of cause, renal biopsy is indicated only when the results would change therapy or prognosis. The benefit should also be weighed against the risks of biopsy. An ultrasound-guided biopsy performed under injectable anesthesia may be the safest for the animal, although biopsies obtained via laparoscopy or laparotomy are also options. A renal aspirate is useful only when lymphosarcoma is suspected, although false-negative results may occur even in the presence of malignancy.[1]

TREATMENT

Treatment of AKI consists of specific therapy for the cause, as well as supportive therapy based on the stage of acute renal failure and the animal's fluid, electrolyte, and acid-base status.

Specific Therapy

Specific therapy to correct or eliminate the cause of AKI should be instituted if the cause is known or suspected. Vomiting should be induced in animals with known recent toxin ingestion, such as ethylene glycol, or lilies in cats. Animals that have been exposed to toxins should receive an antidote if available. Those that have ingested ethylene glycol should receive 4-methylpyrazole or ethanol to prevent the metabolism of ethylene glycol to its toxic components. The renal excretion of intact ethylene glycol can be enhanced by intravenous fluid diuresis. Intact ethylene glycol and its metabolite glycolic acid can be removed by hemodialysis.[26] In geographic areas where leptospirosis occurs, all dogs with presumed AKI should receive antibiotics effective against leptospires (penicillin, amoxicillin, or doxycycline). Empiric therapy with an antibiotic that is primarily excreted by the kidneys is indicated until pyelonephritis is ruled out.

Supportive Therapy

Fluid therapy

Correction and maintenance of the animal's hydration, acid-base, and electrolyte status are the mainstays of treatment of AKI. Intravenous (IV) fluid therapy is almost always required. Placement of a catheter in the jugular vein allows monitoring of central venous pressure and more precise assessment of intravascular volume status. However, if hemodialysis is a treatment option, the jugular veins should not be used for IV catheters or even venipuncture for blood samples; rather, they should be preserved for placement of the hemodialysis catheter. Frequent monitoring is essential for making appropriate adjustments in therapy, including clinical assessment of hydration, mucous membrane capillary refill time, heart and respiratory rate, arterial blood pressure, packed cell volume and plasma total solids, and serum chemistry parameters, including BUN, creatinine, sodium, potassium, chloride, and phosphorus.

The initial volume of fluid to be administered should be calculated based on the animal's body weight and degree of hydration. Water deficits should be replaced within 4 to 6 hours to restore RBF to normal as soon as possible. Maintenance fluid requirements must be met (44–66 mL/kg/d), as well as estimated fluid losses from causes such as vomiting and diarrhea. An isotonic, polyionic fluid, such as lactated Ringer's solution (LRS) or Plasma-Lyte A (Baxter, Deerfield, IL, USA) may be administered initially. If hyperkalemia is present or suspected because of oliguria or anuria, a potassium-free fluid, such as 0.9% sodium chloride, may be indicated. Following rehydration, the type of fluid should be adjusted based on the animal's fluid and electrolyte status.[1,2,27,28] Continued administration of fluids high in sodium relative to maintenance needs may lead to hypernatremia, especially in cats. Fluids containing less sodium, such as half-strength LRS or 0.45% sodium in 2.5% dextrose, may be used in these animals for longer maintenance therapy.[28] Traditionally, IV fluids have been administered at as high a rate as the animal can tolerate without adverse signs, with the goal of maximizing GFR and RBF and increasing elimination of metabolic waste products. However, increasing fluid administration does not necessarily equate to increased urinary excretion of such substances. In humans, recent studies have concluded that fluid overload is associated with adverse consequences and decreased survival; mortality decreased when fluid overload was corrected by dialysis.[29,30] Although similar studies in clinical veterinary patients have not been published, it would seem reasonable that avoiding fluid overload would similarly be beneficial, especially because dialysis is not readily available to many practices. The primary reason for fluid overload is failure to adjust the fluid administration rate in the face of decreased urine production.

Assessing urine output is one of the most important and probably the most neglected aspects of monitoring animals with AKI. Placement of an indwelling urinary catheter is the most accurate method for monitoring urine volume. However, the benefits of an indwelling catheter must be weighed against the risks of ascending infection, and in cats, sedation or anesthesia to place the catheter.[31] The risk of infection can be reduced by scrupulous attention to sterile placement of the catheter, maintenance of a closed collection system, and daily cleaning of the visible portions of the catheter with disinfectant. Because the incidence of catheter-induced infections increases rapidly after 3 days, changing the urinary catheter every 2 to 3 days may be beneficial.[31]

Management of oliguria or anuria

Once the animal has been hydrated, urine flow should rapidly increase to 2 to 5 mL/kg/h, depending on the rate of IV fluid administration. If urine production is not sufficient, the following steps should be taken. First, the clinician should reassess the animal's hydration status, including arterial blood pressure and central venous pressure (jugular catheters should be avoided if hemodialysis is a possibility). Decreased circulating blood volume can result in decreased GFR and an appropriate decrease in urine volume. If the animal is normally hydrated or volume overloaded, the rate of fluid administration should be slowed to prevent further fluid overload and associated adverse effects. An indwelling urinary catheter should be placed if not already present. Calculation of the "ins and outs" can then be used to provide appropriate quantities of IV fluids to match urine output. The maintenance fluid requirement (estimated at 22 mL/kg/d for insensible losses) is calculated for a short interval of time, typically 4 hours. An estimate of the amount of fluid lost due to vomiting, diarrhea, or other loss is added. The volume of urine produced during the previous time interval is added to the maintenance amount, giving the volume of IV fluids to be administered over the subsequent 4-hour period. This regimen helps maintain hydration while minimizing the risk of fluid overload.[1,2]

Specific therapy to increase urine flow is the next step (**Table 1**). Furosemide, a loop diuretic, is the first drug to be administered. Although furosemide may increase urine output by acting on renal tubules, it does not increase GFR or improve outcome. Its value lies in increasing urine output so that IV fluid therapy to correct acid-base and electrolyte imbalances can continue. Traditionally, furosemide has been administered as a bolus at an initial dose of 2 mg/kg IV, with escalating doses to 4–6 mg/kg at hourly intervals if the initial dose fails to increase urine production. However, a loading dose of 0.66 mg/kg followed by continuous rate infusion (CRI) at 0.66 mg/kg/h has been shown to be more effective in producing diuresis in normal dogs.[32] A CRI of 0.5 to 1.0 mg/kg/h is the currently recommended protocol.[1,2]

If furosemide administration fails to increase urine production, osmotic diuresis can be attempted. A 20% mannitol solution can be given as a bolus dose of 0.5 to 1.0 g/kg body weight over 15 to 20 minutes. If effective, urine flow increases within one hour. Repeat bolus doses can then be administered every 4 to 6 hours, or it can be administered as a CRI at a dosage of 1–2 mg/kg/min. Dosages greater than 2 to 4 gm/kg/d can actually cause AKI and should be avoided. Mannitol may have additional beneficial effects in addition to its action as a diuretic. It inhibits renin release because of its hyperosmolar effect on tubular luminal filtrate. Also, it acts as a free radical scavenger, blunts damaging increases in intramitochondrial calcium, and may result in a beneficial release of atrial natriuretic peptide.[1,2,28,33,34] Because mannitol is not metabolized, its effects remain in the intravascular space longer than those of dextrose. Administration of hypertonic solutions are contraindicated in oliguric animals that are volume overloaded because they result in increased serum osmolality, circulating blood volume, and blood pressure. Alternatively, a 20% dextrose solution can be given at 2 to 10 mL/min for the first 10 to 15 minutes, followed by a rate of 1 to 5 mL/min for a total daily dose of 22 to 66 mL/kg. Administration of hypertonic dextrose should be alternated with a polyionic solution to prevent dehydration from osmotic diuresis. Urine should be monitored for glucose to determine the effectiveness of this therapy.[1]

Administration of dopamine has traditionally been recommended for oliguric or anuric animals. Dopamine stimulates 2 types of dopamine receptors (DA-1 and DA-2) as well as α- and β-adrenergic receptors. In normal dogs, it causes an increase in RBF and urine volume; GFR increases or is unchanged. Studies in experimental models of canine AKI have shown conflicting results regarding improvement in RBF and/or sodium excretion.[35] In normal cats, increased urine production can occur in the absence of increases in RBF or GFR, possibly due to α-adrenergic stimulation that increases cardiac output and blood pressure and induces natriuresis.[28] Although it was thought for some time that cats lacked renal dopamine receptors, one study detected a putative DA-1 receptor in the feline renal cortex.[36] Dopamine is no longer considered to have a role in the prevention or treatment of AKI in humans based on several meta-analyses that failed to show a clinical benefit in survival or need for dialysis.[37,38] There is little or no documentation on the efficacy of dopamine in dogs and cats with AKI, and its routine use to increase urine production in oliguric or anuric AKI cannot be justified.

In contrast, fenoldopam, a selective DA-1 agonist, has been found to be renoprotective in humans. A meta-analysis of humans undergoing cardiovascular surgery found that fenoldopam consistently and significantly reduced the need for renal replacement therapy and in-hospital death.[39] Another study found that humans who received fenoldopam while undergoing complex cardiac surgical procedures had a significantly lower rate of postsurgery AKI than those who received a placebo.[40] In animals, one experimental study in healthy cats found that an infusion of 0.5 mcg/kg/min produced more diuresis than dopamine.[41] However, a study in experimental dogs undergoing nephrotomy showed no difference in GFR or urine volume between dogs receiving fenoldopam or saline.[42] No clinical studies have been reported in dogs or cats with AKI, and its role in the management of oliguric AKI is not yet known.

One study reported that administration of diltiazem for therapy of dogs with AKI from leptospirosis resulted in increased urine output and more rapid reduction of serum creatinine, although the differences were not statistically significant.[43] The rationale for using diltiazem is that it is thought to reverse renal vasoconstriction via preglomerular vasodilation, inhibit tubuloglomerular-feedback-induced preglomerular vasoconstriction, and cause natriuresis independent of GFR. In humans, diltiazem has been used to treat or prevent AKI associated with cardiovascular surgery and renal transplantation.

If pharmacologic measures fail to increase urine output or improve azotemia and uremia, renal replacement therapy is indicated.

Management of polyuria
Animals that recover from the oliguric or anuric phase of AKI or those that have milder renal injury and do not become azotemic often have profound polyuria for days to weeks. These animals can develop electrolyte abnormalities, especially hyponatremia and hypokalemia, that need to be corrected with IV or, sometimes, oral therapy. Frequent monitoring of serum electrolytes and adjustment of therapy should be performed until urine output decreases and renal function and serum electrolyte concentrations stabilize.

Correction of acid-base and electrolyte abnormalities
Metabolic acidosis may occur in animals with AKI. Alkalinizing therapy is not recommended unless the blood pH level is less than 7.2 or the serum bicarbonate level is less than 14 mEq/L after correcting fluid deficits. Such therapy can result in significant complications, including paradoxical CSF acidosis, decreased ionized serum calcium level, and hypernatremia. If necessary, the bicarbonate deficit is calculated as follows:

Body weight (kg) x 0.3 x (24: measured bicarbonate) = mEq bicarbonate deficit. One-quarter of the deficit is administered over 12 hours and acid-base status reassessed before further administration.

Moderate to severe, life-threatening hyperkalemia may occur if the animal is oliguric or anuric. The first and most important step in therapy for hyperkalemia is to ensure urine production and excretion. Animals with severe hyperkalemia or those with persisting oliguria may benefit from additional specific therapy, such as with sodium bicarbonate, regular insulin and glucose, or, in life-threatening situations, calcium gluconate.

Treatment of other uremic complications

Vomiting Vomiting is one of the most common signs of uremia in animals with AKI. The cause of vomiting is multifactorial; it is centrally mediated by uremic toxins that act on the chemoreceptor trigger zone and locally mediated by uremic gastritis. Hypergastrinemia occurs in animals with decreased renal function and may contribute to increased gastric acidity and associated inflammation.[44] Drugs that inhibit gastric acid production may be beneficial, including histamine receptor antagonists, such as famotidine (0.5–1.0 mg/kg every 24 hours [q24h] by mouth [PO]), and proton pump inhibitors, such as omeprazole (Prilosec; 0.7 mg/kg q24h PO), or lansoprazole (Prevacid; 0.6–1.0 mg/kg q24h IV). Centrally acting antiemetics may also be necessary in some animals. Maropitant (Cerenia) is a neurokinin-1 (NK-1) receptor antagonist that has efficacy against peripheral and centrally mediated vomiting. The dose is 1 mg/kg subcutaneous (SQ) or 2 mg/kg PO once daily for up to 5 days. Metoclopramide, a dopamine antagonist, may be given as intermittent therapy at a dose of 0.2 to 0.5 mg/kg every 8 hours [q8h] IV or as a CRI at 1-2 mg/kg/d IV. Other centrally acting drugs include dolasetron (Anzemet; 0.6 mg/kg q24h PO or SQ or diluted in compatible IV fluid and administered over 15 minutes IV) and ondansetron (Zofran; 0.1–0.2 mg/kg q8h SQ or 0.5 mg/kg IV loading dose, then 0.5 mg/kg/h CRI). Phenothiazine-derivative antiemetics, such as chlorpromazine (0.2–0.5 mg/kg every 6–8 hours SQ, intramuscular, or IV) can be tried if vomiting persists despite other therapy. Side effects of phenothiazines include sedation and decreased blood pressure.

Hypertension Arterial hypertension is common in animals with AKI and may be exacerbated by overhydration.[26] Treatment includes reducing the rate of IV fluid administration, administration of diuretics, and dialysis to remove excess fluid if the animal is oliguric or anuric. Pharmacologic treatment is limited because most antihypertensive drugs are only available in oral formulations, and the vomiting associated with AKI often precludes oral medication. If hypertension is severe, parenteral antihypertensives may be necessary; however, these require very close monitoring of blood pressure. Such drugs include nitroprusside (initial dose 1–2 mcg/kg/min CRI IV; titrating the dose up every 5 minutes to achieve desired blood pressure) or hydralazine (0.5–3 mg/kg every 12 hours IV or 0.1 mg/kg loading dose IV, then 1.5–5 mcg/kg/min CRI IV). In the blood, nitroprusside releases cyanide through a nonenzymatic breakdown process. Cyanide is metabolized by the liver to form additional toxic metabolites (eg, thiocyanate) that must be cleared by the kidney. Seizures, coma, permanent neurologic dysfunction, and death have been documented in human AKI patients treated with nitroprusside. Oral antihypertensives include amlodipine (Norvasc; 0.1–0.25 mg/kg every 12–24 hours [q12–24h] PO in dogs, 0.625–1.25 mg/kg q24h PO in cats) and angiotensin-converting enzyme (ACE) inhibitors, such as enalapril (0.25–0.5 mg/kg q12–24h PO) or benazepril (Lotensin; 0.25–0.5 mg/kg q24h, PO). ACE inhibitors have been associated with worsening of renal function in humans.[1]

Nutritional management Animals with AKI that are anorexic are at risk of becoming malnourished if the lack of food intake persists beyond several days. Adverse consequences associated with malnutrition include immunosuppression, decreased tissue synthesis and repair (including renal tubular cells), and altered drug metabolism.[45] Enteral nutrition, using a nasogastric esophagostomy or gastrostomy tube can be used if the animal is not vomiting; otherwise, parenteral nutrition is indicated. Detailed information on enteral and parenteral nutrition can be found elsewhere.[45–47] A recent review and meta-analysis concluded that there was insufficient evidence to support the effectiveness of nutritional support in humans with AKI.[48] However, the number of people included in this review was small (257), making it difficult to draw conclusions.

Prognosis and duration of treatment The prognosis for dogs and cats with AKI has been reported to be highly correlated with the cause.[1,2] Overall, the reported mortality rate in dogs with AKI is approximately 53% to 60%[3,4,49] and in cats, 50%.[50] Dogs with leptospirosis have a good prognosis, with reported survival of 85%. Conversely, dogs with ethylene glycol toxicity that are already azotemic when diagnosed have been shown to have a poor-to-grave prognosis, even with therapy[3,4] Other criteria that have been shown to confer a poor prognosis for dogs with AKI include severe azotemia (serum creatinine >10 mg/dL), hypocalcemia, anemia, decreased urine production, hyperphosphatemia, lack of improvement or worsening of azotemia with appropriate fluid and supportive therapy, and comorbid disorders, such as pancreatitis or sepsis.[3,4,49] For cats with AKI, hyperkalemia, hypoalbuminemia, and decreased serum bicarbonate levels at presentation were associated with decreased survival. In contrast to dogs, the degree of azotemia and serum phosphate and calcium concentrations did not predict survival.[50]

Supportive and specific treatment should be continued until one of the following occurs: (1) renal function returns to normal; (2) renal function improves and stabilizes, although not to normal levels and the animal is doing well clinically; (3) renal function worsens, fails to improve, or does not improve sufficiently for the animal to be managed medically at home for the resulting renal insufficiency. In the first 2 scenarios, fluid therapy can be tapered off and other supportive medications adjusted in response to the animal's clinical signs. In the third scenario, dialysis may be considered to support the animal for a period of time to see if renal function improves. If dialysis is not an option, euthanasia may be indicated at this point.

SUMMARY

AKI is characterized by the rapid loss of nephron function, resulting in azotemia and/or fluid, electrolyte, and acid-base abnormalities. The decrease in renal function that occurs with AKI is multifactorial and includes decreased intrarenal blood flow and cellular damage. There are many potential causes of AKI in dogs and cats.

The prognosis for dogs and cats with AKI has been correlated with the cause. Overall, the reported mortality rate in dogs with AKI is approximately 53% to 60% and in cats, 50% . If medical management fails to increase urine output or improve azotemia, renal replacement therapy is indicated.

REFERENCES

1. Ross L. Acute renal failure. In: Bonagura JD, Twedt DC, editors. Current Veterinary Therapy XIV. St. Louis (MO): Saunders Elsevier; 2009. p. 879–82.
2. Langston C. Acute uremia. In: Ettinger S, Feldman EC, editors. Textbook of Veterinary Internal Medicine. 7th edition. St. Louis (MO): Saunders Elsevier; 2010. p. 1969–85.

3. Vaden SL, Levine J, Breitschwerdt EB. A retrospective case-control of acute renal failure in 99 dogs. J Vet Intern Med 1997;11:58–64.
4. Segev G, Kass PH, Francey T. A novel clinical scoring system for outcome prediction in dogs with acute kidney injury managed by hemodialysis. J Vet Intern Med 2008;22(2):301–8.
5. Abuelo JG. Normotensive ischemic acute renal failure. N Engl J Med 2007; 357(8):797–805.
6. Devarajan P. Update on mechanisms of ischemic acute kidney injury. J Am Soc Nephrol 2006;17(6):1503–20.
7. Goligorsky MS, Noiri E. Duality of nitric oxide in acute renal injury. Seminars in Nephrology 1999;18:263–71.
8. Clarkson MR, Friedewald John J, Eustace JA, et al. Acute kidney injury. In: Brenner BM, editor. The Kidney. 8th edition. Philadelphia: Saunders Elsevier; 2008. p. 943–86.
9. Awad AS, Rouse M, Huang L, et al. Compartmentalization of neutrophils in the kidney and lung following acute ischemic kidney injury. Kidney International 2009;75:689–98.
10. Bolisetty S, Agarwal A. Neutrophils in acute kidney injury: not neutral any more. Kidney International 2009;75:674–6.
11. Akcay A, Nguyen Q, Edelstein CL. Mediators of inflammation in acute kidney injury. Mediators of Inflammation 2009;2009:137072.
12. Li X, Hassoun HT, Santora R, et al. Organ crosstalk: the role of the kidney. Curr Opin Crit Care 2009;15(6):481–7.
13. Hoke TS, Douglas IS, Klein CL, et al. Acute renal failure after bilateral nephrectomy is associated with cytokine-mediated pulmonary injury. J Am Soc Nephrol 2007;18:155–64.
14. Hassoun HT, Grigoryev DN, Lie ML, et al. Ischemic acute kidney injury induces a distant organ functional and genomic response distinguishable from bilateral nephrectomy. Am J Physiol Renal Physiol 2007;293:F30–40.
15. Grigoryev DN, Liu M, Hassoun HT, et al. The local and systemic inflammatory transcriptome after acute kidney injury. J Am Soc Nephrol 2008;19:5457–556.
16. Liu M, Liang Y, Chigurupati S, et al. Acute kidney injury leads to inflammation and functional changes in the brain. J Am Soc Nephrol 2008;19(7):1360–70.
17. Vanholder R, De Deyn PP, Van Biesen W, et al. Marconi revisited: From kidney to brain – two organ systems communicating at long distance. J Am Soc Nephrol 2008;7:1253–5.
18. Herget-Rosenthal S, Glorieux G, Jankowski J, et al. Uremic toxins in acute kidney injury. Seminars in Dialysis 2009;22(4):445–8.
19. Price PM, Safirstein RL, Megyesi J. The cell cycle and acute kidney injury. Kid Intern 2009;76(6):604–13.
20. Bellomo R, Ronco C, Kellum JA, et al. Acute renal failure—definition, outcome measures, animal models, fluid therapy and information technology needs: the Second International Consensus Conference of the Acute Dialysis Quality Initiative (ADQI) Group. Crit Care 2004;8:R204–12.
21. Waldrop JE. Urinary electrolytes, solutes, and osmolality. Vet Clin North Am Small Anim Pract 2008;38(3):503–12.
22. PRN Pharmacal. http://www.prnpharmacal.com/react/index.php. Updated 2010. Accessed August 6, 2010.
23. Gautam R, Wu CC, Guptill LE, et al. Detection of antibodies against *Leptospira* serovars via microscopic agglutination tests in dogs in the United States, 2000–2007. J Am Vet Med Assoc 2010;3:293–8.

24. Greene CE, Sykes JE, Brown CA, et al. Leptospirosis. In: Greene CE, editor. Infectious Diseases of the Dog and Cat. 3rd edition. St. Louis, MO: Saunders Elsevier; 2006. p. 402–17.
25. Online web site. IDEXX Laboratories. http://www.idexx.com/pubwebresources/pdf/en_us/smallanimal/reference-laboratories/diagnostic-updates/realpcr-canine-leptospirosis.pdf. Updated August 2009. Accessed August 6, 2010.
26. Cowgill LD, Francey T. Hemodialysis. In: DiBartola SP, editor. Fluid, electrolyte, and acid-base disorders in small animal practice. 3rd edition. St. Louis (MO): Saunders Elsevier; 2006. p. 650–77.
27. Langston C. Managing fluid and electrolyte disorders in renal failure. Vet Clin North Am Small Anim Pract 2008;38(3):677–97.
28. Chew DJ, Gieg JA. Fluid therapy during intrinsic renal failure. In: DiBartola SP, editor. Fluid, Electrolyte, and Acid-Base Disorders in Small Animal Practice. 3rd edition. St. Louis (MO): Saunders Elsevier; 2006. p. 518–40.
29. Bouchard J, Soroko SB, Chertow GM, et al. Fluid accumulation, survival, and recovery of kidney function in critically ill patients with acute kidney injury. Kidney Int 2009;76(5):422–7.
30. Prowle JR, Echeverri JE, Ligabo EV, et al. Fluid balance and acute kidney injury. Nature Reviews Nephrol 2010;6(2):107–15.
31. Barsanti JA. Urinary tract catheterization and nosocomial infections in dogs and cats. In: Proceedings of the ACVIM Forum. Anaheim CA 2010;445–7.
32. Adin DB, Taylor AW, Hill RC, et al. Intermittent bolus injection versus continuous infusion of furosemide in normal adult greyhound dogs. J Vet Intern Med 2003;17:632–6.
33. Better OS, Rubinstein RE, Winaver JM, et al. Mannitol therapy revisited (1940–1997). Kidney Int 1997;51:886–94.
34. Cowgill LD, Francey T. Acute uremia. In: Ettinger SF, Feldman EC, editors. Textbook of Veterinary Internal Medicine. 6th edition. St. Louis (MO): Elsevier Saunders; 2005. p. 1731–51.
35. Sigrist NE. Use of dopamine in acute renal failure. J Vet Emerg Crit Care 2007;17(2):117–26.
36. Flournoy WS, Wohl JS, Albrecht-Schmitt, et al. Pharmacologic identification of putative D1 dopamine receptors in feline kidneys. J Vet Pharmacol Therap 2003;26(4):283–90.
37. Kellum JA, Decker JM. Use of dopamine in acute renal failure: a meta-analysis. Crit Care Med 2001;29:1526–31.
38. Friedrich JO, Adhikari N, Herridge MS, et al. Meta-analysis: low-dose dopamine increases urine output but does not prevent renal dysfunction or death. Ann Intern Med 2005;142(7):510–24.
39. Landoni G, Biondi-Zoccai GG, Marino G, et al. Fenoldopam reduces the need for renal replacement therapy and in-hospital death in cardiovascular surgery: a meta-analysis. J Cardiothorac Vasc Anesth 2008;22(1):27–33.
40. Ranucci M, De Benedetti D, Bianchini C, et al. Effects of fenoldopam infusion in complex cardiac surgical operations: a prospective, randomized, double-blind, placebo-controlled study. Minerva Anestesiol 2010;76(4):249–59.
41. Simmons JP, Wohl JS, Schwartz DD, et al. Diuretic effects of fenoldopam in healthy cats. J Vet Emerg Crit Care 2006;16(2):96–103.
42. Zimmerman-Pope N, Waldron DR, Barber DL, et al. Effect of fenoldopam on renal function after nephrotomy in normal dogs. Vet Surg 2003;32:566–73.
43. Mathews KA, Monteith G. Evaluation of adding diltiazem therapy to standard treatment of acute renal failure caused by leptospirosis: 18 dogs (1998–2001). J Vet Emerg Crit Care 2007;17:149–58.

44. Grauer GF. Acute renal failure and chronic kidney disease. In: Nelson RW, Couto CG, editors. Small Animal Internal Medicine. 4th edition. St. Louis (MO): Mosby Elsevier; 2009. p. 645–59.

45. Saker KE, Remillard RL, et al. Critical care nutrition and enteral-assisted feeding. In: Hand MS, Thatcher CD, Remillard RL, et al, editors. Small animal clinical nutrition. 5th edition. Topeka: Kansas:Mark Morris Institute; 2010. p. 439–76.

46. Remillard RL, Saker KE. Parenteral-assisted feeding. In: Hand MS, Thatcher CD, Remillard RL, et al, editors. Small animal clinical nutrition. 5th edition. Topeka (KS): Mark Morris Institute; 2010. p. 477–98.

47. Thomovsky E, Reniker A, Backus R, et al. Parenteral nutrition: uses, indications, and compounding. Compend Contin Educ Pract Vet 2007;29(2):76–85.

48. Li Y, Tang X, Zhang J, et al. Nutritional support for acute kidney injury. Cochrane Database Syst Rev 2010;1:CD005426.

49. Behrend E, Grauer GF, Mani I, et al. Hospital-acquired acute renal failure in dogs: 29 cases (1983–1992). J Am Vet Med Assoc 1996;208:537–41.

50. Worwag S, Langston CE. Feline acute intrinsic renal failure: 32 cats (1997–2004). J Am Vet Med Assoc 2008;232:728–32.

Chronic Kidney Disease in Small Animals

David J. Polzin, DVM, PhD

KEYWORDS

• Renal failure • Chronic kidney disease • Uremia • Anemia

Chronic kidney disease (CKD) is defined as the presence of structural or functional abnormalities of one or both kidneys that have been present for an extended period, usually 3 months or longer. As is apparent from this definition, CKD may be characterized by a wide spectrum of disease, ranging from a minor structural lesion in a single kidney to extensive loss of nephrons affecting both kidneys. Thus, the clinical presentation and diagnostic and therapeutic challenges presented by patients with CKD may vary greatly from patient to patient.

RECOGNIZING AND DIAGNOSING KIDNEY DISEASE

Recognizing kidney disease requires consideration of evidence from multiple sources, including renal function tests, serum electrolyte concentrations and acid-base status, urinalysis, and renal imaging studies. Kidney disease is usually suspected on the basis of reduced kidney function or *markers* of kidney disease. Markers of kidney disease may be recognized from hematologic or serum biochemical evaluations, urinalysis, or imaging or pathology studies (**Table 1**). Findings suggestive of kidney disease may also be found by physical examination or from the medical history (eg, changes in kidney size or shape, changes in urine volume). Markers of kidney disease should be viewed as hints that kidney disease may be present and should be pursued diagnostically; they do not necessarily confirm the presence of kidney disease.

ACUTE VERSUS CHRONIC KIDNEY DISEASE

Because they differ in diagnostic, therapeutic, and prognostic implications, acute kidney injury (AKI) and CKD must be diagnostically discriminated. However, AKI and CKD may occur together in some patients (so-called acute on chronic kidney disease). In general, CKD is viewed as an irreversible disease that is often progressive, whereas AKI may be reversible.

The authors have nothing to disclose.
Department of Veterinary Clinical Sciences, Veterinary Internal Medicine, College of Veterinary Medicine, University of Minnesota, 1352 Boyd Avenue, Room 432 VMC, St Paul, MN 55108, USA
E-mail address: polzi001@umn.edu

Vet Clin Small Anim 41 (2011) 15–30
doi:10.1016/j.cvsm.2010.09.004   **vetsmall.theclinics.com**

Table 1	
Markers of kidney damage[a]	
Blood Markers	**Urine Markers**
Elevated blood urea nitrogen concentration	Impaired urine concentrating ability
Elevated serum creatinine concentration	Proteinuria
Hyperphosphatemia	Cylindruria
Hyperkalemia or hypokalemia	Renal hematuria
Metabolic acidosis	Inappropriate urine pH level
Hypoalbuminemia	Inappropriate glucosuria
Imaging markers–abnormalities in kidney:	Cystinuria
Size	Density
Shape	Number
Location	Mineralization

[a] Markers must be confirmed to be of renal origin to be evidence of kidney damage. For example, hypoalbuminemia due to urinary protein loss is evidence of kidney disease, whereas hypoalbuminemia due to hepatic failure is not.

Data from Polzin D. Chronic kidney disease. In: Ettinger S, Feldman E, editors. Textbook of veterinary internal medicine. Saunders; 2010. p. 2036–67.

CKD is defined as kidney disease that has been present for an extended period. Kidney disease that has been present 3 months or longer may be considered to be chronic.[1] Duration of CKD may be estimated from the medical history or inferred from physical examination findings or renal structural changes identified through imaging studies or renal pathology (**Table 2**).

Staging CKD

Dogs and cats with CKD are staged according to guidelines developed by the International Renal Interest Society (IRIS) and accepted by the American and European

Table 2		
Physical and laboratory characteristics of AKI and CKD		
Characteristics of CKD	**Characteristics of AKI**	**Reliability for Differentiation**[a]
Weight loss >3 mo	Normal BCS	++
Reduced appetite >3 mo	Recent reduction of appetite	++
Poor hair coat	Healthy hair coat	+
PU/PD >3 mo	Recent change in urine volume	++
Uremic breath >3 mo		+
Small kidney size	Normal/large kidneys	+++
Renal osteodystrophy		+++
Clinical signs mild despite marked azotemia		++
Hypoproliferative anemia		++

Abbreviations: BCS, body condition score; PU/PD, polyuria-polydipsia.
[a] Reliability: + = weak; ++ = moderate; +++ = strong.

Societies of Veterinary Nephrology and Urology. The 4-tier staging system is based on renal function, proteinuria, and blood pressure (**Tables 3–5**). Staging CKD in this fashion facilitates application of appropriate clinical practice guidelines for diagnosis, prognosis, and treatment.

The stage of CKD is based on the level of kidney function as measured by the patient's serum creatinine concentration. Staging should be based on a minimum of 2 serum creatinine values obtained when the patient has been fasted and is well hydrated. Also, creatinine values should ideally be determined over several weeks to assess stability of CKD.

The stage of CKD is further characterized by the magnitude of proteinuria, as measured by the urine protein-to-creatinine ratio (UPC) and arterial blood pressure. Before determining the UPC, the urine sediment should be confirmed to be inactive and urine culture, sterile.[2] Unless the UPC is markedly elevated or less than 0.2, persistence of proteinuria should be confirmed by reexamining the UPC 2 to 3 times over at least 2 weeks. The average of these determinations should be used to classify the patient as nonproteinuric; borderline proteinuric, or proteinuric (see **Table 4**).

As with proteinuria, arterial pressure (AP) should ideally be determined 2 to 3 times over several weeks to establish the blood pressure classification. The AP classification should be based on the lowest repeatable blood pressure values obtained.

Conservative Management of CKD

Conservative medical management of CKD includes therapies other than treatment of active renal diseases (eg, pyelonephritis, urinary obstruction), dialysis, or transplantation. The therapies are designed to (1) prevent and/or treat complications of decreased kidney function, (2) manage comorbid conditions that accompany kidney disease (see **Table 5**), and (3) slow down loss of kidney function. In planning conservative medical management, it is important to recognize and specifically treat active renal diseases in the patient.

Dietary Therapy of CKD

No other single therapeutic modification is more likely to enhance the long-term outcome for patients with CKD stages 3 and 4 than a renal diet. As a consequence, the standard of care is to recommend feeding a renal diet to dogs with CKD stages 3 and 4 and cats with CKD stages 2 to 4. Results of several clinical trials strongly support the beneficial effect of renal diets in preventing or delaying the onset of uremia and premature death due to complications of CKD.[3–6] Also, renal diets have been shown to maintain or improve nutrition, and owners report higher quality-of-life scores than with maintenance diets.[1,3]

Table 3		
IRIS[a] stages of CKD in dogs and cats		
	Serum Creatinine Values (mg/dL/μmol/L)	
Stage	Dogs	Cats
Stage 1	<1.4/<125	<1.6/<140
Stage 2	1.4–2.0/125–179	1.6–2.8/140–249
Stage 3	2.1–5.0/180–439	2.9–5.0/250–439
Stage 4	>5.0/>440	>5.0/>440

[a] http://www.iris-kidney.com.

Table 4
Classification of proteinuria by urine

Protein/Creatinine Ratio[a]

Classification	Urine Protein/Creatinine Ratio	
	Dogs	Cats
Proteinuric (P)	>0.5	>0.4
Borderline proteinuric (BP)	0.2–0.5	0.2–0.4
Nonproteinuric (NP)	<0.2	<0.2

[a] Based on the American College of Veterinary Internal Medicine (ACVIM) Consensus Statement on Proteinuria (Lees, 2005).

The term *renal diet* has been misinterpreted to mean just restricting dietary protein intake; however, renal diets include other diet modifications that are probably as important and effective as protein restriction or more so. Consequently, substituting maintenance or senior diets that are lower in protein content than the pet's usual diet is not a satisfactory substitute for feeding diets specifically formulated for dogs and cats with CKD. Diets specifically designed for dogs and cats with CKD are modified from typical maintenance diets in several ways, including reduced protein, phosphorus, and sodium content, increased B-vitamin and soluble fiber content, increased caloric density, neutral effect on acid-base balance, supplementation of omega-3 polyunsaturated fatty acids, and addition of antioxidants. Feline renal diets are supplemented with potassium.

Although some dogs and a few cats readily accept the change to a renal diet, in many pets, a more gradual approach should be used. A 7- to 10-day gradual switch from the old diet to the renal diet is appropriate for dogs, and a transition period of several weeks may be needed for some cats. The transition may be made by gradually mixing increasing amounts of the renal diet into the old food. Alternately, both the old and renal diet may be made available while gradually reducing the amount of the old diet. It is important to be certain that metabolic, gastrointestinal, and dental complications are well controlled before introducing the renal diet. Introducing a renal diet to a patient with uremia or experiencing any medical issue that may promote a dietary aversion is likely to be doomed to failure.

The nutritional response to diet therapy should be regularly evaluated by monitoring body weight, body condition score, food intake (calorie intake), serum albumin concentration, packed cell volume, and quality of life. The primary goal is to assure adequate food intake, stable body weight, and body condition score at or near 5 out of 9. Patients not meeting nutritional goals should be evaluated for uremic complications, dehydration,

Table 5
IRIS[a] Arterial pressure (AP) stages for dogs and cats

AP Stage	Systolic Blood Pressure	Diastolic Blood Pressure
Stage 0	<150 mm Hg	<95 mm Hg
Stage I	150 to 159 mm Hg	95–99 mm Hg
Stage II	160 to 179 mm Hg	100–119 mm Hg
Stage III	≥180 mm Hg	≥120 mm Hg

[a] http://www.iris-kidney.com.

and progression of CKD, metabolic acidosis, anemia, electrolyte abnormalities, urinary tract infection, and non-urinary tract diseases. Also, feeding practices should be examined.

When patients fail to spontaneously consume adequate quantities of food, placing a feeding tube should be seriously considered. Feeding via gastrostomy or esophagostomy tubes is a simple and effective way to provide an adequate intake of calories and water. Also, feeding tubes simplify drug administration.

MANAGING GASTROINTESTINAL SIGNS OF UREMIA

Gastrointestinal complications of CKD, including reduced appetite with reduced food intake, nausea, vomiting, uremic stomatitis and halitosis, gastrointestinal hemorrhage, diarrhea, and hemorrhagic colitis, are common in dogs and cats with CKD stages 3 and 4. Treatment for these complications of CKD is largely symptomatic. Diet therapy, and specifically protein restriction, may limit or ameliorate many of the gastrointestinal signs of uremia. Although a link between the products of protein metabolism/catabolism and clinical signs of uremia is clear, the precise toxins remain unknown, and improvement in clinical signs often correlates with a reduction in blood urea nitrogen (BUN) as protein intake is reduced. Thus, the presence of gastrointestinal complications of CKD is sufficient justification to warrant reducing dietary protein intake.

Management of anorexia, nausea, and vomiting typically includes (1) limiting gastric acidity using H_2 blockers, (2) suppressing nausea and vomiting using antiemetics, and (3) providing mucosal protection using sucralfate. Of these treatments, H_2 blockers are the most commonly used and few adverse effects have been attributed to their use. The most commonly used H_2 blockers include famotidine and ranitidine. However, their efficacy remains unproven.

Antiemetics are typically added when anorexia, nausea, or vomiting persist despite the use of an H_2 blocker. Antiemetics commonly used in patients with CKD include metoclopramide, 5-HT_3 receptor antagonists, such as ondansetron hydrochloride or dolasetron mesylate and maropitant citrate, the neurokinin (NK_1) receptor antagonist. Studies in uremic humans have shown the 5-HT_3 receptor antagonist ondansetron to be twice as effective as metoclopramide in reducing uremic nausea and vomiting.[7,8] Sucralfate should be added when gastrointestinal ulcerations and hemorrhage are suspected.

Managing Hyperphosphatemia

Retention of excess phosphorus in the body can promote renal secondary hyperparathyroidism, mineralization of tissues, and progression of CKD. Increased serum phosphorus concentrations (P_s) have been linked to increased mortality in humans, cats, and dogs with CKD, and consuming diets high in phosphorus has been shown to increase mortality in dogs with induced CKD.[9-13] Therefore, minimizing phosphorus retention and hyperphosphatemia is an important therapeutic goal in dogs and cats with CKD.

Because the kidneys are the primary route of phosphorus excretion, declining kidney function results in phosphorus retention and its consequences. However, reducing phosphorus intake in proportion to the decline in kidney function largely prevents retention of phosphorus and its adverse consequences.

In patients with CKD stages 1 and 2, P_s typically remain within the normal range because of a compensatory reduction in phosphorous reabsorption in surviving nephrons, thereby enhancing phosphaturia. This compensatory adaptation is a consequence of the phosphaturic effects of fibroblast growth factor 23 (FGF-23) and parathyroid hormone (PTH). Increases in FGF-23 and PTH levels occur after phosphorus retention, even though P_s initially remain within the normal range. The trade-offs or consequences of ameliorating development of hyperphosphatemia include renal secondary hyperparathyroidism and impaired production of calcitriol. In dogs and cats with CKD stages 3 and 4, the usual compensatory mechanisms typically fail to prevent hyperphosphatemia.

At some point in the development of CKD, presumably during CKD stage 2, phosphorus retention and hyperphosphatemia begin to promote progression of CKD. In humans with early CKD, plasma FGF-23 concentrations, an early measure of phosphorus retention, have been shown to predict progression of CKD.[14] The association between phosphorus retention and progression of CKD provides the basis of the recommendations for managing P_s in dogs and cats with CKD.

Therapeutic management of P_s is indicated for dogs and cats with CKD stages 2 to 4. The goal of therapy is to maintain P_s within specific target ranges, which vary according to the stage of CKD (**Table 6**). Target ranges were established based on expert opinion and have not been evaluated in clinical trials.[13] The P_s target ranges are less than the upper limits of many established laboratory normal ranges, because the stated goal is to limit phosphorus retention, which precedes overt hyperphosphatemia.

The first step in minimizing P_s is a diet reduced in phosphorus content (typically, a renal diet). Manufactured renal diets are substantially reduced in phosphorus content and are often successful in achieving serum phosphorus targets in CKD stage 3. Approximately 4 to 6 weeks after initiating dietary therapy, P_s should be measured to determine whether the treatment target has been met. Samples obtained for determinations of P_s should be collected after a 12-hour fast to avoid postprandial hyperphosphatemia. If after 4 to 8 weeks, the target P_s has not been achieved, adding an intestinal phosphate-binding agent should be considered.

Intestinal phosphate-binding agents induce formation of nonabsorbable salts of phosphorus within the lumen of the gastrointestinal tract, thus rendering phosphorus contained in the diet poorly absorbable. Because dietary phosphorus is the target of such therapy, it is essential that phosphate-binding agents be given at or around meal-time. If the patient is fed more than once daily, the total daily dose of phosphate binder should be divided and a portion administered with every meal. Administering the binders away from mealtime markedly reduces their effectiveness.

The most commonly used intestinal phosphate-binding agents in dogs and cats contain aluminum as hydroxide, oxide, or carbonate salts. Various salts of calcium (acetate, carbonate, citrate) and lanthanum (carbonate) have also been used. Because of concern about aluminum toxicity in humans, aluminum-containing binding agents are becoming more difficult to obtain. Although aluminum-containing binding agents usually seem to be well tolerated and safe in dogs and cats, aluminum toxicity characterized by neurologic signs and microcytosis has been reported in dogs with

Table 6	
Recommended serum phosphorus concentrations target	
Ranges Adjusted for CKD Stages[a]	
CKD Stage	Target Serum Phosphorus Range
Stage 2	3.5–4.5 mg/dL
Stage 3	3.5–5.0 mg/dL
Stage 4	3.5–6.0 mg/dL

[a] *Ref.*[13]

advanced CKD treated with high doses of aluminum-containing phosphate-binding agents.[15]

The risk of inducing aluminum toxicity may be minimized by adding calcium- or lanthanum-containing intestinal phosphate binders to minimize the amount of aluminum that may be required for effective phosphorus binding. Experience with these drugs in dogs and cats is limited, but hypercalcemia may be a problem with the calcium-based products, particularly when administered with calcitriol or between meals. The newest product, lanthanum carbonate, and other salts of lanthanum seem to be quite effective and are associated with minimal side effects.

Phosphorus binders should be dosed "to effect," meaning the dose is adjusted to assure that the serum phosphorus target is achieved. Therapy usually begins at the lower end of the recommended dose range and is adjusted upward as needed every 4 to 6 weeks until the therapeutic target is reached.

Recommended starting dosage for aluminum-containing intestinal phosphorus-binding agents (eg, aluminum hydroxide, aluminum carbonate, and aluminum oxide) is 30 to 100 mg/kg/d. Because calcium-based phosphorus-binding agents may promote clinical hypercalcemia, serum calcium concentrations should be monitored when using these drugs. The recommended dosage for calcium acetate is 60 to 90 mg/kg/d and 90 to 150 mg/kg/d for calcium carbonate. The initial dose for lanthanum carbonate is 30 mg/kg/d.

Metabolic Acidosis

The decision to treat metabolic acidosis should be based on laboratory assessment of the patient's acid-base status, preferably based on blood gas analysis. It has been reported that metabolic acidosis occurs in less than 10% of cats with stages 2 and 3 CKD but in nearly 50% of cats with overt signs of uremia.[16] Metabolic acidosis has been incriminated in promoting progression of CKD and impairing protein nutrition.[17–20] Recently, bicarbonate therapy in humans with CKD has been reported to slow progression of CKD and improve nutritional status.[21]

Alkalinization therapy is indicated for dogs and cats with CKD stages 1 to 4 when blood pH level and bicarbonate concentration drop below the normal range. Changing to a renal diet may improve acidosis by providing a pH-neutral diet. When diet alone is insufficient, administration of an alkalinizing salt, usually sodium bicarbonate or potassium citrate, is indicated. Potassium citrate offers the advantage of using a single drug to treat hypokalemia and acidosis. Starting dosages of 40 to 60 mg/kg every 8 to 12 hours are recommended. Dosage of sodium bicarbonate is 8 to 12 mg/kg body weight given orally every 8 to 12 hours. It is available as 5- and 10-grain tablets. Response to alkalinization therapy should be assessed by performing blood gas analysis 10 to 14 days after initiating therapy and dosage adjusted until normalized. Urine pH level is an unreliable means of assessing the need for or response to treatment.

Hypokalemia and Hyperkalemia

Hypokalemia and potassium depletion are fairly common in cats with CKD stages 2 and 3, but they are recognized less commonly in CKD stage 4, because the marked reduction in glomerular filtration rate is more likely to promote potassium retention and hyperkalemia. The prevalence of hypokalemia in cats with CKD stages 2 and 3 is reportedly in the range of 20% to 30%.[16,20,22] The cause of hypokalemia in cats with CKD has not been fully elucidated, but inadequate potassium intake, increased urinary loss, and enhanced activation of the renin-angiotensin-aldosterone system due to dietary salt restriction may play a role.[23] Also, amlodipine may promote hypokalemia in cats with CKD.[24]

Hypokalemia may be associated with hypokalemic myopathy, progressive renal injury, polyuria, and polydipsia. Increasing the potassium content of renal diets has reduced the incidence of overt clinical signs of hypokalemia, but hypokalemia remains a common laboratory finding in cats with CKD.

Cats with hypokalemia should receive potassium supplementation. Oral replacement is the safest and preferred route for administering potassium; parenteral therapy is generally reserved for patients requiring emergency reversal of hypokalemia or when they cannot or will not accept oral therapy. Up to 30 mEq/L of potassium chloride may be added to fluids to be administered subcutaneously.

Potassium gluconate or citrate are good choices for oral supplementation; however, potassium chloride is not recommended because it is acidifying and unpalatable. Depending on the size of the cat and severity of hypokalemia, the dosage for potassium gluconate (Tumil-K) ranges from 2 to 6 mEq per cat per day. Potassium citrate solution (Polycitra-K Syrup) is an excellent alternative that has the advantage of providing simultaneous alkalinization therapy. Potassium citrate is initially given at a dosage of 40 to 60 mg/kg/d divided into 2 or 3 doses. If hypokalemic myopathy is present, it usually resolves within 1 to 5 days after initiating parenteral or oral potassium supplements. Thereafter, potassium dosage should be adjusted based on the clinical response of the patient and serum potassium determinations. Serum potassium concentration should be monitored every 7 to 14 days and the dosage adjusted accordingly to establish the final maintenance dosage. It is unclear whether all cats require or benefit from long-term potassium supplementation; however, preliminary evidence suggests that such therapy may be required, at least by some older cats with CKD.

Diets low in potassium and high in acid content have been implicated in impairing renal function and promoting development of lymphoplasmacytic tubulointerstitial lesions in cats.[25–29]

Consequently, prophylactic supplementation of low oral daily dosages of potassium (2 mEq/d) has been recommended for cats with CKD.[30] This recommendation seems to be based on the as yet unproven hypothesis that in some cats with CKD, hypokalemia and potassium depletion might promote a self-perpetuating cycle of declining renal function, metabolic acidosis, and continuing potassium losses. It is proposed that supplementation may stabilize renal function before potassium depletion exacerbates the disease. However, the value of prophylactic potassium supplementation in normokalemic cats has yet to be established.

Maintaining Hydration

Dehydration is a common complication of CKD and is often responsible for deterioration in kidney function and episodes of acute uremia. Because compensatory polydipsia prevents dehydration, lack of access to good quality drinking water, certain environmental conditions, and intercurrent illnesses limiting fluid intake or facilitating fluid losses (eg, pyrexia, vomiting, or diarrhea) promote dehydration. Cats with CKD seem to be particularly susceptible to chronic dehydration, perhaps because they fail to achieve an adequate compensatory polydipsia. Withholding water from patients with CKD is inappropriate and potentially dangerous.

Chronic dehydration may promote anorexia, lethargy, weakness, constipation, and prerenal azotemia and may predispose to AKI. Additional loss of kidney function due to AKI is an important cause of CKD progression. Owners of pets with CKD should be taught that vomiting or diarrhea or inadequate access to water may lead to dehydration, which may promote deterioration in kidney function or precipitate uremic crisis.

Fluid therapy is indicated for clinically dehydrated patients. The goal is to correct and prevent dehydration and its clinical effects. Acute correction of fluid needs may be done through intravenous or subcutaneous administration depending on the severity of dehydration and the specific needs of the patient. Long-term administration of subcutaneous fluid therapy may be considered for patients with signs consistent with chronic or recurrent dehydration. The principal benefits of subcutaneous fluid therapy may include improved appetite and activity and reduced constipation. Not every patient with CKD requires or benefits from fluid therapy; the decision to recommend administration of subcutaneous fluids should be made on a case-by-case basis. Cats seem more likely to benefit than dogs.

For long-term administration, a balanced electrolyte solution (eg, lactated Ringer's solution) is administered subcutaneously every 1 to 3 days as needed. The volume to be administered depends on patient size; a typical cat requires about 75 to 100 mL per dose. If the clinical response of the patient is suboptimal, the dose may be increased cautiously. However, overzealous fluid administration may subject the patient to fluid overload. Balanced electrolyte solutions do not provide electrolyte-free water; a more physiologically appropriate approach is to provide water via a feeding tube. Furthermore, evidence suggests that excessive sodium intake may be harmful to the kidneys, and excessive salt intake may impair effectiveness of antihypertensive therapy.[31]

Response to long-term subcutaneous fluid therapy should be monitored by serially assessing hydration status, clinical signs, and renal function. If a detectable improvement in clinical signs and or renal function does not accompany fluid therapy, the need for long-term therapy should be reassessed.

Management of Anemia of CKD

Anemia of CKD is common in dogs and cats with CKD stages 3 and 4. It results primarily from impaired ability of the kidneys to produce a sufficient quantity of erythropoietin; however, iatrogenic and spontaneous blood loss, poor nutrition, and reduced red blood cell lifespan may also contribute. Optimal response to therapy requires recognition of all causes contributing to anemia.

Chronic, low-grade gastrointestinal hemorrhage often contributes to anemia in CKD. Key signs suggesting gastrointestinal hemorrhage include an anemia that is disproportionately severe relative to the level of azotemia, an unusually rapid decline in hematocrit, and an elevation in the BUN/creatinine ratio. Iron deficiency may provide indirect evidence of occult gastrointestinal blood loss. Gastrointestinal signs or melena are inconsistently present in these patients. A therapeutic trial with an H_2-receptor antagonist and sucralfate may support the diagnosis. An increase in hematocrit supports the diagnosis.

Options for treating anemia of CKD include hormone replacement therapy, anabolic steroids, and correcting factors promoting red blood cell loss or impairing red blood cell production. Erythropoietin therapy is generally the most effective therapy, but optimal therapeutic response requires all factors contributing to the patient's anemia to be addressed.

Erythropoietin products most commonly used in dogs and cats include the recombinant human erythropoietin Epogen (EPO) and darbepoetin alpha (DPO). Administration of EPO has been shown to result in a dose-dependent increase in hematocrit, resulting in correction of anemia and its associated clinical signs within approximately 2 to 8 weeks.[32] Although EPO is usually effective in correcting anemia of CKD, initially; development of antibodies directed at EPO may render it ineffective. Furthermore, continued administration despite development of anti-EPO antibodies may render the patient's own endogenously produced erythropoietin largely ineffective as well, leaving the patient potentially transfusion-dependent. Hence, EPO use has usually been reserved for patients with advanced CKD requiring correction of anemia to maintain a satisfactory quality of life. Thus, erythropoietin therapy is recommended only for dogs and cats with fairly advanced CKD, clinical signs attributable to anemia, and hematocrit values less than about 22 vol%. Hormone replacement therapy with recombinant human erythropoietin (rHuEPO) is described elsewhere.[1]

DPO (Aranesp), a longer-acting form of erythropoietin, has supplanted EPO as the product currently recommended for use in dogs and cats. The duration of action of DPO is approximately 3 times longer than EPO. Preliminary, uncontrolled observations on the use of DPO in dogs and cats with anemia of CKD suggest that it may be substantially less likely to induce antierythropoietin antibodies, perhaps because of the structural modifications responsible for its longer duration of action. Unlike EPO, DPO is supplied in micrograms rather than units, with 1 μg of DPO being the equivalent of 200 units of EPO. Patients currently receiving EPO may be switched to an EPO-equivalent dosage of DPO (the product package insert should be consulted for details), but with a dosing interval that is extended threefold.

Therapy with DPO includes an induction and a maintenance phase. The induction phase is designed to correct anemia and the maintenance phase sustains the normal hematocrit for the remainder of the pet's life. In the induction phase, DPO is administered at a dosage of 1.5 μg/kg subcutaneous once weekly. Higher doses may accelerate the response to therapy, whereas lower doses may slow the response. It is critical that the hematocrit be measured weekly during this phase to prevent overdosing. When the hematocrit reaches the lower end of the normal range, the frequency of administration of DPO is reduced to every other week to transition the patient to the maintenance phase.

During the early part of the maintenance phase, the hematocrit should be measured monthly and either the dose or the frequency of administration of DPO adjusted to maintain the hematocrit in the normal range. Although the optimal therapeutic target hematocrit has not been established for dogs and cats with CKD, a reasonable cost-effective target would be the lower end of the normal range. Studies in humans have suggested that maintaining hematocrit values at the lower end of the normal range may be as effective as and possibly safer than maintaining higher hematocrit values.[33] Once the hematocrit has been stabilized within the target range, it should be monitored approximately every 3 months. Maintenance of a normal hematocrit requires ongoing hormone therapy and monitoring. Failure to monitor the hematocrit and adjust the dose of DPO can result in severe polycythemia and death, particularly during the induction phase.

The demand for iron associated with stimulated erythropoiesis is high, and human patients without preexisting iron overload exhaust iron storage during erythropoietin therapy. The same seems true of dogs and cats. Iron supplementation is therefore recommended for all patients receiving erythropoietin therapy. At a minimum, an intramuscular injection of iron dextran (50–300 mg) should be provided at the time that EPO or DPO are initiated.

The most important complications associated with hormone replacement therapy are refractory anemia and hypoplasia of the erythroid bone marrow associated with formation of neutralizing antierythropoietin antibodies.[32] A test for antierythropoietin antibodies is not currently available. However, in the absence of an identifiable cause for treatment failure, the failure of an increase in EPO or DPO dosage to increase hematocrit strongly suggests development of antierythropoietin antibody formation. Demonstrating an increase in the bone marrow myeloid/erythroid ratio provides further support that erythropoietin resistance results from antibody formation. If antierythropoietin antibody formation is suspected, EPO or DPO therapy should be terminated immediately. Because antierythropoietin antibodies may interfere with administered and endogenous erythropoietin, anemia may become worse than before initiation of erythropoietin therapy. However, antibody titers typically decline with cessation of therapy, and early recognition of the development of antierythropoietin antibodies minimizes the extent and duration of bone marrow suppression. Persistent administration of EPO despite formation of antibodies may result in persistence of antibodies. After therapy is stopped and antibody titers decline, suppressed erythropoiesis may be reversible and pretreatment levels of erythropoiesis may be attained.

Calcitriol Therapy

Patients with CKD typically have reduced levels of calcitriol. With mild CKD, the decline in calcitriol production may be ameliorated by limiting phosphorus intake. However, as CKD progresses, calcitriol supplementation becomes necessary to maintain normal levels.[34]

It has generally been believed that the effects of calcitriol therapy in patients with CKD are mediated by its effects on PTH and mineral metabolism.[35] However, various important renal effects unrelated to PTH and mineral metabolism have recently been recognized, including suppression of activity of the renin-angiotensin system, systemic activation of vitamin D receptors, and reducing podocyte loss associated with glomerular hypertrophy.[36–38] These effects seem likely to be important in mediating the recently recognized benefits of calcitriol for limiting progression of CKD and improving survival of patients with CKD. A masked, randomized controlled clinical trial (RCCT) performed on dogs with CKD stages 3 and 4 indicated that calcitriol therapy increased survival time by slowing progression of CKD (Polzin, unpublished data, 2006). These findings are consistent with the results of recent studies in human patients with CKD that demonstrated a similar survival benefit of calcitriol therapy.[39,40] However, an RCCT performed in cats failed to reveal similar benefits for calcitriol in altering the course of feline CKD (Polzin, unpublished data, 2006). The reason for these divergent results in cats are unclear but may relate to the fairly indolent course of CKD in many cats.

Calcitriol therapy is indicated for dogs with CKD stages 3 and 4 (and possibly CKD stage 2) to slow progressive deterioration in renal function. A recommendation for or against use of calcitriol in cats with CKD cannot be supported at this time. In preparation for calcitriol therapy, serum phosphorus should be managed to achieve the treatment targets described previously, and absence of hypercalcemia should be confirmed by measuring ionized calcium levels. Serum phosphorus and (ideally) ionized calcium concentrations should be monitored during calcitriol therapy. Total serum calcium values may not accurately portray ionized calcium levels in dogs with CKD.[41]

Calcitriol should initially be provided at a dosage of 2.0 to 2.5 ng/kg every 24 hours.[1] Ionized calcium and PTH levels should be monitored to establish the proper dose. The goal is to minimize PTH without inducing hypercalcemia. Because it enhances intestinal absorption of calcium and phosphorus, calcitriol should not be given with meals; administration in the evening on an empty stomach reduces the risk of hypercalcemia. When calcitriol therapy is associated with hypercalcemia, the daily dose may be doubled and given every other day, thereby reducing calcitriol-induced intestinal absorption.[42] Calcitriol dosage should not exceed about 5.0 ng/kg/d. Lifelong treatment is necessary to achieve the desired effect of reduced renal mortality. Details on dosing and monitoring are available elsewhere.[1]

Managing Proteinuria

Proteinuria is associated with CKD progression in dogs and cats.[43,44] Reducing proteinuria slows CKD progression in humans; however, evidence supporting this benefit in dogs and cats is scant.[45–47] Nonetheless, therapy designed to reduce proteinuria is recommended for dogs and cats in CKD stages 2, 3 and 4 when urine protein/creatinine ratios exceed 0.5 and 0.4, respectively and for dogs and cats with CKD stage 1 and protein/creatinine ratios greater than 2.0.[2]

The standard management of proteinuria in dogs and cats with CKD is to initiate therapy with a renal diet and administer an angiotensin-converting enzyme inhibitor (ACEI) with the therapeutic goal of at least halving the urine protein/creatinine ratio or, ideally, bringing it into the normal range. Initial dosage for the ACEIs enalapril and benazepril in dogs and cats with CKD is 0.25 to 0.5 mg/kg given orally every 12 to 24 hours.[48] Benazepril has been preferred to enalapril, because it is cleared largely by hepatic rather than renal excretion. Occasionally ACEI therapy is associated with a marked decline in kidney function; therefore, serum creatinine levels should be measured before and 1 to 2 weeks after initiating therapy. Large or progressive increases in serum creatinine levels should prompt reassessment of therapy. Dosage of ACEIs should be cautiously increased to maximize the impact on proteinuria. A beneficial effect of enalapril on progression of CKD in dogs has been reported using a dosage of 2.0 mg/kg/d.[47] Serum potassium levels should be monitored, because hyperkalemia is a recognized side effect of ACEI therapy that may limit the dosage increases.

Managing Arterial Hypertension

Arterial hypertension is a common complication of CKD in dogs and cats and has been linked to renal, ocular, neurologic, and cardiac complications. Because no generally agreed value to define arterial hypertension in dogs and cats exists, APs are classified into 4 stages (see **Table 5**).

The diagnosis of arterial hypertension must be based on measuring blood pressure. Unless there is evidence of retinal lesions or neurologic signs or the systolic blood pressure is greater than 200 mm Hg, the decision to initiate antihypertensive therapy should generally not be considered an emergency. Blood pressure should be confirmed by at least 3 independent measurements, ideally collected over several days to several weeks.[49]

Patients with CKD stages 2 to 4 having arterial blood pressures persistently exceeding 160 over 100 (AP stage II) are candidates for treatment. Treatment should be considered for CKD stage 1 with arterial blood pressures persistently exceeding 180 over 100 (AP stage III).

The optimal endpoint for antihypertensive therapy has not been established for dogs and cats with CKD. Without such information, treatment for arterial hypertension should be initiated cautiously, with the goal of reducing blood pressure to at least below 160 over 100 mm Hg. Except in patients with ocular or neurologic lesions, rapid reduction in blood pressure is not necessary. Particularly in dogs, it may take weeks to months to achieve satisfactory blood pressure control.

ACEIs (eg, enalapril and benazepril) and calcium channel blockers (eg, amlodipine) are the preferred antihypertensive drugs for dogs and cats with CKD, because they have potential renoprotective benefits. Although ACEIs generally produce fairly small reductions in blood pressure, their beneficial role in altering intraglomerular hemodynamics, proteinuria, and profibrotic effects of the intrarenal renin-angiotensin system have been demonstrated. ACEIs may have renoprotective effects, even in the absence of achieving adequate blood pressure control. Dosing of ACEIs for antihypertensive effects is the same as for proteinuria (see earlier discussion).

Clinical experience has shown amlodipine to be an effective antihypertensive agent in dogs and cats with CKD. Also, it has few side effects and relatively rapid onset. In cats, amlodipine may reduce proteinuria. It is prescribed at a dose of 0.625 mg for cats lighter than 5 kg and 1.25 mg for cats heavier than 5 kg. Dosage may be doubled if needed. In dogs, amlodipine dosage ranges from 0.1 to 0.5 mg/kg given every 24 hours and it should be combined with an ACEI.

PROGNOSIS OF CKD

In dogs with CKD stages 3 and 4, the disease tends to be progressive. Most dogs with CKD of this severity die or are euthanized because of their disease. Dogs typically survive for months to a year or two depending on the severity of their kidney disease. Furthermore, proteinuria and arterial hypertension are associated with poorer prognoses, although this may be modifiable to some degree with therapy.[43,50]

Cats with CKD vary in their clinical course. Some cats have progressive disease similar to dogs, but typically CKD progresses more slowly in cats. Also, some cats with CKD seem to have stable kidney function for many months to years, often dying of causes unrelated to CKD.[5] As with dogs, proteinuria heralds a poorer prognosis. Also, the stage of CKD has been shown to be related to outcome.

FOLLOW-UP MONITORING OF PATIENTS WITH CKD

Because CKD tends to be progressive, patient needs may change with time. Consequently, regular monitoring of patients is an essential component of the treatment plan. Treatment goals should be clearly recorded and compared with regular measurement of the patient's progress. Patients in CKD stages 3 and 4 should typically be evaluated every 3 to 4 months approximately. Patients in CKD stages I and II often require less frequent monitoring, every 4 to 6 months approximately, once stable renal function has been established. However, patients with progressive CKD, proteinuria, or arterial hypertension should be monitored more frequently. A typical monitoring visit should include a medical history at least, with medication review, physical examination, body weight and nutritional assessment, hematocrit, chemistry profile, urinalysis, and blood pressure. Depending on the patient and results of the urinalysis, the urine protein/creatinine ratio and a urine culture may also be included.

REFERENCES

1. Polzin D. Chronic kidney disease. In: Ettinger S, Feldman E, editors. Textbook of veterinary internal medicine. Saunders; 2010. p. 2036–67.
2. Lees GE, Brown SA, Elliott J, et al. Assessment and management of proteinuria in dogs and cats: 2004 ACVIM forum consensus statement (small animal). J Vet Intern Med 2005;19:377–85.
3. Jacob F, Polzin DJ, Osborne CA, et al. Clinical evaluation of dietary modification for treatment of spontaneous chronic renal failure in dogs. J Am Vet Med Assoc 2002;220(8):1163–70.
4. Elliott J, Rawlings JM, Markwell PJ, et al. Survival of cats with naturally occurring chronic renal failure: effect of dietary management. J Small Anim Pract 2000;41: 235–42.
5. Ross SJ, Osborne CA, Kirk CA, et al. Clinical evaluation of dietary modification for treatment of spontaneous chronic kidney disease in cats. J Am Vet Med Assoc 2006;229:949–57.
6. Plantinga EA, Everts H, Kastelein AMC, et al. Retrospective study of the survival of cats with acquired chronic renal insufficiency offered different commercial diets. Vet Rec 2005;157:185–7.

7. Israel R, O'Mara V, Meyer BR. Metoclopramide decreases renal plasma flow. Clin Pharmacol Ther 1986;39:261–4.
8. Perkovic LD, Rumboldt D, Bagatin Z, et al. Comparison of ondansetron with metoclopramide in the symptomatic relief of uremia-induced nausea and vomiting. Kidney Blood Press Res 2002;25:61–4.
9. Boyd LM, Langston C, Thompson K, et al. Survival in cats with naturally occurring chronic kidney disease (200–2002). J Vet Intern Med 2008;22:1111–7.
10. King JN, Tasker S, Gunn-More DA, et al. Prognostic factors in cats with chronic kidney disease. J Vet Intern Med 2007;21:906–16.
11. Block G, Hulbert-Shearon T, Levin N, et al. Association of serum phosphorus and calcium X phosphate product with mortality risk in chronic hemodialysis patients: a national study. Am J Kidney Dis 1998;31:607–17.
12. Finco D, Brown S, Crowell W, et al. Effects of dietary phosphorus and protein in dogs with chronic renal failure. Am J Vet Res 1992;53:2264–71.
13. Elliot J, Brown S, Cowgill L, et al. Symposium on phosphatemia management in the treatment of chronic kidney disease. Louisville (KY): Vetoquinol; 2006.
14. Fliser D, Koleritis B, Neyer U, et al. Fibroblast growth factor 23 (FGF23) predicts progression of chronic kidney disease: The mild to moderate kidney disease (MMKD) study. J Am Soc Nephrol 2007;18:2601–8.
15. Segev G, Bandt C, Francey T, et al. Aluminum toxicity following administration of aluminum-based phosphate binders in 2 dogs with renal failure. J Vet Intern Med 2008;22:1432–5.
16. Elliot J, Barber P. Feline chronic renal failure: Clinical findings in 80 cases diagnosed between 1992 and 1995. J Small Anim Pract 1998;39:78–85.
17. Nath K. The tubulointerstitium in progressive renal disease. Kidney Int 1998;54: 992–4.
18. Wesson DE, Simoni J. Increased tissue acid mediates a progressive decline in glomerular filtration rate of animals with reduced nephron mass. Kidney Int 2009;75:929–35.
19. Mitch W. Mechanisms causing loss of lean body mass in kidney disease. Am J Clin Nutr 1997;67:359–66.
20. DiBartola S, Rutgers H, Zack P, et al. Clinicopathologic findings associated with chronic renal disease in cats: 74 cases (1973–1984). J Am Vet Med Assoc 1987; 190:1196–202.
21. de Brito-Ashurst I, Varagunam M, Raftery MJ, et al. Bicarbonate supplementation slows progression of CKD and improves nutritional status. J Am Soc Nephrol 2009;20:2075–84.
22. Buranakarl C, Mathur S, Brown SA. Effects of dietary sodium chloride intake on renal function and blood pressure in cats with normal and reduced renal function. Am J Vet Res 2004;65:620–7.
23. Lulich J, Osborne C, O'Brien T, et al. Feline renal failure: questions, answers, questions. Compendium on Continuing Education for the Practicing Veterinarian 1992;14:127–52.
24. Henik R, Snyder P, Volk L. Treatment of systemic hypertension in cats with amlodipine besylate. J Am Anim Hosp Assoc 1997;33:226–34.
25. Dow S, Fettman M, LeCouteur R, et al. Potassium depletion in cats: renal and dietary influences. J Am Vet Med Assoc 1987;191:1569–75.
26. Dow S, Fettman M, Smith K, et al. Effects of dietary acidification and potassium depletion on acid-base balance, mineral metabolism and renal function in adult cats. J Nutr 1990;120:569–78.

27. Theisen S, DiBartola S, Radin M, et al. Muscle potassium content and potassium gluconate supplementation in normokalemic cats with naturally occurring chronic renal failure. J Vet Intern Med 1997;11:212–7.
28. Adams L, Polzin D, Osborne C, et al. Correlation of urine protein/creatinine ratio and twenty-four-hour urinary protein excretion in normal cats and cats with surgically induced chronic renal failure. J Vet Intern Med 1992;6:36–40.
29. DiBartola S, Buffington C, Chew D, et al. Development of chronic renal disease in cats fed a commercial diet. J Am Vet Med Assoc 1993;202:744–51.
30. Dow S, Fettman M. Renal disease in cats: the potassium connection. In: Kirk R, editor. Current veterinary therapy xi. Philadelphia: WB Saunders; 1992. p. 820–2.
31. Weir M, Fink JC. Salt intake and progression of chronic kidney disease: an overlooked modifiable exposure? a commentary. Am J Kidney Dis 2005;45:176–88.
32. Cowgill L, James K, Levy J, et al. Use of recombinant humans erythropoietin for management of anemia in dogs and cats with renal failure. J Am Vet Med Assoc 1998;212:521–8.
33. Singh AK, Szczech L, Tang KL, et al. Correction of anemia with epoetin alfa in chronic kidney disease. N Engl J Med 2006;355:2085–98.
34. Gutierrez O, Isakova T, Rhee E, et al. Fibroblast growth factor-23 mitigates hyperphosphatemia but accelerates calcitriol deficiency in chronic kidney disease. J Am Soc Nephrol 2005;16:2205–15.
35. Nagode L, Chew D, Podell M. Benefits of calcitriol therapy and serum phosphorus control in dogs and cats with chronic renal failure: both are essential to prevent or suppress toxic hyperparathyroidism. Vet Clin North Am 1996;26: 1293–330.
36. Andress DL. Vitamin D in chronic kidney disease: a systemic role for selective vitamin receptor activation. Kidney Int 2006;69:33–43.
37. Pörsti IH. Expanding targets of vitamin D receptor activation: downregulation of several RAS components in the kidney. Kidney Int 2008;74:1371–3.
38. Freundlich M, Quiroz Y, Zhang Z, et al. Suppression of renin-angiotensin gene expression in the kidney by paracalcitol. Kidney Int 2008;74:1394–402.
39. Shoben AB, Rudser KD, de Boer IA, et al. Association of oral calcitriol with improved survival in nondialyzed CKD. J Am Soc Nephrol 2008;19:1613–9.
40. Cheng S, Coyne D. Vitamin D and outcomes in chronic kidney disease. Curr Opin Nephrol Hypertens 2007;16:77–82.
41. Schenck PA, Chew DJ. Determination of calcium fractionation n dogs with chronic renal failure. Am J Vet Res 2003;64:1181–4.
42. Hostutler RA, DiBartola SP, Chew DJ, et al. Comparison of the effects of daily and intermittent-dose calcitriol on serum parathyroid hormone and ionized calcium concentrations in normal cats and cats with chronic renal failure. J Vet Intern Med 2006;20:1307–13.
43. Jacob F, Polzin DJ, Osborne CA, et al. Evaluation of the association between initial proteinuria and morbidity rate or death in dogs with naturally occurring chronic renal failure. J Am Vet Med Assoc 2005;226:393–400.
44. Syme HM, Markwell PJ, Pfeiffer D, et al. Survival of cats with naturally occurring chronic renal failure is related to severity of proteinuria. J Vet Intern Med 2006;20:528–35.
45. King JN, Gunn-Moore DA, Séverine Tasker S, et al. Tolerability and efficacy of benazepril in cats with chronic kidney disease. J Vet Intern Med 2006;20:1054–64.
46. Grauer G, Greco D, Getzy D, et al. Effects of enalapril versus placebo as a treatment for canine idiopathic glomerulonephritis. J Vet Intern Med 2000; 14:526–33.

47. Grodecki KM, Gains MJ, Baumal R, et al. Treatment of X-linked hereditary nephritis in Samoyed dogs with angiotensin converting enzyme (ACE) inhibitor. J Comp Pathol 1997;117:209–25.
48. Plumb DC. Plumb's veterinary drug handbook. 6th edition. Ames(IA): Blackwell Publishing; 2008. p. 130–1.
49. Brown SA, Atkins C, Bagley R, et al. Guidelines for the identification, evaluation, and management of systemic hypertension in dogs and cats. J Vet Intern Med 2007;21:542–58.
50. Jacob F, Polzin D, Osborne C, et al. Association between initial systolic blood pressure and risk of developing a uremic crisis or of dying in dogs with chronic renal failure. J Am Vet Med Assoc 2003;222:322–9.

Protein-losing Nephropathy in Small Animals

Meryl P. Littman, VMD

KEYWORDS

- Proteinuria • Glomerular disease • Glomerulonephritis
- Glomerulosclerosis • Amyloidosis

The prevalence of protein-losing nephropathy (PLN) in the general population is much greater in dogs than cats but is largely unknown and probably higher than currently recognized.[1–3] Renal failure is arguably the most common organ failure in dogs and cats. The prevalence of glomerular lesions, mostly immune-mediated glomerulonephritis (IMGN), was found in 43% to 90% of random dogs.[1,3] Increased urine protein/creatinine ratio (UPC), as an indicator of glomerular disease, is a negative predictor of outcome.[4–7] Microalbuminuria (MA) is detected in about 25% of all dogs and cats, increasing with age (36% in dogs 9–11 years, 49% in dogs $\geq$12 years, 39% in cats $\geq$12 years, and 65% of cats $\geq$16 years),[8] but its clinical significance is not known. When the first insult to the nephron is at the glomerulus, proteinuria occurs, which ultimately damages the rest of the nephron. By the time end-stage renal disease (ESRD) is discovered, the initiating glomerular cause may go undetected. Because proteinuria decreases with nephron dropout and decreased glomerular filtration, hypoalbuminemia may no longer exist or it may be masked by dehydration. Therefore, glomerular disease as the initiating cause of ESRD may go unrecognized.

Renal biopsy results may not settle the question of chicken-or-egg regarding whether glomerular versus tubular damage (chronic interstitial nephritis) was the primary cause, because both are often seen in end-stage kidney samples. Even when renal biopsies are taken earlier in the disease process, pathologists' interpretations using routine histopathology techniques do not necessarily agree.[9] There is inherent subjectivity with visual analysis of membrane thickening or mesangial cell numbers present. Tissue sections traditionally cut at 5 to 6 μm for light microscopy are too thick for careful examination of renal lesions. Therefore, the incidence of subtypes of glomerulonephritis reported may not be accurate, and treatment protocols that might work for a particular subset (for instance, steroids or cyclosporine) may not seem beneficial because these cases were not properly identified.

Clinical Studies-Philadelphia, University of Pennsylvania School of Veterinary Medicine, 3900 Delancey Street, Philadelphia, PA 19104-6010, USA
E-mail address: merylitt@vet.upenn.edu

Vet Clin Small Anim 41 (2011) 31–62
doi:10.1016/j.cvsm.2010.09.006
0195-5616/11/$ – see front matter © 2011 Elsevier Inc. All rights reserved.

With the advancement of technology, there are now sensitive and specific methods to detect and monitor proteinuria and abnormalities can be identified earlier in the disease process. The source of proteinuria can be localized and the cause characterized via diagnostic tests; the trend can be followed and stability or disease progression can be monitored. Kidney biopsies can be safely taken percutaneously with ultrasound guidance, sophisticated methodology can be used with light microscopy (LM) examination of thin (3–4 μm) tissue sections, and the glomerular lesions can be characterized by transmission electron microscopy (TEM), immunofluorescence (IF), and immunohistochemistry (IHC). Specific treatments may be recommended for specific causes, as well as symptomatic and supportive therapies to reduce proteinuria, hypertension, risk of thromboembolic events, edema/effusions, and progression of renal failure.

NORMAL GLOMERULAR STRUCTURE AND FUNCTION

The normal glomerulus is a complicated, elegant sieve, filtering 20% of the cardiac output, producing liters of ultrafiltrate per day, allowing water and small molecules to cross the fenestrated vascular endothelial barrier by the force of transcapillary pressure, to penetrate the glomerular basement membrane (GBM), traverse the podocyte slit diaphragm (SD), and enter into the glomerular filtrate while holding back larger molecules based on their size and electrical charge. The endothelial cell glycocalyx is negatively charged; the underlying supportive GBM is made up of collagen type IV, laminins, nidogen, and negatively charged glycosaminoglycans.[10] Podocyte foot processes are attached to the GBM via cell membrane receptors (α3β1 integrans linked to talin, vinculin, and paxillin, and α- and β-dystroglycans linked to utrophin).[10] Recently the structure and function of a myriad of molecules in the glomerular filtration barrier of the SD (ie, the 25- to 40-nm wide pore between the foot processes) have been reviewed (**Fig. 1**).[11] Produced by podocytes, these molecules work in concert to form a dynamic three-dimensional complex at the SD; they translate outside-inside signaling, control calcium influx, and rearrange the actin cytoskeleton within the podocytes to cause their contraction and modification of their morphology as well as the intricate architecture of their interdigitating foot processes and SD aperture, thus sensing and reacting to a changing environment. Normally very few proteins with molecular weight of albumin (69,000 Da) or higher get passed into glomerular filtrate, especially if they are negatively charged as is albumin. The few proteins that do pass through into the glomerular filtrate are normally reabsorbed and degraded by tubular cells and their lysosomes, but this work can cause tubular cell damage.[12]

GENETIC ABNORMALITIES ASSOCIATED WITH PLN

Genetic mutations producing 1 or more abnormal molecules at the SD or GBM may lead to immediate malfunction of the integrity of the permselective barrier, or to a susceptibility to injury by environmental triggers, or allow increased entrapment of circulating immune complexes (CIC), which may cause later onset proteinuria. Although not yet discovered in dogs and cats, more than 100 different mutations have been identified in NPHS1, the gene for *nephrin* (the major SD transmembrane adhesion protein of the immunoglobulin superfamily)[13]; more than 40 mutations in NPHS2, the gene for *podocin* (a stomatin family member closely associated with nephrin at the SD); and various mutations in other genes including NPHS3 (phospholipase Cε1), ACTN4 (α-actinin 4), CD2AP (CD-2 associated protein), TRPC6 (transient receptor potential cation channel 6), WT 1 (WT 1 protein), LAMB2 (laminin β-2), the NEPH 1-3 complex, several mitochondrial genes, MYH9 (nonmuscle myosin11A

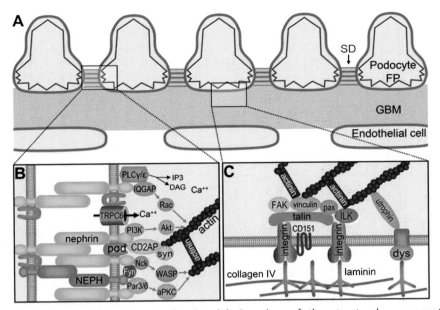

Fig. 1. The glomerular filtration barrier. (*A*) Overview of the structural components, including capillary endothelial cells, GBM, and podocyte foot processes (FP). The SD connects neighboring foot processes. Blue lines within the podocytes symbolize their actin cytoskeleton. (*B*) Molecules related to the nephrin-NEPH-podocin complex at the SD. Green arrows indicate effector pathways that have been proposed to be involved in the regulation of actin cytoskeleton reorganization. Only a subset of known molecules and interactions are shown. (*C*) Molecules at the podocytes-GBM interface and linkage to the FP actin cytoskeleton. Adhesion receptors expressed at the basal site of FP include integrin α3β1 and dystroglycan. Only a subset of known molecules and interactions are shown. DAG, diacylglycerol; dys, dystroglycan; FAK, focal adhesion kinase; ILK, integrin-linked kinase; IP3, inositol 1,4,5-triphosphate; pax, paxillin; PI3K, phosphoinositide-3 kinase; pod, podocin; syn, synaptopodin. (*From* Zenker M, Machuca E, Antignac C. Genetics of nephrotic syndrome: new insights into molecules acting at the glomerular filtration barrier. J Mol Med 2009;87:850; with permission.)

heavy chain), and many more (too numerous to mention here).[11,14] Genetic abnormalities of the SD have been associated with many types of phenotypic expression (ie, mild to severe proteinuria); histopathology showing minimal change disease to severe focal segmental glomerulosclerosis (FSGS); onset that is congenital/infantile, childhood, or adult onset; inheritance that is autosomal recessive, dominant, possibly with low, medium, or high penetrance; and some genetic abnormalities include extrarenal abnormalities (eg, neurologic, orthopedic, or genital).[11,15] At times complex inheritance such as a triple hit (homozygosity for 1 allele and heterozygosity for another) or a 4-allelic hit (homozygosity at 2 sites) might be involved for phenotypic expression.[14,15] The expression of the phenotype may not be easily explained by just the presence of 1 or more genetic mutations but by the interplay of the entire molecular background.[14]

Genetic causes of PLN are usually steroid-resistant. Many breeds are predisposed to PLN (**Table 1**), and their genetic defects may someday be discovered to involve podocytopathies that interfere with the normal development and maintenance of the structure and function of the GBM or SD. Onset of PLN because of genetic causes

Table 1
Breeds predisposed to glomerular pathogenic proteinuria

Breed	Disease	Characterization
American foxhound[16–19]	MPGN secondary to leishmaniasis	Breed is at risk for leishmaniasis
Basenji[20,21]	Glomerulopathy with SIIPD	DDX, Fanconi syndrome
Beagle[22,23]	Primary glomerulopathy[22] Amyloidosis[23]	May present up to 8 y, at least 5 to 11 y
Bernese mountain dog[24–27]	MPGN	AR ± sex-linked modifier gene, F/M ~4, 2–5 y of age
Boxer[28]	Reflux nephropathy with segmental hypoplasia	Onset <5 y of age
Brittany spaniel[29]	Primary glomerulopathy	AR, associated with complement deficiency
Bull terrier[30–35]	Primary glomerulopathy	AD model of Alport syndrome, average 3.5 y, up to 10 y DDX, polycystic kidney disease (also AD)
Bullmastiff[36]	FSGS	AR, 2.5–11 y
Dalmatian[37]	Hereditary nephropathy	AD model of Alport syndrome, onset 18 mo (8 mo to 7 y)
Doberman pinscher	Primary glomerulopathy[38,39] Also IMGN caused by sulfa[40–42]	<3 y
English cocker spaniel[43–46]	Hereditary nephropathy	AR model of Alport syndrome, 10–24 mo Allele-specific PCR test to identify carrier dogs, OptiGen
English foxhound[47]	Amyloidosis	4 to 8 y
French mastiff (Bordeaux)[48]	Juvenile glomerulopathy	Cystic glomerular atrophy, glomerular hypercellularity, <2 y
German shepherd[49–52]	IMGN (MCD) secondary to *Ehrlichia canis* infection	Cell-mediated immunity abnormality Experimental Beagle model is not as severely affected
Golden retriever[53–59]	IMGN caused by Lyme nephritis (*Borrelia burgdorferi*)[53–57] JRD[58,59]	Most Lyme-positive dogs, even retrievers, do not get Lyme nephritis; average age 5.6 ± 2.6 y Experimental beagle model does not get Lyme nephritis JRD, <3 y of age, may have proteinuria, hypoalbuminemia, hypercholesterolemia
Gordon setter[60]	Juvenile nephropathy	May have proteinuria, hypoalbuminemia, <3 y
Greyhound[61–64]	GN vasculopathy (skin, renal)	6 mo to 6 y

Breed	Disease	Comments
Labrador retriever[53-57]	IMGN caused by Lyme nephritis (*Borrelia burgdorferi*)	Most Lyme-positive dogs, even retrievers, do not get Lyme nephritis; average age 5.6 ± 2.6 y; Experimental beagle model does not get Lyme nephritis
Mixed Navasota dog and kindred[65,66]	Primary glomerulopathy	X-linked dominant Alport syndrome, 6 to 18 mo
Newfoundland[67]	Glomerulosclerosis	AR, 2 to 12 mo; DDX, cystinuria (post-renal proteinuria, AR− DNA marker available)
Norwegian elkhound[68,69]	Periglomerular fibrosis plus tubulointerstitial disease	Mode of inheritance not known 3 mo to 4 y
Pembroke Welsh corgi[70]	Primary glomerulonephropathy	Littermates presented at 3 and 5 months of age; similar to Doberman
Rottweiler[71]	Primary glomerulopathy	<1 y of age, atrophic glomerulopathy, massive proteinuria
Samoyed and kindred[72-78]	Primary glomerulopathy	Alport syndrome, X-linked recessive (an allele-specific PCR test is available for carrier Samoyeds, VetGen) Males die at 2–15 mo; carrier females: high urinary protein at 2–3 mo of age but do not progress
Shar pei[79-83]	Amyloidosis	Mean 4.1 y; M/F 1:2.5
Shetland sheepdog[53-57]	IMGN caused by Lyme nephritis (*Borrelia burgdorferi*)	Most Lyme-positive dogs do not get Lyme nephritis; average age 5.6 ± 2.6 y; Experimental beagle model does not get Lyme nephritis
Soft-coated wheaten terrier[84-91]	FSGS vs IMGN[84-89] JRD[90,91]	Unknown inheritance, F/M = 1.6:1 PLN average 6.3 ± 2.0 y; PLE/PLN combined average 5.9 ± 2.2 y 2/12 dogs with JRD had proteinuria
Abyssinian and Siamese cats[92-97]	Amyloidosis	1–5 y Proteinuria variable (medullary vs glomerular involvement)

Abbreviations: AD, autosomal dominant; AR, autosomal recessive; DDX, differentiate this from another type of renal proteinuria seen in this breed (as noted); FSGS, focal segmental glomerulosclerosis; GN, glomerulonephritis; IMGN, immune-mediated glomerulonephritis; JRD, juvenile renal disease (renal dysplasia); MCD, minimal change disease; MPGN, membranoproliferative glomerulonephritis; PCR, polymerase chain reaction; PLE, protein-losing enteropathy; SIIPD, small intestinal immunoproliferative disease.

Data from Lees GE. Familial renal disease in dogs. In: Ettinger SJ, Feldman EC, editors. Textbook of veterinary internal medicine. 7th edition. St. Louis (MO): Saunders (Elsevier); 2010. p. 2058–62.

is usually young to middle age,[98] but variable expression and incomplete penetrance modes of inheritance may allow for later onset. For most breeds, specific genetic mutations are yet to be identified. It is hoped that, using DNA saved from animals with well-characterized phenotypes, future genome-wide association studies (GWAS) with new SNP chip technology followed by fine mapping (gene sequencing) of areas of interest that are found, specific markers for these defects will be discovered so that by a simple polymerase chain reaction (PCR) test, carriers of at-risk genes will be identified and breeding of a dominant individual or 2 at-risk recessive carriers may be avoided. By identifying genes involved and realizing their function, the underlying physiologic defects will be better understood and appropriate therapeutic protocols can be planned.

Alport syndrome (hereditary nephritis) affects the production and maintenance of the GBM as a result of abnormal collagen IV production and assembly. Normally collagen IV is made up of heterotrimers of different types of chains, numbered α1-6. In Alport syndrome, there may be insufficient amounts or abnormalities in subtypes α3-5 chains produced. Various mutations of the encoding genes (COL4A3, COL4A4, and COL4A5) lead to nanomechanic GBM failure, and in humans may affect the inner ear and eye as well. The abnormal GBM thickening or basket weave appearance and ultrastructural splitting of the lamina densa is seen by TEM, often with intramembranous electron dense deposits. With light microscopy alone, these cases may be misinterpreted as a type of glomerulonephritis (eg, membranoproliferative) or renal cortical hypoplasia. In humans, more than 350 mutations have been found affecting COL4A5 (coding for α5) on the X-chromosome.[65] Mutations on the autosomal genes COL4A3 and COL4A4 are usually recessive. The primary glomerulopathies affecting bull terrier, Dalmatian, English cocker spaniel, Samoyed and Navasota mixbreed dogs are types of Alport syndrome and their mode of inheritance has been identified (see **Table 1**). By gene sequencing, carrier Samoyeds were found to have a premature stop codon caused by a single nucleotide substitution in exon 35 on the gene COL4A5 on the X-chromosome that codes for the α5 chain. In X-linked recessive Alport syndrome in Samoyeds, affected males have proteinuria by 4 months and ESRD at 8 to 10 months; carrier females are proteinuric early but do not progress to renal failure. In contrast, mixed breed dogs from Navasota, Texas, were found to have an X-linked dominant COL4A5 defect as a result of a 10-bp deletion on exon 9 that causes a frame shift and premature stop codon in exon 10; carriers of both sexes show early onset of proteinuria by 6 months and ESRD at 6 to 18 months.[65] There has been high clinical variability found in autosomal dominant types of Alport syndrome in humans.[99] Treatment is nonspecific (see later discussion). DNA screening tests exist for Samoyed and English cocker spaniel breeds. Early screening by MA, and early treatment may slow progression. Progression to renal failure occurs before age 2 years in affected Samoyed and English cocker spaniel dogs, but is more variable (up to 10 years) in Dalmatians and bull terriers.

Familial renal amyloidosis in Shar pei, beagles, English foxhounds, and Abyssinian and Siamese cats is often primarily medullary without gross proteinuria but progresses to renal failure. Medullary renal biopsies are not recommended because of the risk of hemorrhage. Familial amyloidosis in Shar pei has earlier onset than reactive amyloidosis (mean age 4.1 years, M/F = 1:2.5); only 25% to 43% have proteinuria but 64% had some glomerular involvement, thus renal cortical biopsies are still helpful (amyloid stains with Congo Red). Recurrent fever/swollen hock syndrome/increased interleukin (IL)-6 is seen in Shar pei, similar to familial Mediterranean fever.

Several hereditary types of collagenofibrotic nephropathies (type I, type III, periodic acid-Schiff [PAS] negative) and fibronectin glomerulopathies (PAS positive) have been described in humans with PLN associated with massive infiltration of collagen or fibronectin fibrils in the mesangium and subendothelium.[100] Collagenofibrotic glomerulonephropathy (collagen III) has been described in 2 unrelated young dogs with PLN[101,102] and nonamyloid fibrillary glomerulonephritis in a nephrotic cat and a young dog.[103,104] Without special stains and EM, these biopsies would have been misread as other forms of glomerular disease.

Many dog breeds[98] are predisposed to juvenile renal disease (renal dysplasia), polycystic renal disease, Fanconi syndrome, and so forth, which are not primary glomerulopathies but in some dogs cause proteinuria, possibly hypoalbuminemia, and/or hypercholesterolemia, mimicking changes seen with primary glomerular disease. Breeds predisposed to primary glomerulopathies as well as other familial renal diseases that need to be differentiated include the bull terrier, golden retriever, and soft-coated wheaten terrier (SCWT) (see **Table 1**). Also listed are breeds with higher risk for immune-mediated glomerular disease, possibly triggered by infection (eg, Lyme nephritis in retrievers, leishmaniasis in American foxhounds, ehrlichiosis in German shepherds), by drugs (eg, sulfa in Doberman pinschers), or by other hypersensitivities (possibly food allergies in SCWT).

ACQUIRED CAUSES OF GLOMERULAR LEAKAGE OF PROTEIN

Acquired PLN is sporadically seen in any breed and is often caused by IMGN, reactive amyloidosis, or glomerulosclerosis (GS). Comprehensive descriptions (TEM and/or IF in addition to LM analysis) of renal lesions in several hundred clinical cases of PLN were described 17 to 40 years ago.[1-3,105-114] Because newly emerging infectious diseases (especially tick-borne) and new genetic predispositions may change the spectrum of disease with time, comprehensive examinations of renal cortical biopsies on our current patients with PLN need to be done so that predominant types of glomerular lesions as presented to veterinarians in various locations are known, treatment protocols for properly identified subsets of PLN can be investigated, and individuals treated appropriately.

In general, glomerular lesions are common. In dogs with and without clinical signs of renal disease, 90% had glomerular lesions in 1 study.[107] Among dogs with renal disease, 52% had glomerular lesions in another study.[106] The population at risk for PLN was middle-aged to older dogs, with slightly more males represented. Glomerulonephritis and amyloidosis were described more often than other types of glomerular lesions in dogs and cats.[1-3,105-116] Membranoproliferative glomerulonephritis (MPGN) was common in dogs (presumably immune-mediated, and possibly postinfectious, as is seen in people in developing countries). Membranous nephropathy (MN) was the most common lesion in cats with PLN, but in general, PLN is not common in cats.[113,114]

IMGN

Pathologists describe lesions depending on how much of each glomerulus is involved (eg, segmental, global), how many glomeruli are involved in the sample (eg, focal, diffuse), and whether there is inflammatory cell infiltration or mesangial cellular proliferation. Immune complex (antigen-antibody) deposits can involve immunoglobulin (Ig) A, IgG, and/or IgM, with or without complement (C3). The complexes can be CIC or be formed in situ as antigens are caught and bind antibody secondarily. The antigens involved are rarely identified but are sought indirectly by history, clinical presentation, by serologic tests for antibodies, by using culture, cytology, and PCR for antigens associated with infections, and by searching for inflammatory disease and neoplasia.

The true cause is often unproved because immunohistochemistry or elution studies on the glomerular complexes are rarely done. Immune complex deposition causes inflammation (glomerulonephritis) through a variety of mediators, inflammatory cells, complement and platelet activation, renin-angiotensin-aldosterone (RAA) system activation, and numerous humoral and cellular responses that influence the progression versus resolution by mesangial phagocytosis.[1,3,117]

MPGN is the most common form of IMGN in dogs with a mean age of 10.5 years and no sex predilection.[110] It is uncommon in the cat.[118] Most common in dogs is type 1 MPGN with immune complexes seen as lumpy-bumpy deposits by EM and IF on the subendothelial side of the GBM (mesangiocapillary GN) and/or in the mesangium. Linear deposits that would indicate true autoimmune disease (systemic lupus erythematosus) have not been described in dogs and cats. The granular deposits of IMGN may stain positive for complement and IgA, IgG, and/or IgM combinations. By LM, the complexes make the GBM appear thickened or duplicated (railroad) but if tissue sections are cut thickly at 5 to 6 μm, MPGN may be overdiagnosed.

MPGN has been associated with sulfa drugs (mostly in Dobermans[40–42]), neoplasia, inflammatory diseases, and with many types of infectious diseases, such as chronic bacterial infection (endocarditis, bartonellosis,[119] brucellosis[120]), arthropod-borne (anaplasmosis [suspected],[121] babesiosis,[122–126] Lyme borreliosis,[53–57] ehrlichiosis,[49–52] hepatozoonosis,[127,128] leishmaniasis,[16–19] Rocky Mountain spotted fever (RMSF)[129]), viral diseases (canine adenovirus I,[130] feline leukemia virus,[131] feline immunodeficiency virus [suspected],[132–134] feline infectious peritonitis [FIP][135]) or parasitic diseases (Dirofilaria/Wolbachia,[136–140] heterobilharziasis [schistosomiasis],[141] trypanosomiasis[1,3]) in which carrier status and chronic immune stimulation from antigenic variation occurs. In leishmaniasis, high antihistone antibodies are present and associated with MPGN[142]; histones are cationic and are implicated in binding the CIC to the GBM, perhaps as a planted antigen. Some diseases may cause proteinuria as a result of vasculitis (RMSF, anaplasmosis, bartonellosis, ehrlichiosis, greyhound vasculopathy, leptospirosis, FIP) or renal infiltration (toxoplasmosis, cryptococcosis, systemic fungal infections, neoplasia), and not necessarily IMGN.

Although dogs seropositive for leptospirosis were described as having IMGN,[143] coinfections (eg, heartworms, leishmaniasis, and so forth) may have played a role; leptospirosis is generally considered to cause tubular rather than glomerular proteinuria, or vasculitis.[144–146] Another spirochetal disease, Lyme borreliosis, has been associated with MPGN involving Lyme-specific immune complexes, accompanied by tubular necrosis/regeneration and interstitial nephritis, sometimes with glycosuria caused by tubular disease.[53–56] Lyme nephritis may be seen in any breed but mostly in Labrador and golden retrievers and Shetland sheepdogs, and has a younger onset at 5.6 ± 2.6 years compared with other dogs with PLN at 7.1 ± 3.6 years. There may be specific Borrelia strains or genetic predispositions for this form of Lyme disease because most Lyme-positive dogs (even retrievers) remain asymptomatic and do not show proteinuria or PLN.[57] Thus, when a dog with PLN happens to be Lyme positive, it should be checked for coinfections and other causes of PLN, because Lyme seropositivity indicates tick exposure and not necessarily a diagnosis of Lyme nephritis.[54]

Bernese mountain dogs have a genetic predisposition (see **Table 1**) for MPGN that is no longer believed to be associated with Lyme seropositivity. The mode of inheritance is autosomal recessive, possibly with an X-linked modifier (M/F ratio = 1:4).[24–27] Another type of MPGN is seen in congenital complement deficiency in Brittany spaniels[29]; normal complement levels were found in 49 other dogs with acquired PLN.[147]

Treatment of type I MPGN involves treating the underlying infectious, inflammatory, or neoplastic disease process. Antiplatelet drugs may also be tried to decrease platelet activation, which seems to be involved in the inflammatory cascade. Sometimes IMGN is also treated with immunosuppressive protocols (see later discussion).

Membranous nephropathy (MN) is a form of IMGN characterized by severe proteinuria (similar to that seen with reactive amyloidosis) and seen more often in males. The glomerular damage is caused by complement-dependent mechanisms and not inflammatory cell infiltration because the immune complexes are found on the subepithelial (podocyte) side of the GBM, away from the capillaries. Unbound circulating antibody may react to antigens that are fixed on the urinary side of the GBM. It may be a true autoimmune disease; in humans it is associated with underlying immunologic defects. It is the second most common lesion in dogs (M/F = 1.75:1, mean age 8 years, range 1–14 years). Because of the severe proteinuria, it is often accompanied by the nephrotic syndrome, identified in 14 (30%) of 46 proteinuric dogs (mean 6.5 years). Survival times for dogs with MN ranged from 4 days to 3 years. In cats with PLN, MN is the most common lesion (M/F = 6:1, mean age 3.6 years, range 1–7 years). In a study of 24 cats with MN, 46% died or were euthanized shortly after diagnosis; 17% survived 4 to 10 months, 33% survived 2.5 to 6 years (3/8 of the long-term survivors were given steroids). Cats with only IgG and/or C3 deposits had longer survival than those that had IgA or IgM deposits. Spontaneous remissions have been reported but more study needs to be done to validate treatment regimes and prognostic factors. In MN in human patients, immunosuppressive treatment with pulse or alternate-day steroids and alkylating agents (cyclophosphamide, chlorambucil) for 6 months helps, although relapses are common. Cyclosporine also helps in two-thirds of cases.[1,112–114]

Familial MN is seen in Doberman pinschers (<3 years old). By LM the GBM looks thickened, possibly showing spikes on the epithelial side that do not take up silver stain. Deposits are seen by IF and TEM and the granularity may be so intense that the beaded pattern almost seems linear. Mesangia may also stain for IgG and C3, which are more common than IgM and/or IgA in dogs. TEM can stage the engulfment and resolution process.

Proliferative glomerulonephritis (PGN), also known as endocapillary or mesangial PGN, has been described in 2% to 16% of dogs with PLN (mean 7–9 years).[1] It is seen in humans with lupus, IgA nephropathy, or as a postinfectious GN (eg, after streptococcal or staphylococcal infection) in which GN follows an infection without a carrier status, which may be why there is no membranous component. The mesangial proliferation is defined as 4 or more mesangial or mononuclear cells per area, often with increased mesangial matrix seen. By IF and TEM there are fine granular deposits of IgG and/or IgM, subepithelial in the BM and in the mesangium. Treatment is to remove the source antigen.

IgA nephropathy may appear just as mesangial proliferative GN by LM but the immune deposits are seen by TEM and stain for IgA (more than for IgG or IgM) by IF.[148] Because IgA is dimeric in dogs, it may be trapped nonspecifically in the mesangium in 47% to 85% of normal dogs.[109,149,150] IgA nephropathy may be associated with hepatic and gastrointestinal disease[149]; treatment may depend on removing the underlying cause. IgA positivity (and less so IgM) was seen in some glomeruli in SCWT with protein-losing enteropathy (PLE)/PLN and food allergies,[87] but it is not yet proved whether the glomerular lesions in that breed are primarily immune mediated or sclerotic (FSGS) with secondary deposition of immune complexes.

Minimal change disease (MCD) is common in children (often steroid responsive but relapses are common) but rarely described in veterinary literature.[151] Ehrlichiosis and the drug masitinib were shown to cause MCD.[49,152] This nil disease shows no morphologic lesions by LM, but there is foot process effacement seen by TEM examination, and increased vimentin staining by IF. Loss of the anionic charge at the GBM causes massive proteinuria and often nephrotic syndrome.

Reactive Amyloidosis

Reactive amyloidosis may be seen in any breed (dog > cat) and is often associated with glomerular deposition and severe proteinuria caused by extracellular deposition of polymerized serum amyloid A protein (SAA, an acute phase reactant made by the liver) into β-pleated sheets, seen as homogeneous eosinophilic thickening at the GBM and mesangium, staining red with Congo Red stain. This is 1 subset of PLN that can be diagnosed by LM. Other organs may be affected (eg, liver and spleen), becoming friable and hemorrhage easily (biopsy is not recommended). Among dogs with PLN, 23% had amyloidosis in 1 study.[116] Chronic infectious, inflammatory, or neoplastic disease was found in 32% to 53% of cases (mean age 9.2 years, M/F = 1:1.7) with beagles, collies, and Walker hounds predisposed.[153] Nephrotic syndrome is common because proteinuria is severe. Prognosis is poor; 58% of dogs were euthanized or died soon after diagnosis and only 8.5% survived for 1 year or more.[154] Colchicine (0.01–0.03 mg/kg by mouth every 24 hours) may help decrease hepatic production of SAA but may cause gastrointestinal upset. Dimethylsulfoxide (DMSO, 90 mg/kg by mouth 3 times a week or subcutaneous injections diluted 1:4 with sterile water) is antiinflammatory, decreases interstitial fibrosis, and may improve renal function and decrease proteinuria, but it causes garlic breath and may cause nausea/anorexia.[155]

The odorless and tasteless metabolite of DMSO, methylsulfonylmethane (MSM), may be used in place of DMSO.

Glomerulosclerosis

The prevalence of glomerulosclerosis (GS) increases with age.[1] It may be a primary (genetic) disease as in some forms of FSGS or it may be secondary to hypertension (eg, as a result of hyperadrenocorticism or steroid use) or any glomerular injury, such as an end-stage lesion. It may be underdiagnosed and misdiagnosed as MPGN. Nonspecific trapping of complexes in sclerotic/fibrotic areas may be seen by IF. In humans there are 5 subtypes, each with different prognoses, but these are poorly characterized in dogs and cats. Genetic structural defects of the SD or circulating permeability factors may functionally alter the permselectivity of the GBM, and predispose for indolent immune complex deposition, damage, and sclerosis. Glomerulosclerosis secondary to hyperadrenocorticism or hypertension rarely causes severe enough proteinuria to cause hypoalbuminemia.

DETECTING PROTEINURIA, THE HALLMARK OF PLN

Annual screening for proteinuria is recommended in healthy dogs as part of annual health care.[7] In particular, breeds with genetic risks for PLN should be screened early and often, especially if used for breeding. The earliest warning of glomerular disease is microalbuminuria (MA), defined as 1 to 30 mg albumin/dL, which can be detected by species-specific enzyme-linked immunosorbent assays for albuminuria such as the in-house semi-quantitative E.R.D. (HESKA) test or by quantitative MA by a reference laboratory. The sensitive MA test is useful as a first-line screening agent for genetic PLN (eg, SCWT,[89] Samoyeds[74]) or acquired glomerular damage (eg, in Lyme- or heartworm-positive dogs[57,139]).

Microalbuminuria is often associated with age and with systemic diseases.[156,157] In older dogs, MA may be too sensitive to be helpful compared with the UPC test.

Looking for persistence as well as trend of progression or stability is important before assigning clinical significance to MA, because many if not most older dogs have low to moderate positive MA, possibly as a result of normal aging of the kidney or infectious/inflammatory/neoplastic/vascular insults.

Urinary dipstick tests for protein are less sensitive than MA, picking up more than 30 mg/dL, and are less specific for albuminuria, showing false-negative and false-positive results compared with MA. Dipstick false-positive readings may occur with high pH, hematuria, pyuria, and/or bacteriuria, and more often with feline than canine samples.[158] In 1 study, when dipstick and urine specific gravity (USG) were used together, dogs with a USG greater than 1.012 and +1 by dipstick were likely nonproteinuric; but for those with +1 dipstick and USG less than or equal to 1.012, proteinuria should be further assessed by use of the UPC ratio.[159] Both dipstick and urine turbidity with sulfasalicylic acid (SSA) testing for proteinuria were less specific and gave false-positive results, whereas UPC testing showed higher specificity but less sensitivity, with some false-negative results.[160] Multistix PRO dipsticks, read by a Clinitek 50 analyzer (Bayer Corporation), were more sensitive but less specific than SSA testing for proteinuria in dogs (but not a good alternative for cats); manual calculation of the UPC is done with the dipstick's estimated urinary creatinine level.[161] Another in-house analyzer, the IDEXX VetTest, showed strong association for UPC results with the reference Vitros 50 instrument,[162] however not all laboratories use similar methodology, and inter-laboratory comparisons may be difficult.[163] Any UPC test may be increased by Bence Jones and other nonalbumin proteins in the urine. A urine albumin/creatinine ratio can also be done.[164]

Macroproteinuria is generally defined using UPC measurements. Borderline UPC values in nonazotemic animals (0.5–1.0 in dogs and 0.4–1.0 in cats) should be monitored for persistence and trend of progression. Larger amounts (UPC of >1.0) should be investigated and localized as to the source (prerenal, renal, or postrenal); renal proteinuria is then categorized as functional or pathologic (glomerular, tubular, or interstitial).[2,7] Investigation of macroproteinuria is always recommended if azotemia exists. Therapeutic intervention is recommended for nonazotemic animals at UPC greater than or equal to 2.0, but is often started at lower values if a breed-associated cause is suspected and progression is expected without early intervention. For azotemic animals, intervention is recommended at UPC greater than or equal to 0.5 (dogs) and UPC greater than or equal to 0.4 (cats).

Once macroproteinuria is found, UPC is the standard test for quantitation, monitoring, and for comparisons. There was no statistical difference found in the measurement of UPC between free-catch and cystocentesis samples.[165] Day-to-day variation of the UPC was seen in female dogs with stable glomerular proteinuria caused by X-linked hereditary nephropathy.[166] This study showed that significant differences in UPC to indicate progression of disease or failure of intervention would have to be greater than 35% variance at high UPC near 12, and greater than 80% variance at a low UPC near 0.5. This may be true for other forms of PLN (not just mosaics). To minimize costs of averaging results from 3 samples, equal pooling of 3 urine samples for 1 determination was found to be as valid as averaging results from 3 samples ($\pm$ 20%).[167]

Moderate exercise does not cause MA to increase.[168] Contrary to what was seen with another inflammatory marker (C-reactive protein), degree of MA showed no correlation with degree of periodontal disease, and there was no change in USG, MA, or UPC before and after dental treatment[169]; positive MA in 12.4% of dogs needing dental work may be related to their age.

Because whole ejaculate (not just sperm) physically added to urine may increase dipstick proteinuria,[170] it is not recommended to collect urine samples for MA testing immediately after collecting semen. In 1 study, whole blood physically added to urine did not cause UPC greater than 0.4, and abnormal MA greater than 1 mg/dL did not occur until the urine was grossly pink.[171] In experimental dogs, UPC was less than 2.0 even on days 1 to 2 after cystotomy.[172] In dogs with induced bacterial cystitis, UPC ranged from 1.5 to 40.8 but did not correlate with sediment findings.[172] In dogs with spontaneous pyuria, 67% had normal MA and 81% had normal UPC; abnormal MA (but not UPC) was more often seen if pyuria was accompanied by hematuria and bacteriuria.[171]

Cushing's disease,[173–175] exogenous steroids[75,176,177] and hypertension[178] are associated with increased proteinuria. Glomerular damage (glomerulosclerosis) may eventually occur if exposure is severe or prolonged, but the proteinuria is usually mild (UPC <2) and generally not accompanied by hypoalbuminemia. Blood pressure measurements and MA or UPC should be monitored when giving steroids or phenylpropanolamine. Dogs with diabetes mellitus[175,179] may also have proteinuria but these are often accompanied by Cushing's disease and/or hypertension.

Once pre- and postrenal causes for proteinuria are ruled out, renal proteinuria can be further differentiated (glomerular and/or tubular) with the help of sodium dodecyl sulfate-agarose gel electrophoresis (SDS-PAGE) methodology applied to urine samples. High molecular weight proteins (such as albumin at 69,000 Da) indicate glomerular leakage, whereas lower molecular weight proteins are found in urine when tubular cells are not working properly.[17,144,180]

CLINICAL PRESENTATIONS OF PLN: DIAGNOSTIC CLUES

History, physical examination, laboratory tests, imaging, and renal cortical biopsy are used to identify pathologic glomerular proteinuria, search for underlying causes, stage PLN, and classify the subtype of PLN to select specific, supportive, and symptomatic treatments (**Box 1**). The clinicopathologic signs of PLN are initially different from those of whole nephron or primary tubular (interstitial nephritis) causes of renal failure. The mean age at presentation is 5 to 8 years with no sex or slight male predominance.[86,94] Classic signs include proteinuria, hypoalbuminemia and hypercholesterolemia.[1,3,84,105,110–112,116]

The author proposes the following 4 stages of PLN progression.

Stage 1

Persistent glomerular proteinuria (microalbuminuria progressing to macroalbuminuria) begins without other renal signs, but there may be signs from an underlying infectious, inflammatory, immune-mediated, neoplastic, endocrine, or hypertensive disease. For instance, fever, polyarthropathy, vasculitis, uveitis, cytopenias (commonly thrombocytopenia), and/or allergies/hypersensitivities suggest an infectious or immune-mediated cause. Diagnostic clues to identify causes and complications of PLN in the author's geographic area are given in **Box 1**. Because many healthy dogs are Lyme seropositive, finding Lyme seropositivity is not necessarily diagnostic for Lyme nephropathy and a thorough work-up is recommended lest a coinfection go unrecognized (eg, with babesiosis).[125] Depending on geographic area and travel history, tests for additional agents that affect the kidney via vasculitis, immune-mediated mechanisms, or renal invasion may be warranted.[181]

Stage 2

UPC is persistently increased causing serum albumin level to drop. Serum cholesterol level increases as a result of urinary loss of lecithin-cholesterol acyltransferase.

Box 1
Clues to find causes and complications for a dog with PLN in a Lyme-endemic area; treatment ideas

History should include

   Signalment, pedigree, family history, coat or color type (eg, coloring for Labradors: black, yellow, chocolate)

   Travel history, tick exposure

   History of prior treatment of tick-borne disease such as Lyme disease

   Medication exposure (sulfa, masitinib), vaccination exposure

   Polyuria/polydypsia? Vomiting? Appetite? Weight loss?

   History of lower urinary tract signs (pollakiuria, stranguria, accidents)

   History of lameness, dyspnea, blindness, effusions/edema, neurologic events

   History of allergies, inflammatory bowel disease, PLE, Addison disease (SCWT)

Physical examination should include

   Body weight, body condition score, hydration status

   Temperature, femoral pulses, respiration

   Mucous membranes: check for anemia, petechiation

   Ophthalmologic examination including fundic examination

   Peripheral edema? Ascites?

   Ausculation for murmur, dyspnea, muffling

   Lymphadenopathy?

   Abdominal palpation, organomegaly?

   Neurologic examination

   If lameness: joint swelling/effusion? Which joints? Pulses?

   Blood pressure measurements (multiple)

Clinical pathology, microbiology, parasitology, immunology samples

   Blood samples for

      Complete blood count (CBC)

      Biochemical profile

      Coagulation profile, thromboelastography

      Blood cultures if indicated

      SNAP-4Dx (IDEXX) for heartworm antigen and antibodies against *Borrelia burgdorferi* (C6 quantitation if positive), *Ehrlichia canis/chaffeensis, Anaplasma phagocytophilum/ platys*; do additional SNAP test (convalescent) 2 weeks into the illness if the history is acute; get quantitative titers if positive (0 and 6 months after treatment)

      Ehrlichia PCR to check for *Ehrlichia ewingii* antigen, if indicated

      Bartonella Western blot, culture/PCR, titers

      Babesia spp PCR (for novel spp), titers (*B canis, B gibsoni, B microti*); get additional titers (convalescent) 2 weeks into the illness if the history is acute

      Rocky Mountain spotted fever acute/convalescent titers (if the history is acute; RMSF does not cause a carrier status)

Leptospira titers (get additional titer [convalescent] 2 weeks into the illness if the history is acute)

Brucella, Leishmania, Trypanosoma tests, and so forth as indicated

Coombs, antinuclear antibody titer, rheumatoid factor, perinuclear antineutrophil cytoplasmic antibody, and so forth as indicated.

Save additional EDTA whole blood for future PCR testing and for DNA banking or DNA test, if available

Consider samples for antithrombin III, C3, CIC levels, and so forth

Urine samples for

Urinalysis

Urine culture

Urine protein/creatinine ratio (UPC)

Urine SDS-PAGE

Cytology of

Joint fluid cytology/culture

Lymph node aspirate

Bone marrow aspirate

Effusions

Imaging studies

Chest radiographs

Abdominal ultrasound

Echocardiogram if indicated

Radiographs of joints if lameness present

Renal cortical biopsy for TEM, IF, and thin-section LM (via percutaneous ultrasound-guided Tru-cut needle)

Control hypertension if present; discontinue antithrombotics 3–7 days before biopsy

Contact Dr George Lees (email glees@cvm.tamu.edu, tel. 979-845-2351, fax 979-845-6978) at the Texas Veterinary Renal Pathology Service before planning sample collection to get the renal biopsy kit with its special fixatives, tools, and shipment label (if you already have a kit, check that the fixatives are still in date), packing and return shipping instructions, and to coordinate the best date for the procedure to be done because the samples must be received on ice by overnight shipment. Dr George Lees, Building 508, Room 120, Veterinary Teaching Hospital, Texas A&M University, College Station, TX 77843

Consider saving a frozen kidney sample for future elution studies

Therapeutic considerations

Standard therapy

Doxycycline 10 mg/kg/d, pending infectious disease results (1 month; longer for Lyme nephritis)

Angiotensin-converting enzyme (ACE) inhibition: enalapril (Enacard) 0.5–1.0 mg/kg every 12 to 24 hours, or benazepril (Lotensin) 0.25–0.5 mg/kg every 12 to 24 hours

Low antithrombotic dose of aspirin if albumin ≤2.5 g/dL, 1.0 mg/kg every 24 hours

Omega-3 fatty acid supplement

Antihypertensives are added to ACE inhibitor if dog is still hypertensive (eg, amlodipine [Norvasc] 0.2–0.4 mg/kg every 12 hours)

Other therapies for renal disease (eg, dietary modification, phosphate binder, gastroprotectant, antiemetic, and so forth)

Immunosuppressive therapy

If biopsy results (TEM, IF, thin-section LM) show compelling evidence of active immune complex deposition and inflammation, then immunosuppressive medications should be considered

As a rule-of-thumb, if <50% of the glomeruli are open and/or >50% show glomerular obsolescence, and if the tubulointerstitial lesion is characterized by diffuse fibrotic changes (as opposed to cellular inflammatory changes), immunosuppressive protocols may be ineffective and possibly contraindicated

If the patient is decompensating rapidly, consider starting a protocol while renal biopsy results are pending

There are no blinded treatment studies; the following protocols are offered anecdotally depending on owner considerations, patient tolerance, and so forth. Continue to monitor blood pressure, UPC, CBC, chemistry panel, and so forth. every 1–4 weeks, depending on the severity/stability of clinical signs, and continue to look for an underlying cause that may present itself with time or as a result of immunosuppression

Protocol 1: Methylprednisolone sodium succinate (Solu-Medrol) 5 mg/kg intravenously every 24 hours × 2 days; cyclophosphamide (Cytoxan) 200 mg/m^2 intravenous bolus first day. Check white blood cells in 1 week; cyclophosphamide is repeated every 2 weeks for a maximum of 6 cycles; Solu-Medrol is only used when the first cycle of cyclophosphamide is given

Protocol 2 (barring financial constraints): Methylprednisolone sodium succinate as protocol 1; mycophenolate mofetil (CellCept) 10 mg/kg intravenously or by mouth every 12 hours long-term

Protocol 3: Methylprednisolone sodium succinate as protocols 1 and 2; azathioprine (Imuran) 2 mg/kg by mouth every 24 hours × 7 days, then every 48 hours long-term

With thanks, **Box 1** is derived from discussions with Drs Nicola Mason, Reid Groman, and Tabitha Hutton at the University of Pennsylvania School of Veterinary Medicine.

The dyslipidemia occurring with hypoalbuminemia also includes increased hepatic activity of several enzymes leading to decreased high-density lipoprotein and increased low-density lipoprotein and triglycerides.[182] Serious events caused by complications of PLN can occur before azotemia or polyuria/polydipsia exist and are more common in Stage 2 than Stage 1 PLN (eg, hypertension, thromboembolic events, and/or nephrotic syndrome with ascites/edema).

Causes of hypertension are multifactorial and include activation of the RAA system, abnormal salt and water handling, decreased renal production of vasodilatory prostaglandins and kinins, and increased arteriolar sensitivity to circulating vasoconstrictors.[183] Hypertensive target organ damage may be the reason for presentation to the veterinarian. Damage includes blindness caused by retinal hemorrhage/detachment, cardiovascular disease (left ventricular hypertrophy, epistaxis, arteriosclerosis/atherosclerosis), neurologic abnormalities (cerebrovascular accidents or stroke), and renal changes (glomerulosclerosis, proteinuria, pressure diuresis). Self-perpetuation of hypertension is caused by glomerulosclerosis and increased total peripheral resistance as a result of vascular damage (arteriosclerosis/atherosclerosis). Risk for hypertensive target organ damage increases as blood pressure increases; severe risk is seen at blood pressure measurements (BPM) greater than or equal to 180/120 mm Hg, moderate risk at 160 to 179/100 to 119 mmHg, mild risk at 150 to 159/95 to 99 mm Hg, and minimal risk at less than 150/95 mm Hg.[183] Roughly 60%

to 90% of dogs and cats with renal disease are hypertensive and it is associated with poor outcome.[5,183,184]

The risk for thromboembolic events in patients with PLN is well recognized.[1,3,84,116] Mechanisms causing hypercoagulability in patients with PLN include urinary loss of antithrombin (AT, which has similar size and charge as albumin) and platelet hypersensitivity as a result of hypoalbuminemia.[185–188] Spontaneous vascular damage caused by hypertension or vasculitis and iatrogenic damage caused by venipuncture and catheter placement may initiate thrombus formation. Both arterial and venous thromboembolic (TE) events have been associated with PLN. Life-threatening TE events may affect the heart, central nervous system, lung, aortic bifurcation (saddle thrombus), portal/mesenteric/splenic veins, and so forth, causing dyspnea, lameness, abdominal distress, collapse, or sudden death. One report found 22% of dogs with PLN had TE events.[116] In SCWT, 10/84 dogs (12%) with PLN and 11/62 dogs (18%) with combined PLE/PLN were believed to have TE events.[84]

The drop in plasma colloid oncotic pressure caused by hypoalbuminemia allows vascular fluid to be lost to the interstitium (as a result of Starling forces), perhaps leading to peripheral edema and signs of third spacing (dyspnea from pleural effusion; ascites from abdominal effusion; tamponade from pericardial effusion). Arterial hypertension and/or vasculitis from associated infectious, inflammatory, or immune-mediated disease may increase the risk for edema/effusions. Nephrotic syndrome (proteinuria, hypoalbuminemia, hypercholesterolemia, and edema/effusions)[1,3,105,112] may be seen in cases of Stage 2 PLN, and although dramatic, has not been associated with decreased survival compared with cases of non-nephrotic canine PLN.[189] In SCWT, 9/67 dogs (13%) with PLN and 23/58 (40%) of dogs with PLE/PLN had effusions.[84]

Stage 3

Risks continue as in Stage 2, but now azotemia begins. As a result of glomerulotubular imbalance, there may be little or no concentrating defect and therefore no perceived polyuria/polydipsia (PU/PD). In SCWT dogs with PLN (or PLE/PLN), average biochemical findings were serum creatinine = 5.4 ± 4.1 mg/dL (4.6 ± 3.3), BUN = 95 ± 73 mg/dL (86 ± 61), albumin = 2.2 ± 0.4 g/dL (1.8 ± 0.4), cholesterol = 399 ± 126 mg/dL (311 ± 128), phosphorus = 8.9 ± 6.3 mg/dL (8.4 ± 4.6), UPC = 5.3 ± 3.1 (7.1 ± 4.7), and the average USG was $1.023 \pm .011$ (1.022 ± 0.012).[84] The UPC may decrease with increasing azotemia, but this is not necessarily a good sign, because there are fewer working nephrons leaking protein.

Stage 4

ESRD now includes isosthenuria and PU/PD, vomiting, weight loss, and other signs of chronic renal failure, or in some acute cases (eg, Lyme nephritis), possibly oliguria/anuria. The UPC may drop further because of fewer working nephrons. Serum albumin may normalize or hypoalbuminemia may be masked by dehydration. There may be glycosuria and/or renal tubular acidosis as a result of tubular damage and decreased reabsorption of glucose and bicarbonate from the glomerular filtrate.

RENAL CORTICAL BIOPSY

To characterize the type of glomerular damage causing PLN, it is recommended to take renal cortical samples early in the process, before fibrosis or end-stage changes obscure the original lesion. By TEM examination, glomerular basement membrane ultrastructural (hereditary) defects can be seen and not misdiagnosed as acquired

MN or MPGN. With TEM, immune complex deposits can be seen and localized as subendothelial versus subepithelial versus mesangial. With IF and special stains, complexes can be associated with C3 or immunoglobulin subtypes IgA, IgG, and/or IgM. Without knowing what types of subsets are being treated, which protocols work for which disease cannot be studied. Perhaps various subtypes of glomerular disease can be associated with specific prognoses and response to treatments; for example, IMGN and MCD may respond to steroids and/or immunosuppressives, whereas hereditary nephritis and FSGS may not. In human adults, although complete and partial remissions were seen with advocated alternate-day steroid/alkylating agents, a Cochrane systematic review of 18 randomized trials with 1025 patients showed no long-term benefit for the use of immunosuppressives for idiopathic MN[190] but found that immunosuppressives (especially steroids) helped decrease progression to renal failure in 13 studies with 623 people with IgA nephropathy.[191] Such information is not yet available in veterinary medicine. Only 1 controlled study (with cyclosporine) has been done, and the statistics were unable to show a response in dogs with PLN to cyclosporine probably because subtypes were not differentiated adequately or in high enough numbers.[9] Pathologists often disagree about light microscopic evaluations, especially when sections are cut too thickly as they are for other routine histopathology. For breeds with inherited forms of PLN, characterization of phenotype subtype is important to decrease the risk that sporadic (nongenetic) PLN cases are admixed into genome-wide association studies. The challenge for progress in veterinary medicine demands that comprehensive diagnostic testing is done to fully characterize and classify PLN subtypes, and to validate or negate the use of specific treatment protocols for specific entities.[192]

The when, why, and how of procuring renal cortical biopsies are described in detail elsewhere.[193–199] The procedure involves planning several days beforehand. Hypertension should be controlled and antithrombotics should be stopped at least a few days, preferably a week, before to avoid hemorrhage. Contact the Texas Veterinary Renal Pathology Service (glees@cvm.tamu.edu, tel 979-845-2351, fax 979-845-6978) to receive instructions and special materials (see **Box 1**). With anesthesia and ultrasound guidance, 2 to 4 Tru-cut renal cortical biopsies are taken percutaneously, checked by magnification for evidence of glomeruli, and prepared properly for TEM (1-mm cubes in chilled 3% glutaraldehyde), IF (1-mm cubes in chilled Michel transport medium), and for thin-section LM (longer core in 10% formalin). As more information is obtained and shared, more will be learned about PLN subtypes and their response to various treatment protocols. Until then, results will help us make logical choices based on what is known in other species.

MANAGEMENT OF PLN

Specific therapy may include antibiotics for bacterial or rickettsial infections, antiprotozoals for babesiosis, treatment of heartworm infection, chemotherapy or debulking for neoplasia, and so forth (if the underlying cause of PLN is known), and avoidance of possible trigger antigens (eg, sulfa in Dobes, food allergies in SCWT) (see **Box 1**). In our area, doxycycline 10 mg/kg/d is often given for 1 month even without firm cause; Lyme-positive dogs may be given doxycycline much longer (because only 85%–90% are cleared in 1 month).

Nonspecific but standard of care for all patients with PLN includes use of an ACE inhibitor to decrease proteinuria[77,200–204] and a low antithrombotic dose of aspirin[205–207] to help lower the risk of serious TE events and perhaps decrease inflammation and progression to renal failure.

An ACE inhibitor such as enalapril (Enacard) or benazepril (Lotensin) decreases proteinuria by dilating both the efferent as well as afferent arterioles at the glomerulus, thereby lowering the glomerular filtration pressure. The ACE inhibitor therapy should be given to all cases of PLN, whether they are hypertensive or not. If the animal is also hypertensive, the ACE inhibitor may also help decrease the blood pressure a bit, but if needed, a calcium channel blocker (eg, amlodipine [Norvasc]) may be added to further lower BPM. When ACE inhibitors are used for cardiac patients, there is concern that increased azotemia may occur; this is because cardiac patients often have low cardiac output and poor renal perfusion, which can drop further with ACE inhibitor drugs. However, in cases of PLN, when cardiac output is normal and blood pressure is normal or often high, the use of ACE inhibitors is actually renoprotective, and even higher doses of ACE inhibitors can be used without impairing GFR. Another past question was whether to avoid enalapril in cases of azotemic PLN because it is cleared by the kidney, and whether to use benazepril instead which is cleared by the liver. There seems to be no clinical advantage; having an increased blood level and activity of enalapril may be a good thing for these cases. Other drugs that might be added if proteinuria is not responding include angiotensin II receptor blockers (ARB) such as losartan (Cozaar) or telmisartan (Micardis), an aldosterone receptor antagonist such as spironolactone (Aldactone), or a renin inhibitor such as aliskiren (Tekturna).[204] Although these inhibitors of the RAA system may help the kidney by decreasing proteinuria as well as by decreasing inflammation and fibrosis,[3,204] they may increase the serum potassium level, which in 50% of renal cases may already be increased when eating renal diets. If potassium levels do not lower after changing to another renal diet formulation then a home-prepared reduced-potassium diet may be useful, especially for patients needing these drugs.[205]

An antithrombotic dose of aspirin is important for all animals with hypoalbuminemia because of the risk for thromboembolism. Aspirin decreases production of thromboxane A2, which not only helps inhibit platelet aggregation to decrease the risk of thromboembolism[206–208] but because platelet activation is part of the inflammatory process that increases renal damage, aspirin may help decrease proteinuria and fibrosis, as did a thromboxane synthase inhibitor in studies of heartworm-induced PLN.[209–211] The lowest dose for inhibition of platelet function in dogs seems to be 1.0 mg/kg/d.[207,208] The recommended dose for cats is 5 mg per cat every 72 hours.[212] Other TE preventive drugs to be studied include clopidogrel (Plavix) and the anticoagulant warfarin (Coumadin). Heparin (fractionated or unfractionated) is less useful in patients with PLN because heparin works by binding to AT, which is low in cases of PLN because of urinary loss. Thrombolytics that have been used when TE events occur include streptokinase (Streptase)[213] and tissue plasminogen activator.[214]

Samoyed dogs with X-linked hereditary PLN lived 53% longer when fed a diet restricted in protein, lipid, calcium, and phosphorus.[78] Sodium restriction is recommended because dogs with PLN are at risk for hypertension and may be salt sensitive.[3] Omega-3 fatty acids are antiinflammatory and were found to be renoprotective, decreasing the progression of renal failure.[215] Anecdotally, the immunomodulating Chinese herb Astragalus membranaceus (Astragalus propinquus or huang qi) helped 2 people with idiopathic MN and nephrotic syndrome achieve complete remission, after little or no response for years trying more standard treatments (ACE inhibitors, ARB, spironolactone, aliskiren, prednisone, cyclosporine, mycophenolate).[216,217] In 1 patient, nephrosis returned on stopping the herb, and complete remission was achieved again on its reintroduction.[216] She took the herb for 1 year and has remained in remission for 4 years. This herb warrants further investigation.

Especially before and during intravenous therapy and anesthesia to get renal cortical biopsy samples, an animal with low colloid osmotic pressure may require crystalloid therapy for dehydration and also colloid therapy, such as hydroxyethyl starch (Hetastarch), to decrease risk of edema/effusions. Other therapies for renal disease (phosphate binder, gastroprotectant, antiemetic, appetite stimulant, and so forth) are used as needed (see articles by Linda Ross; and David J. Polzin elsewhere in this issue for further exploration of this topic). Recently the use of sodium bicarbonate was shown to slow progression of hypertensive nephropathy, even if the patient was not acidotic.[218] Studies in veterinary medicine need to be done.

Perhaps the most controversial topic is whether (and when) to use immunosuppressive therapy for dogs and cats with PLN. There are no controlled studies that show benefit; there is only 1 randomized study done in canine field cases (and none in cats) that actually showed decreased survival in the cyclosporine-treated group (11 months) compared with placebo (16 months).[9] However, side effects, small numbers, and incomplete subtyping of phenotypes may have played a role, so perhaps cyclosporine could be of benefit in some cases. The immunosuppressants cyclosporine (Neoral, Sandimmune, Atopica) and tacrolimus (FK506 or Prograf) are calcineurin inhibitors that inhibit T-lymphocyte signal transduction and the transcription of IL-2 and related cytokines. Cyclosporine slowed disease progression in hereditary X-linked PLN in Samoyeds.[76] This is possible because in addition to its immunosuppressive properties, calcineurin inhibitors act to stabilize the actin cytoskeleton of the podocyte via synaptopodin and TRPC6 regulation.[10,11] Other drugs used for nephrotic syndrome may also have actions at the podocyte level (eg, corticoids, ACE inhibitors, COX2 inhibitors, and mizoribine).[10] A case report did show benefit of use of mycophenolate (CellCept) in a dog with IMGN.[219] Mycophenolate, a product of the fungus *Penicillium*, is an immunosuppressant (not a calcineurin inhibitor) that acts by reducing guanine nucleotides in lymphocytes, thereby inhibiting DNA synthesis and guanosine triphosphate-dependent metabolism.

The most commonly used immunosuppressant/antiinflammatory combinations in veterinary medicine are corticosteroids, which suppress T- and B-cell proliferation, cell-mediated/humoral immunity, inflammatory mediator/cytokine production, phagocytosis, respiratory burst, and neutrophil/macrophage emigration and function. Steroids are beneficial for human patients with IgA nephropathy,[191] MCD,[1] and children with MPGN,[220,221] however, solid evidence is lacking for the use of steroids for adults with MN.[190] If renal biopsy shows active inflammation and immune-mediated disease, steroids may have a role in veterinary patients with PLN. However, the blind use of steroids for PLN cannot be recommended, because steroids increase proteinuria,[75,173–177] and increase the risk for TE events, hypertension, glomerulosclerosis, and gastric ulceration, all of which may already exist in the patient with PLN. Controlled studies of steroid use in patients with known subtypes of PLN need to be done.

Immunosuppressive alkylating agents such as cyclophosphamide (Cytoxan) and chlorambucil (Leukeran) are used for humans with IgA nephropathy[191] and pulse therapy with steroids for MPGN,[221] lupus, and MN.[1] Alkylating agents interfere with DNA/RNA replication/transcription. They decrease white blood cells and antibody production, but the exact mechanisms are still unclear.

Other immunosuppressive medications such as azathioprine (Imuran, a purine antagonist), sirolimus (Rapamune), methotrexate (MTX), interferon, tumor necrosis factor α antibodies such as inflixamab (Remicade) or etanercept (Enbrel), IV-IgG, and monoclonal antibodies (eg, directed against IL-2) are not generally used for human patients with PLN and have not been studied in veterinary cases of PLN.

Apheresis or plasmapheresis has been advocated to remove antibodies, CIC, and circulating permeability factors that may cause PLN, for instance, in MCD.[222]

Although colchicine and DMSO may be suggested for treatment of amyloidosis, there are no veterinary studies to support their benefit.[155]

If dogs with PLN have renal transplants, they may need 1 or both kidneys removed to help lessen loss of proteins. They could have relapse disease in the transplanted kidney, or if they have an inherited SD defect, they may produce antibodies to the new antigens they are not tolerant to (eg, nephrin if they did not make nephrin before).[10] Patients with PLN having hemodialysis require higher doses of heparin because of their low antithrombin levels.

Monitoring of blood pressure, UPC, CBC, and biochemical parameters is important every 1 to 4 weeks, depending on the severity or stability of signs. With time, or because of immunosuppressive therapy, infectious/inflammatory/neoplastic diseases may reveal themselves and the clinician needs to be watchful for the underlying cause to be unmasked or for an additional diagnosis (eg, urinary tract infection) while on immunosuppressive therapy. If the dog has been treated for an infectious disease such as Lyme disease, C6 antibody quantitation at 6 months is done to compare with the previous baseline, and to get a new baseline for comparison in the future should the dog show lameness or recurrence of signs. If relapse or reinfection is suspected based on an increase in C6 Quant, then doxycycline may need to be repeated.

PREVENTION

As genetic predispositions are discovered for early or late-onset PLN, breeding questions will arise. DNA banking will be helpful along with classification of PLN subtypes, to find genetic marker tests by GWA studies and avoid breeding carriers with one another (for recessive traits). Even without knowing the mode of inheritance, early detection by frequent screening of dogs (by MA or UPC) before breeding is most important. In some cases DNA tests are already available (see **Table 1**). In SCWT dogs, annual screening tests are recommended whether bred or not, including at least MA and serum albumin, and if the owners can afford it, more thorough screening of CBC, Chemscreen, urinalysis, UPC, ± fecal alpha-1 protease inhibitor testing (for PLE). Starting ACE inhibitors early is recommended if the MA or UPC is found with an inactive urinary sediment. Tick control is advocated for all dogs that live or travel to areas with tick-borne diseases that can cause illness.

SUMMARY

Genetic and acquired defects of glomerular permselectivity allow for proteinuria and may lead to PLN. The clinicopathologic abnormalities (proteinuria, hypoalbuminemia, hypercholesterolemia) seen with this type of nephron dysfunction are initially different from those seen with whole nephron loss or primary tubular disease. Morbidity and mortality from complications of PLN may be severe even before progression to azotemia and renal failure occur, including thromboembolic events, nephrotic syndrome with edema/effusions, and hypertensive target organ damage. Leakage of plasma proteins into the glomerular filtrate can damage tubular cells and eventually affect the function of the entire nephron. Detection, localization, and treatment of proteinuria are important to decrease the clinical signs and complications of PLN and to decrease the likelihood of progression to renal failure. Thorough diagnostic work-ups to characterize the underlying causes and to comprehensively describe glomerular lesions by transmission electron microscopy, immunofluorescence, and thin-section light microscopy help to identify subsets of glomerular disease and study their response to specific treatment protocols.

REFERENCES

1. Vaden SL. Glomerular diseases. In: Ettinger SJ, Feldman EC, editors. Textbook of veterinary internal medicine. 7th edition. St. Louis (MO): Saunders (Elsevier); 2010. p. 2021–36.
2. Vaden SL, Brown CA. Glomerular disease. In: Bonagura JD, Twedt DC, editors. Kirk's current veterinary therapy XIV. St. Louis (MO): Saunders (Elsevier); 2009. p. 863–8.
3. Grauer GF. Glomerulonephropathies. In: Nelson RW, Couto CG, editors. Small animal internal medicine. 4th edition. St. Louis (MO): Mosby (Elsevier); 2009. p. 637–44.
4. Jacob F, Polzin DJ, Osborne CA, et al. Evaluation of the association between initial proteinuria and morbidity rate or death in dogs with naturally occurring chronic renal failure. J Am Vet Med Assoc 2005;226(3):393–400.
5. Wehner A, Hartmann K, Hirschberger J. Associations between proteinuria, systemic hypertension and glomerular filtration rate in dogs with renal and non-renal diseases. Vet Rec 2008;162(5):141–7.
6. Syme HM, Markwell PJ, Pfeiffer D, et al. Survival of cats with naturally occurring chronic renal failure is related to severity of proteinuria. J Vet Intern Med 2006; 29(3):528–35.
7. Lees GE, Brown SA, Elliott J, et al. Assessment and management of proteinuria in dogs and cats: 2004 ACVIM Forum Consensus Statement (Small Animal). J Vet Intern Med 2005;19(3):377–85.
8. Heska Corporation data. Prevalence of microalbumuminuria in veterinary clinic staff-owned dogs, 2003. Available at: http://www.heska.com/Documents/RenalHealthScreen/erd_data.aspx; Prevalence of microalbuminuria in cats, 2003. Available at: http://www.heska.com/Documents/RenalHealthScreen/erd_datacat.aspx. Accessed July 24, 2010.
9. Vaden SL, Breitschwerdt EB, Armstrong PJ, et al. The effects of cyclosporine versus standard care in dogs with naturally occurring glomerulonephritis. J Vet Intern Med 1995;9(4):259–66.
10. Lowik MM, Groenen PJ, Levtchenko EN, et al. Molecular genetic analysis of podocyte genes in focal segmental glomerulosclerosis – a review. Eur J Pediatr 2009;168(11):1291–304.
11. Zenker M, Machuca E, Antignac C. Genetics of nephrotic syndrome: new insights into molecules acting at the glomerular filtration barrier. J Mol Med 2009;87(9):849–57.
12. Russo LM, Bakris GL, Comper WD, et al. Renal handling of albumin: a critical review of basic concepts and perspective. Am J Kidney Dis 2002;39(5):899–919.
13. Schoeb DS, Chernin G, Heeringa SF, et al. Nineteen novel NPHS1 mutations in a worldwide cohort of patients with congenital nephrotic syndrome (CNS). Nephrol Dial Transplant 2010;25(9):2970–6.
14. Caridi G, Trivelli A, Sanna-Cherchi S, et al. Familial forms of nephrotic syndrome. Pediatr Nephrol 2010;25(2):241–52.
15. Santin S, Garcia-Maset R, Ruiz P, et al. Nephrin mutations cause childhood- and adult-onset focal segmental glomerulosclerosis. Kidney Int 2009;76(12):1268–76.
16. Gaskin AA, Schantz P, Jackson J, et al. Visceral leishmaniasis in a New York foxhound kennel. J Vet Intern Med 2002;16(1):34–44.

17. Zatelli A, Borgarelli M, Santilli R, et al. Glomerular lesions in dogs infected with *Leishmania* organisms. Am J Vet Res 2003;64(5):558–61.
18. Poli A, Abramo F, Mancianti F, et al. Renal involvement in canine leishmaniasis. A light microscopic, immunohistochemical and electron-microscopy study. Nephron 1991;57(4):444–52.
19. Costa FAL, Goto H, Saldanha LCB, et al. Histopathologic patterns of nephropathy in naturally acquired canine visceral leishmaniasis. Vet Pathol 2003; 49(6):677–84.
20. Breitschwerdt EB. Immunoproliferative enteropathy of Basenjis. Semin Vet Med Surg (Small Anim) 1992;7(2):153–61.
21. Bartges JW. Gee – It's GN: proteinuria. In: Proceedings of the Atlantic Coast Veterinary Conference. Available at: http://www.vin.com/Members/Proceedings/Proceedings.plx?CID=ACVC2006&PID=pr14336&Print=1&O=VIN. Accessed July 14, 2010.
22. Rha JY, Labato MA, Ross LA, et al. Familial glomerulonephropathy in a litter of beagles. J Am Vet Med Assoc 2000;216(1):46–50.
23. Bowles MH, Mosier DA. Renal amyloidosis in a family of beagles. J Am Vet Med Assoc 1992;201(4):569–74.
24. Reusch C, Hoerauf A, Lechner J, et al. A new familial glomerulonephropathy in Bernese mountain dogs. Vet Rec 1994;134(16):411–5.
25. Minkus G, Breuer W, Wanke R, et al. Familial nephropathy in Bernese Mountain Dogs. Vet Pathol 1994;31(4):421–8.
26. Gerber B, Eichenberger S, Haug K, et al. Association of urine protein excretion and infection with *Borrelia burgdorferi* sensu lato in Bernese Mountain dogs. Vet J 2009;182(3):487–8.
27. Gerber B, Haug K, Eichenberger S, et al. Follow up of Bernese Mountain dogs and other dogs with serologically diagnosed *Borrelia burgdorferi* infection: what happens to seropositive animals? BMC Vet Res 2009;5:18.
28. Chandler ML, Elwood C, Murphy KF, et al. Juvenile nephropathy in 37 boxer dogs. J Small Anim Pract 2007;48(12):690–4.
29. Cork LC, Morris JM, Olson JL, et al. Membranoproliferative glomerulonephritis in dogs with a genetically determined deficiency of the third component of complement. Clin Immunol Immunopathol 1991;60(3):455–70.
30. Hood JC, Savige J, Hendtlass A, et al. Bull terrier hereditary nephritis: a model for autosomal dominant Alport syndrome. Kidney Int 1995;47:758–65.
31. Hood JC, Robinson WF, Clark WF, et al. Proteinuria as an indicator of early renal disease in bull terriers with hereditary nephritis. J Small Anim Pract 1991;32(5): 241–8.
32. Hood JC, Savige JA, Dowling J, et al. Ultrastructural appearance of renal and other basement membranes in the bull terrier model of autosomal dominant hereditary nephritis. Am J Kidney Dis 2000;36(2):378–91.
33. Hood JC, Dawling J, Bertram JF, et al. Correlation of histopathological features and renal impairment in autosomal dominant Alport syndrome in Bull terriers. Nephrol Dial Transplant 2002;17(11):1897–908.
34. Burrows AK, Malik R, Hunt GB, et al. Familial polycystic kidney disease in bull terriers. J Small Anim Pract 1994;35(7):364–9.
35. O'Leary CA, MacKay BM, Malik R, et al. Polycystic kidney disease in Bull Terriers: an autosomal dominant inherited disorder. Aust Vet J 1999;77(6): 361–6.
36. Casal ML, Dambach DM, Meister T, et al. Familial glomerulonephropathy in the Bullmastiff. Vet Pathol 2004;41(4):319–25.

37. Hood JC, Huxtable C, Naito I, et al. A novel model of autosomal dominant Alport syndrome in Dalmatian dogs. Nephrol Dial Transplant 2002;17(12):2094–8.
38. Wilcock BP, Patterson JM. Familial glomerulonephritis in Doberman Pinscher dogs. Can Vet J 1979;20(9):244–9.
39. Picut CA, Lewis RM. Juvenile renal disease in the Doberman pinscher: ultra-structural changes of the glomerular basement membrane. J Comp Pathol 1987;97(5):587–96.
40. Giger U, Werner LL, Millichamp NJ, et al. Sulfadiazine-induced allergy in six Doberman Pinschers. J Am Vet Med Assoc 1985;186(5):479–84.
41. Vasilopulos RJ, Mackin A, Lavergne SN, et al. Nephrotic syndrome associated with administration of sulfadimethoxine/ormetoprim in a dobermann. J Small Anim Pract 2005;46(5):232–6.
42. Trepanier LA. Idiosyncratic toxicity associated with potentiated sulfonamides in the dog. J Vet Pharmacol Ther 2004;27(3):129–38.
43. Lees GE, Wilson PD, Helman RG, et al. Glomerular ultrastructural findings similar to hereditary nephritis in four English cocker spaniels. J Vet Intern Med 1997;11(2):80–5.
44. Lees GE, Helman RG, Homco LD, et al. Early diagnosis of familial nephropathy in English cocker spaniels. J Am Anim Hosp Assoc 1998;34(3):189–95.
45. Lees GE, Helman RG, Kashtan CE, et al. A model of autosomal recessive Alport syndrome in English cocker spaniel dogs. Kidney Int 1998;54(3):706–19.
46. Davidson AG, Bell RJ, Lees GE, et al. Genetic cause of autosomal recessive hereditary nephropathy in the English cocker spaniel. J Vet Intern Med 2007; 21(3):394–401.
47. Mason NJ, Day MJ. Renal amyloidosis in related English foxhounds. J Small Anim Pract 1996;37(6):255–60.
48. Lavoue R, van der Lugt JJ, Day MJ, et al. Progressive juvenile glomerulonephropathy in 16 related French Mastiff (Bordeaux) dogs. J Vet Intern Med 2010; 24(2):314–22.
49. Codner EC, Caceci T, Saunders GK, et al. Investigation of glomerular lesions in dogs with acute experimentally induced *Ehrlichia canis* infection. Am J Vet Res 1992;53(12):2286–91.
50. Codner EC, Maslim WR. Investigation of renal protein loss in dogs with acute experimentally induced *Ehrlichia canis* infection. Am J Vet Res 1992; 53(3):294–9.
51. Nyindo M, Huxsoll DL, Ristic M, et al. Cell-mediated and humoral immune responses of German shepherd dogs and beagles to experimental infection with *Ehrlichia canis*. Am J Vet Res 1980;41(2):250–4.
52. de Castro MB, Machado RZ, de Aquino LP, et al. Experimental acute canine monocytic ehrlichiosis: clinicopathological and immunopathological findings. Vet Parasitol 2004;119(1):73–86.
53. Dambach DM, Smith CA, Lewis RM, et al. Morphologic, immunohistochemical, and ultrastructural characteristics of a distinctive renal lesion in dogs putatively associated with *Borrelia burgdorferi* infection: 49 cases (1987–1992). Vet Pathol 1997;34(2):85–96.
54. Littman MP, Goldstein RE, Labato MA, et al. ACVIM small animal consensus statement on Lyme disease in dogs: diagnosis, treatment, and prevention. J Vet Intern Med 2006;20(2):422–34.
55. Chou J, Wunschmann A, Hodzic E, et al. Detection of *Borrelia burdorferi* DNA in tissues from dogs with presumptive Lyme borreliosis. J Am Vet Med Assoc 2006;229(8):1260–5.

56. Sanders NA. Canine Lyme nephritis. In: Proceedings of the 18th ACVIM Forum. Seattle (WA), May 25–28, 2000. p. 627–8.

57. Goldstein RE, Cordner AP, Sandler JL, et al. Microalbuminuria and comparison of serologic testing for exposure to *Borrelia burgdorferi* in nonclinical Labrador and Golden Retrievers. J Vet Diagn Invest 2007;19(3):294–7.

58. Kerlin RL, Van Winkle TJ. Renal dysplasia in golden retrievers. Vet Pathol 1995; 32(3):327–9.

59. de Morais HS, DiBartola SP, Chew DJ. Juvenile renal disease in golden retrievers: 12 cases (1984–1994). J Am Vet Med Assoc 1996;209(4):792–7.

60. Reilly CM, Munson L, Bell JS. Progressive juvenile nephropathy in Gordon Setters. Vet Pathol 2007;44(5):740.

61. Carpenter JL, Andelman NC, Moore FM, et al. Idiopathic cutaneous and renal glomerular vasculopathy of greyhounds. Vet Pathol 1988;25(6):401–7.

62. Hertzke DM, Cowan LA, Schoning P, et al. Glomerular ultrastructural lesions of idiopathic cutaneous and renal glomerular vasculopathy of greyhounds. Vet Pathol 1995;32(5):451–9.

63. Cowan LA, Hertzke DM, Fenwick BW, et al. Clinical and clinicopathologic abnormalities in greyhounds with cutaneous and renal glomerular vasculopathy: 18 cases (1992–1994). J Am Vet Med Assoc 1997;210(6):789–93.

64. Bjotvedt G, Hendricks GM, Brandon TA. Hemodynamic basis of renal arteriosclerosis in young greyhounds. Lab Anim Sci 1988;38(1):62–7.

65. Cox ML, Lees GE, Kashtan CE, et al. Genetic cause of X-linked Alport syndrome in a family of domestic dogs. Mamm Genome 2003;14(6):396–403.

66. Lees GE, Helman RG, Kashtan CE, et al. New form of X-linked dominant hereditary nephritis in dogs. Am J Vet Res 1999;60(3):373–83.

67. Koeman JP, Biewenga WJ, Gruys E. Proteinuria associated with glomerulosclerosis and glomerular collagen formation in three Newfoundland dog littermates. Vet Pathol 1994;31(2):188–93.

68. Finco DR. Familial renal disease in Norwegian elkhound dogs: physiologic and biochemical examinations. Am J Vet Res 1976;37(1):87–91.

69. Finco DR, Duncan JD, Crowell WA, et al. Familial renal disease in Norwegian elkhound dogs: morphologic examinations. Am J Vet Res 1977;38(7):941–7.

70. McKay LW, Seguin MA, Ritchey JW, et al. Juvenile nephropathy in two related Pembroke Welsh corgi puppies. J Small Anim Pract 2004;45(11):568–71.

71. Cook SM, Dean DF, Golden DL, et al. Renal failure attributable to atrophic glomerulopathy in four related rottweilers. J Am Vet Med Assoc 1993;202(1): 107–9.

72. Zheng K, Thorner PS, Marrano P, et al. Canine X chromosome-linked hereditary nephritis: a genetic model for human X-linked hereditary nephritis resulting from a single base mutation in the gene encoding the $\alpha5$ chain of collagen type IV. Proc Natl Acad Sci U S A 1994;91(9):3989–93.

73. Jansen B, Valli VE, Thorner P, et al. Samoyed hereditary glomerulonephropathy: serial clinical and laboratory (urine, serum biochemistry and hematology) studies. Can J Vet Res 1987;51(3):387–93.

74. Lees GE, Jensen WA, Simpson DF, et al. Persistent albuminuria precedes onset of overt proteinuria in male dogs with X-linked hereditary nephropathy. J Vet Intern Med 2002;16(3):353.

75. Lees GE, Willard MD, Dziezyc J. Glomerular proteinuria is rapidly but reversibly increased by short-term prednisone administration in heterozygous (carrier) female dogs with X-linked hereditary nephropathy. J Vet Intern Med 2002; 16(3):352.

76. Chen D, Jefferson B, Harvey SJ, et al. Cyclosporine A slows the progressive renal disease of Alport syndrome (X-linked hereditary nephritis): results from a canine model. J Am Soc Nephrol 2003;14(3):690–8.

77. Grodecki KM, Gains MJ, Baumal R, et al. Treatment of X-linked hereditary nephritis in Samoyed dogs with angiotensin-converting enzyme (ACE) inhibitor. J Comp Pathol 1997;117(3):209–25.

78. Valli VE, Baumal R, Thorner P, et al. Dietary modification reduces splitting of glomerular basement membranes and delays death due to renal failure in canine X-linked hereditary nephritis. Lab Invest 1991;65(1):67–73.

79. DiBartola SP, Tarr MJ, Webb DM, et al. Familial renal amyloidosis in Chinese Shar Pei dogs. J Am Vet Med Assoc 1990;197(4):483–7.

80. May C, Hammill J, Bennett D. Chinese Shar Pei fever syndrome: a preliminary report. Vet Rec 1992;131(25–26):586–7.

81. Rivas AL, Tintle L, Kimball ES, et al. A canine febrile disorder associated with elevated interleukin-6. Clin Immunol Immunopathol 1992;64(1):36–45.

82. Rivas AL, Tintle L, Meyers-Wallen V, et al. Inheritance of renal amyloidosis in Chinese Shar Pei dogs. J Hered 1993;84(6):438–42.

83. Johnson KH, Sletten K, Hayden DW, et al. AA amyloidosis in Chinese Shar Pei dogs: immunohistochemical and amino acid sequence analysis. Int J Exp Clin Invest 1995;2(2):92–9.

84. Littman MP, Dambach DM, Vaden SL, et al. Familial protein-losing enteropathy and protein-losing nephropathy in soft-coated wheaten terriers: 222 cases (1983–1997). J Vet Intern Med 2000;14(1):68–80.

85. Vaden SL, Hammerberg B, Davenport DJ, et al. Food hypersensitivity reactions in soft-coated wheaten terriers with protein-losing enteropathy or protein-losing nephropathy or both: gastroscopic food sensitivity testing, dietary provocation, and fecal immunoglobulin E. J Vet Intern Med 2000;14(1):60–7.

86. Vaden SL, Sellon RK, Melgarejo LT, et al. Evaluation of intestinal permeability and gluten sensitivity in soft-coated wheaten terriers with familial protein-losing enteropathy, protein-losing nephropathy, or both. Am J Vet Res 2000;61(5): 518–24.

87. Afrouzian M, Vaden SL, Harris T, et al. Immune complex mediated proliferative and sclerosing glomerulonephritis in Soft Coated Wheaten Terriers (SCWT): is this an animal model of IgA nephropathy or IgM mesangial nephropathy? J Am Soc Nephrol 2001;12:670A.

88. Allenspach K, Lomas B, Wieland B, et al. Evaluation of perinuclear anti-neutrophilic cytoplasmic autoantibodies as an early marker of protein-losing enteropathy and protein-losing nephropathy in Soft Coated Wheaten Terriers. Am J Vet Res 2008;69(10):1301–4.

89. Vaden SL, Jensen W, Longhofer S, et al. Longitudinal study of microalbuminuria in soft-coated wheaten terriers. J Vet Intern Med 2001;15(3):300.

90. Nash AS, Kelly DF, Gaskell CJ. Progressive renal disease in soft-coated wheaten terriers: possible familial nephropathy. J Small Anim Pract 1984;25(8):479–87.

91. Eriksen K, Grondalen J. Familial renal disease in soft-coated wheaten terriers. J Small Anim Pract 1984;25(8):489–500.

92. Chew DJ, DiBartola SP, Boyce JT, et al. Renal amyloidosis in related Abyssinian cats. J Am Vet Med Assoc 1982;181(2):139–42.

93. DiBartola SP, Benson MD, Dwulet FE, et al. Isolation and characterization of amyloid protein AA in the Abyssinian cat. Lab Invest 1985;52(5):485–9.

94. DiBartola SP, Tarr MJ, Benson MD. Tissue distribution of amyloid deposits in Abyssinian cats with familial amyloidosis. J Comp Pathol 1986;96(4):387–98.

95. Boyce JT, DiBartola SP, Chew DJ, et al. Familial renal amyloidosis in Abyssinian cats. Vet Pathol 1984;21(1):33–8.
96. Niewold TA, van der Linde-Sipman JS, Murphy C, et al. Familial amyloidosis in cats: Siamese and Abyssinian AA proteins differ in primary sequence and pattern of deposition. Amyloid 1999;6(3):205–9.
97. Godfrey DR, Day MJ. Generalised amyloidosis in two Siamese cats: spontaneous liver haemorrhage and chronic renal failure. J Small Anim Pract 1998; 39(9):442–7.
98. Lees GE. Familial renal disease in dogs. In: Ettinger SJ, Feldman EC, editors. Textbook of veterinary internal medicine. 7th edition. St. Louis (MO): Saunders (Elsevier); 2010. p. 2058–62.
99. Pescucci C, Mari F, Longo I, et al. Autosomal-dominant Alport syndrome: natural history of a disease due to COL4A3 or COL4A4 gene. Kidney Int 2004;65(5): 1598–603.
100. Herrera GA, Turbat-Herrera EA. Renal diseases with organized deposits: an algorithmic approach to classification and clinicopathologic diagnosis. Arch Pathol Lab Med 2010;134(4):512–31.
101. Kamile J, Yasuno K, Ogihara K, et al. Collagenofibrotic glomerulonephropathy with fibronectin deposition in a dog. Vet Pathol 2009;46(4):688–92.
102. Kobayashi R, Yasuno K, Ogihara K, et al. Pathological characterization of collagenofibrotic glomerulonephropathy in a young dog. J Vet Med Sci 2009;71(8): 1137–41.
103. Cavana P, Capucchio MT, Bovero A, et al. Noncongophilic fibrillary glomerulonephritis in a cat. Vet Pathol 2008;45(3):347–51.
104. Brown PJ, Skuse AM, Tappin SW. Pulmonary haemorrhage and fibrillary glomerulonephritis (pulmonary-renal syndrome) in a dog. Vet Rec 2008;162(4):486–7.
105. Center SA, Smith CA, Wilkinson E, et al. Clinicopathologic, renal immunofluorescent, and light microscopic features of glomerulonephritis in the dog: 41 cases (1975–1985). J Am Vet Med Assoc 1987;190(1):81–90.
106. Macdougall DF, Cook T, Steward AP, et al. Canine chronic renal disease: prevalence and types of glomerulonephritis in the dog. Kidney Int 1986;29(6): 1144–51.
107. Muller-Peddinghaus R, Trautwein G. Spontaneous glomerulonephritis in dogs. I. Classification and immunopathology. Vet Pathol 1977;14(1):1–13.
108. Muller-Peddinghaus R, Trautwein G. Spontaneous glomerulonephritis in dogs. II. Correlation of glomerulonephritis with age, chronic interstitial nephritis and extrarenal lesions. Vet Pathol 1977;14(2):121–7.
109. Koeman JP, Biewenga WJ, Gruys E. Proteinuria in the dog: a pathomorphological study of 51 proteinuric dogs. Res Vet Sci 1987;43(3):367–78.
110. Vilafranca M, Wohlsein P, Trautwein G, et al. Histological and immunohistological classification of canine glomerular disease. Zentralbl Veterinarmed A 1994; 41(8):599–610.
111. Biewenga WJ, Gruys E. Proteinuria in the dog: a clinicopathological study in 51 proteinuric dogs. Res Vet Sci 1986;41(2):257–64.
112. Jaenke RS, Allen TA. Membranous nephropathy in the dog. Vet Pathol 1986; 23(6):718–33.
113. Nash AS, Wright NG, Spencer AJ, et al. Membranous nephropathy in the cat: a clinical and pathological study. Vet Rec 1979;105(4):71–7.
114. Wright NG, Nash AS, Thompson H, et al. Membranous nephropathy in the cat and dog: a renal biopsy and follow-up study of sixteen cases. Lab Invest 1981;45(3):269–77.

115. Grauer GF. Canine glomerulonephritis: new thoughts on proteinuria and treatment. J Small Anim Pract 2005;46(10):469–78.
116. Cook AK, Cowgill LD. Clinical and pathological features of protein-losing glomerular disease in the dog: a review of 137 cases (1985–1992). J Am Anim Hosp Assoc 1996;32(4):313–22.
117. Nangaku M, Couser WG. Mechanisms of immune-deposit formation and the mediation of immune renal injury. Clin Exp Nephrol 2005;9(3):183–91.
118. Asano T, Tsukamoto A, Ohno K, et al. Membranoproliferative glomerulonephritis in a young cat. J Vet Med Sci 2008;70(12):1373–5.
119. Breitschwerdt EB, Maggi RG, Chomel BB, et al. Bartonellosis: an emerging infectious disease of zoonotic importance to animals and human beings. J Vet Emerg Crit Care 2010;20(1):8–30.
120. Margolis G, Forbus WD, Kerby GP, et al. Glomerulonephritis occurring in experimental brucellosis in dogs. Am J Pathol 1947;23(6):983–93.
121. Granick JL, Armstrong PJ, Bender JB. *Anaplasma phagocytophilum* infection in dogs: 34 cases (2000–2007). J Am Vet Med Assoc 2009;234(12):1559–65.
122. Pomianowski A, Lew S, Kuleta Z, et al. Peritoneal dialysis in a dog with acute renal failure caused by the infection with *Babesia canis*. Pol J Natur Sc 2008;23(1):257–67.
123. Cavalcante LFH, Neuwald EB, Mello FP, et al. Nephrotic syndrome in dog associated *Babesia canis*. Acta Scientiae Veterinariae 2006;34(3):335–8.
124. Camacho AT, Guitian FJ, Pallas E, et al. Azotemia and mortality among *Babesia microti*-like infected dogs. J Vet Intern Med 2004;18(2):141–6.
125. Slade DJ, Lees GE, Berridge BR, et al. Resolution of a proteinuric nephropathy associated with *Babesia gibsoni* infection in a dog. J Am Anim Hosp Assoc, in press.
126. Kim HJ, Park C, Jung DI, et al. A case of protein losing nephropathy in a dog infected with canine *Babesia gibsoni*. Korean J Vet Res 2006;46(1):77–81.
127. Baneth G, Weigler B. Retrospective case-control study of hepatozoonosis in dogs in Israel. J Vet Intern Med 1997;11(6):365–70.
128. Macintire DK, Vincent-Johnson N, Dillon AR, et al. Hepatozoonosis in dogs: 22 cases (1989–1994). J Am Vet Med Assoc 1997;210(7):916–22.
129. Quigg RJ, Gaines R, Wakely PE Jr, et al. Acute glomerulonephritis in a patient with Rocky Mountain Spotted Fever. Am J Kidney Dis 1991;17(3):339–42.
130. Hervas J, Gomez-Villamandos JC, Perez J, et al. Focal mesangial-sclerosing glomerulonephritis and acute-spontaneous infectious canine hepatitis; structural, immunohistochemical and subcellular studies. Vet Immunol Immunopathol 1997;57(1/2):25–32.
131. Glick AD, Horn RG, Holscher M. Characterization of feline glomerulonephritis associated with viral-induced hematopoietic neoplasms. Am J Pathol 1978;92(2):321–32.
132. Poli A, Abramo F, Taccini E, et al. Renal involvement in feline immunodeficiency virus infection: a clinicopathological study. Nephron 1993;64(2):282–8.
133. Baxter KJ, Levy JK, Edinboro CH, et al. Renal disease in cats infected with feline immunodeficiency virus. J Vet Intern Med 2010;24(3):677.
134. Avila A, Reche A Jr, Kogika MM, et al. Occurrence of chronic kidney disease in cats naturally infected with immunodeficiency virus. J Vet Intern Med 2010;24(3):760.
135. Hayashi T, Ishida T, Fujiwara K. Glomerulonephritis associated with feline infectious peritonitis. Nippon Juigaku Zasshi 1982;44(6):909–16.

136. Grauer GF, Culham CA, Cooley AJ, et al. Clinicopathologic and histologic evaluation of *Dirofilaria immitis*-induced nephropathy in dogs. Am J Trop Med Hyg 1987;37(3):588–96.
137. Kramer L, Simon F, Tamarozzi F, et al. Is *Wolbachia* complicating the pathological effects of *Dirofilaria immitis* infections? Vet Parasitol 2005;133(2/3):133–6.
138. Ludders JW, Grauer GF, Dubielzig RR, et al. Renal microcirculatory and correlated histologic changes associated with dirofilariasis in dogs. Am J Vet Res 1988;49(6):826–30.
139. Grauer GF, Oberhauser EB, Basaraba RJ, et al. Development of microalbuminuria in dogs with heartworm disease. J Vet Intern Med 2002;16(3):352.
140. Casey HW, Splitter GA. Membranous glomerulonephritis in dogs infected with *Dirofilaria immitis*. Vet Pathol 1975;12(2):111–7.
141. Ruth J. *Heterobilharzia americana* infection and glomerulonephritis in a dog. J Am Anim Hosp Assoc 2010;46(3):203–8.
142. Ginel PJ, Camacho S, Lucena R. Anti-histone antibodies in dogs with leishmaniasis and glomerulonephritis. Res Vet Sci 2008;85(3):510–4.
143. Ortega-Pacheco A, Colin-Flores RF, Gutierrez-Blanco E, et al. Frequency and type of renal lesions in dogs naturally infected with *Leptospira* species. Ann N Y Acad Sci 2008;1149:270–4.
144. Zaragoza C, Barrera R, Centeno F, et al. Characterization of renal damage in canine leptospirosis by sodium dodecyl sulphate-polyacrylamide gel electrophoresis (SDS-PAGE) and Western blotting of the urinary proteins. J Comp Pathol 2003;129(2–3):169–78.
145. Mastrorilli C, Dondi F, Agnoli C, et al. Clinicopathologic features and outcome predictors of *Leptospira interrogans* Australis serogroup infection in dogs: a retrospective study of 20 cases (2001–2004). J Vet Intern Med 2007;21(1):3–10.
146. Sykes JE, Hartmann K, Lunn KF, et al. 2010 ACVIM/ISCAID Small Animal consensus statement on leptospirosis: diagnosis, epidemiology, treatment, and prevention. Draft is currently on the ACVIM. Available at: http://www.acvim.org/websites/acvim/File/Resources/Lepto_consensus_draft_July11_forcomment_2010.pdf. Accessed July 25, 2010, to be published J Vet Intern Med 2011.
147. Acierno MJ, Labato MA, Stern LC, et al. Serum concentrations of the third component of complement in healthy dogs and dogs with protein-losing nephropathy. Am J Vet Res 2006;67(7):1105–9.
148. Harris CH, Krawiec DR, Gelberg HB, et al. Canine IgA glomerulonephropathy. Vet Immunol Immunopathol 1993;36(1):1–16.
149. Miyauchi Y, Nakayama H, Uchida K, et al. Glomerulopathy with IgA deposition in the dog. J Vet Med Sci 1992;54(5):969–75.
150. Biewenga WJ, Gruys E, Hendriks HG. Urinary protein loss in the dog: nephrological study of 29 dogs without signs of renal disease. Res Vet Sci 1982;33(3):366–74.
151. Vilafranca M, Wohlsein P, Leopold-Temmler B, et al. A canine nephropathy resembling minimal change nephrotic syndrome in man. J Comp Pathol 1993;109(3):271–80.
152. Sum SO, Hensel P, Rios L, et al. Drug-induced minimal change nephropathy in a dog. J Vet Intern Med 2010;24(2):431–5.
153. DiBartola SP, Tarr MJ, Parker AT, et al. Clinicopathologic findings in dogs with renal amyloidosis: 59 cases (1976–1986). J Am Vet Med Assoc 1989;195(3):358–64.

154. DiBartola SP, Benson MD. The pathogenesis of reactive systemic amyloidosis. J Vet Intern Med 1989;3(1):31–41.
155. Pressler BM, Vaden SL. Managing renal amyloidosis in dogs and cats. Vet Med 2003;98(4):320–33.
156. Whittemore JC, Gill VL, Jensen WA, et al. Evaluation of the association between microalbuminuria and the urine albumin-creatinine ratio and systemic disease in dogs. J Am Vet Med Assoc 2006;229(6):958–63.
157. Whittemore JC, Miyoshi Z, Jensen WA, et al. Association of microalbuminuria and the urine albumin-to-creatinine ratio with systemic disease in cats. J Am Vet Med Assoc 2007;230(8):1165–9.
158. Grauer GF, Moore LE, Smith AR, et al. Comparison of conventional urine protein test strip method and quantitative ELISA for the detection of canine and feline albuminuria. J Vet Intern Med 2004;18(3):418–9.
159. Zatelli A, Paltrinieri S, Nizi F, et al. Evaluation of a urine dipstick test for confirmation or exclusion of proteinuria in dogs. Am J Vet Res 2010;7(2):235–40.
160. Lyon SD, Sanderson MW, Vaden SL, et al. Comparison of urine dipstick, sulfosalicylic acid, urine protein-to-creatinine ratio, and species-specific ELISA methods for detection of albumin in urine samples of cats and dogs. J Am Vet Med Assoc 2010;236(8):874–9.
161. Welles EG, Whatley EM, Hall AS, et al. Comparison of Multistix PRO dipsticks with other biochemical assays for determining urine protein (UP), urine creatinine (UC), and UP:UC ratio in dogs and cats. Vet Clin Pathol 2006;35(1):31–6.
162. Kahn M, Fernandes P, Jensen M, et al. Comparison of the Vitros 250 and the IDEXX VetTest chemistry analyzer for urine protein:creatinine ratios in dogs and cats. J Vet Intern Med 2005;19(3):431.
163. Fernandes P, Kahn M, Yang V, et al. Comparison of methods used for determining urine protein-to-creatinine ratio in dogs and cats. J Vet Intern Med 2005;19(3):431.
164. Kuwahar Y, Nishii N, Takasu M, et al. Use of urine albumin/creatinine ratio for estimation of proteinuria in cats and dogs. J Vet Med Sci 2008;70(8):865–7.
165. Beatrice L, Nizi F, Callegari D, et al. Comparison of urine protein-to-creatinine ratio in urine samples collected by cystocentesis versus free catch in dogs. J Am Vet Med Assoc 2010;236(11):1221–4.
166. Nabity MB, Boggess MM, Kashtan CE, et al. Day-to-day variation of the urine protein:creatinine ratio in female dogs with stable glomerular proteinuria caused by X-linked hereditary nephropathy. J Vet Intern Med 2007;21(3):425–30.
167. LeVine DN, Zhang DW, Harris T, et al. The use of pooled vs. serial urine samples to measure urine protein:creatinine ratios. Vet Clin Pathol 2010;39(1):53–6.
168. Gary AT, Cohn LA, Kerl ME, et al. The effects of exercise on urinary albumin excretion in dogs. J Vet Intern Med 2004;18(1):52–5.
169. Rawlinson JE, Goldstein RE, Erb HN, et al. Tracking inflammatory and renal parameters in dogs pre- and post-treatment for periodontal disease. J Vet Intern Med 2005;19(3):430–1.
170. Prober LG, Johnson CA, Olivier NB, et al. Effect of semen in urine specimens on urine protein concentration determined by means of dipstick analysis. Am J Vet Res 2010;71(3):288–92.
171. Vaden SL, Pressler BM, Lappin MR, et al. Effects of urinary tract inflammation and sample blood contamination on urine albumin and total protein concentrations in canine urine samples. Vet Clin Pathol 2004;33(1):14–9.

172. Bagley RS, Center SA, Lewis RM, et al. The effect of experimental cystitis and iatrogenic blood contamination on the urine protein/creatinine ratio in the dog. J Vet Intern Med 1991;5(2):66–70.

173. Ortega TM, Feldman EC, Nelson RW, et al. Systemic arterial blood pressure and urine protein/creatinine ratio in dogs with hyperadrenocorticism. J Am Vet Med Assoc 1996;209(10):1724–9.

174. Hurley KG, Vaden SL. Evaluation of urine protein content in dogs with pituitary-dependent hyperadrenocorticism. J Am Vet Med Assoc 1998;212(3):369–73.

175. Mazzi A, Fracassi F, Dondi F, et al. Ratio of urinary protein to creatinine and albumin to creatinine in dogs with diabetes mellitus and hyperadrenocorticism. Vet Res Commun 2008;32(Suppl 1):S299–301.

176. Waters CB, Adams LG, Scott-Moncrieff JC, et al. Effects of glucocorticoid therapy on urine protein-to-creatinine ratios and renal morphology in dogs. J Vet Intern Med 1997;11(3):172–7.

177. Schellenberg S, Mettler M, Gentillini F, et al. The effects of hydrocortisone on systemic arterial blood pressure and urinary protein excretion in dogs. J Vet Intern Med 2008;22(2):273–81.

178. Bacic A, Kogika MM, Barbaro KC, et al. Evaluation of albuminuria and its relationship with blood pressure in dogs with chronic kidney disease. Vet Clin Pathol 2010;39(2):203–9.

179. Struble AL, Feldman EC, Nelson RW, et al. Systemic hypertension and proteinuria in dogs with diabetes mellitus. J Am Vet Med Assoc 1998;213(6):822–5.

180. Zini E, Bonfanti U, Zatelli A. Diagnostic relevance of qualitative proteinuria evaluated by use of sodium dodecyl sulphate-agarose gel electrophoresis and comparison with renal histologic findings in dogs. Am J Vet Res 2004;65(7):964–71.

181. Littman MP. Diagnosis of infectious diseases of the urinary tract. In: Bartges JW, Polzin DJ, editors. Nephrology and urology of small animals. Ames (IA): Blackwell; 2011. p. 241–52.

182. Laquaniti A, Bolignano D, Donato V, et al. Alterations in lipid metabolism in chronic nephropathies: mechanisms, diagnosis and treatment. Kidney Blood Press Res 2010;33(2):100–10.

183. Brown S, Atkins C, Bagley R, et al. ACVIM consensus statement: guidelines for the identification, evaluation, and management of systemic hypertension in dogs and cats. J Vet Intern Med 2007;21(3):542–58.

184. Finco DR. Association of systemic hypertension with renal injury in dogs with induced renal failure. J Vet Intern Med 2004;18(3):289–94.

185. Green RA, Russo EA, Greene RT, et al. Hypoalbuminemia-related platelet hypersensitivity in two dogs with nephrotic syndrome. J Am Vet Med Assoc 1985;186(5):485–8.

186. Palmer KG, King LG, Van Winkle TJ. Clinical manifestations and associated disease syndromes in dogs with cranial vena cava thrombosis: 17 cases (1989–1996). J Am Vet Med Assoc 1998;213(2):220–4.

187. Greco DS, Green RA. Coagulation abnormalities associated with thrombosis in a dog with nephrotic syndrome. Compend Cont Educ Pract Vet 1987;9(6):653–8.

188. Goncalves R, Penderis J, Chang YP, et al. Clinical and neurological characteristics of aortic thromboembolism in dogs. J Small Anim Pract 2008;49(4):178–84.

189. Klosterman ES, Moore GE, deBrito Galvao JF, et al. A case-control study of nephrotic syndrome in dogs: 78 cases. J Vet Intern Med 2010;24(3):678.

190. Schieppati A, Perna A, Zamora J, et al. Immunosuppressive treatment for idiopathic membranous nephropathy in adults with nephrotic syndrome. Cochrane Database Syst Rev 2004;4:CD004293.

191. Barakat R, Molony DA, Samuels JA. Immunosuppressive agents for treating IgA nephropathy. Cochrane Database Syst Rev 2003;4:CD003965.
192. Cowgill LD. Diagnostic assessment of proteinuric renal disease: the 21st century vision. In: ACVIM Forum Proceedings. 2009. Available at: http://www.vin.com/Members/proceedings/Proceedings.plx?CID=ACVIM2009&Category=&PID=51528&O=VIN. Accessed October 20, 2010.
193. Lees GE, Berridge BR. Renal biopsy – when and why. NAVC Clinician's Brief 2009;7(10):26–8.
194. Lees GE, Berridge BR, Clubb FJ. Evaluation of renal biopsy samples. NAVC Clinician's Brief 2009;7(10):67–9.
195. Lees GE, Berridge BR, Cianciolo RE. Renal biopsy stains. NAVC Clinician's Brief 2010;8(1):27–30.
196. Lees GE, Bahr A, Sanders MH. Performing renal biopsy. NAVC Clinician's Brief 2010;8(4):67–72.
197. Vaden SL, Levine JP, Lees GE, et al. Renal biopsy: a retrospective study of methods and complications in 283 dogs and 65 cats. J Vet Intern Med 2005; 19(6):794–801.
198. Vaden SL. Renal biopsy of dogs and cats. Clin Tech Small Anim Pract 2005; 20(1):11–22.
199. Vaden SL. Renal biopsy: methods and interpretation. Vet Clin North Am Small Anim Pract 2004;34(4):887–908.
200. Brown SA, Finco DR, Brown CA, et al. Evaluation of the effects of inhibition of angiotensin converting enzyme with enalapril in dogs with induced chronic renal insufficiency. Am J Vet Res 2003;64(3):321–7.
201. Lefebvre HP, Laroute V, Concordet D, et al. Effects of renal impairment on the disposition of orally administered enalapril, benazepril, and their active metabolites. J Vet Intern Med 1999;13(1):21–7.
202. Tenhundfeld J, Wefstaedt P, Nolte IJA. A randomized controlled clinical trial of the use of benazepril and heparin for the treatment of chronic kidney disease in dogs. J Am Vet Med Assoc 2009;234(8):1031–7.
203. Grauer GF, Greco DS, Getzy DM, et al. Effects of enalapril versus placebo as a treatment for canine idiopathic glomerulonephritis. J Vet Intern Med 2000; 14(5):526–33.
204. Vaden SL. What's on the horizon for management of proteinuria renal diseases? In: ACVIM Forum Proceedings. 2009. Available at: http://www.vin.com/Members/Proceedings/Proceedings.plx?CID=acvim2009&PID=pr51531&O=VIN. Accessed October 20, 2010.
205. Segev G, Fascetti AJ, Weeth LP, et al. Correction of hyperkalemia in dogs with chronic kidney disease consuming commercial renal diets by potassium-reduced home-prepared diet. J Vet Intern Med 2010;24(3):546–50.
206. Grauer GF, Rose BJ, Toolan LA, et al. Effects of low-dose aspirin and specific thromboxane synthetase inhibition on whole blood platelet aggregation and adenosine triphosphate secretion in healthy dogs. Am J Vet Res 1992;53(9): 1631–5.
207. Rackear D, Feldman B, Farver T, et al. The effect of three different dosages of acetylsalicylic acid on canine platelet aggregation. J Am Anim Hosp Assoc 1988;24(1):23–6.
208. Shearer L, Kruth SA, Wood D. Effects of aspirin and clopidogrel on platelet function in healthy dogs. In: Proceedings of the 19th ECVIM-CA Congress. Available at: http://www.vin.com/Members/Proceedings/Proceedings.plx?CID=ecvim2009&PID=pr52275&O=VIN. Accessed July 10, 2010.

209. Longhofer SL, Frisbie DD, Johnson HC, et al. Effects of thromboxane synthetase inhibition on immune complex glomerulonephritis. Am J Vet Res 1991;52(3): 480–7.

210. Grauer GF, Frisbie DD, Longhofer SL, et al. Effects of a thromboxane synthetase inhibitor on established immune complex glomerulonephritis in dogs. Am J Vet Res 1992;53(5):808–13.

211. Grauer GF, Frisbie DD, Snyder PS, et al. Treatment of membranoproliferative glomerulonephritis and nephrotic syndrome in a dog with a thromboxane synthetase inhibitor. J Vet Intern Med 1992;6(2):77–81.

212. Smith SA, Tobias AH, Jacob KA, et al. Arterial thromboembolism in cats: acute crisis in 127 cases (1992–2001) and long-term management with low-dose aspirin in 24 cases. J Vet Intern Med 2003;17(1):73–83.

213. Ramsey CC, Burney DP, Macintire DK, et al. Use of streptokinase in four dogs with thrombosis. J Am Vet Med Assoc 1996;209(4):780–5.

214. Clare AC, Kraje BJ. Use of recombinant tissue-plasminogen activator for aortic thrombolysis in a hypoproteinemic dog. J Am Vet Med Assoc 1998;212(4): 539–43.

215. Brown SA, Brown CA, Crowell WA, et al. Beneficial effects of chronic administration of dietary omega-3 polyunsaturated fatty acids in dogs with renal insufficiency. J Lab Clin Med 1998;131(5):447–55.

216. Ahmed MS, Hou SH, Battaglia MC, et al. Treatment of idiopathic membranous nephropathy with the herb *Astragalus membranaceus*. Am J Kidney Dis 2007; 50(6):1028–32.

217. Leehey DJ, Casini T, Massey D. Remission of membranous nephropathy after therapy with *Astragalus membranaceus*. Am J Kidney Dis 2010;55(4):772.

218. Mahajan A, Simoni J, Sheather SJ, et al. Daily oral sodium bicarbonate preserves glomerular filtration rate by slowing its decline in early hypertensive nephropathy. Kidney Int 2010;78(3):303–9.

219. Banyard MRC, Hassett RS. The use of mycophenolate mofetil in the treatment of a case of immune-mediated glomerulonephritis in a dog. Aust Vet Pract 2001; 31(3):103–6.

220. Alchi B, Jayne D. Membranoproliferative glomerulonephritis. Pediatr Nephrol 2010;25(8):1409–18.

221. Yagi K, Yanagida H, Sugimoto K, et al. Clinicopathologic features, outcome, and therapeutic interventions in four children with isolated C3 mesangial proliferative glomerulonephritis. Pediatr Nephrol 2005;20(9):1273–8.

222. Yokoyama H, Wada T, Zhang W, et al. Advances in apheresis therapy for glomerular diseases. Clin Exp Nephrol 2007;11(2):122–7.

Hypertension in Small Animal Kidney Disease

Harriet Syme, BVetMed, PhD, FHEA, MRCVS

KEYWORDS

- Sodium retention • Chronic kidney disease
- Renin-angiotensin-system • Hypertension

Kidney disease is an important cause of hypertension in many species. It is often considered separately from primary (so-called essential or idiopathic) hypertension. This approach may be flawed; however, because many of the mechanisms that are proposed to cause hypertension in patients with kidney disease may also play a role in the pathogenesis of primary hypertension, and vice versa. It may also result in renal hypertension being considered as a single pathologic entity, with uniform underlying cause, which is unlikely to be the case.

This article reviews the mechanisms that are currently considered to be of greatest importance in the pathogenesis of hypertension and how best to treat the condition. Methods of blood pressure measurement and descriptions of the end-organ damage that occurs in dogs and cats with hypertension (in organs other than the kidney) are not described in this article. These topics have been the subject of numerous reviews, and readers are referred to those for information on these topics.[1–4]

CONTROL OF BLOOD PRESSURE

The long-term control of blood pressure is possible by a complex mixture of neural, hormonal, and intrinsic factors involving the brain, heart, vasculature, and especially the kidneys. The rudiments of this control mechanism are summarized in **Fig. 1**. Extracellular fluid volume varies in line with total body sodium content. A primary function of the kidneys is to regulate sodium and water excretion, and consequently, they play a dominant role in the long-term control of blood pressure. The 2 predominant mechanisms of renal regulation of blood pressure are pressure natriuresis and the renin-angiotensin-aldosterone system (RAAS). These systems are augmented by the sympathetic nervous system and the influence of numerous vasoactive mediators acting at both local and systemic levels.

Pressure Natriuresis

Pressure natriuresis is a system that regulates the amount of extracellular water by coupling the excretion of salt and water in response to changes in blood volume

Department of Veterinary Clinical Sciences, Royal Veterinary College, Hawkshead Lane, North Mymms, Hatfield, Hertfordshire AL9 7TA, UK
E-mail address: hsyme@rvc.ac.uk

Vet Clin Small Anim 41 (2011) 63–89
doi:10.1016/j.cvsm.2010.11.002
0195-5616/11/$ – see front matter © 2011 Elsevier Inc. All rights reserved.

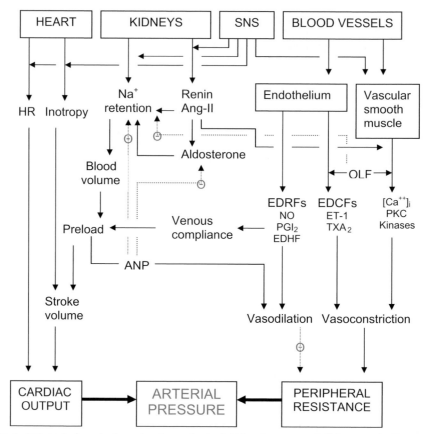

Fig. 1. Integrated control mechanisms of arterial blood pressure. Solid arrows indicate positive effects; dashed arrows, negative effects. Ang-II, angiotensin II; ANP, atrial natriuretic peptide; $[Ca^{++}]_i$, intracellular calcium ion concentration; EDCFs, endothelium-derived constricting factors; EDHF, endothelium-derived hyperpolarizing factor; EDRFs, endothelium-derived relaxing factors; ET-1, endothelin 1; HR, heart rate; NO, nitric oxide; OLF, ouabainlike factor; PGI_2, prostacyclin; PKC, protein kinase C; SNS, sympathetic nervous system; TXA_2, thromboxane A_2.

and cardiac output, which are detected as alterations in renal perfusion pressure. The kidney acts as a servocontroller with infinite negative feedback gain; essentially, when functioning normally, it is able to adjust blood pressure back to a normal level regardless of the magnitude of the initial deviation. Regulation of sodium excretion is achieved through control of glomerular filtration, tubular reabsorption, and tubular secretion, which are processes that are controlled by biophysical characteristics such as transcapillary pressure gradients as well as a variety of hormones and locally acting vasoactive substances.

Disruption of the pressure natriuresis relationship is a fundamental aspect of hypertension in all experimental models of hypertension and in naturally occurring disease. Guyton and colleagues[5] showed in a series of experiments in the 1980s that if the renal arterial pressure was maintained at a normal level (due to a hydraulic occluder placed around the aorta) infusion of vasoactive hormones such as angiotensin II, aldosterone, or vasopressin caused significant increases in systemic pressure and signs of volume overload. When the suprarenal aortic constriction was relieved, natriuresis and diuresis occurred, and the hypertension was ameliorated.

In patients with kidney disease, the capacity of the kidney to excrete sodium may decrease, resulting in an increase in salt sensitivity[6] concomitant with an increasing incidence of hypertension.[7] This mechanism for hypertension is particularly important in patients with end-stage renal disease with extreme reduction in glomerular filtration rate (GFR) resulting in a decrease in the amount of sodium that is filtered at the glomerulus. With lesser degrees of kidney dysfunction, any reduction in the filtered sodium load should be offset by a reduction in tubular sodium reabsorption in any remaining functional nephrons. This suggests that the hypertension in patients with milder forms of chronic kidney disease (CKD) is linked to impairment of sodium handling in the tubules and/or collecting ducts. It is notable that most monogenic causes of hypertension relate to defective sodium handling in the collecting duct,[8] whereas alterations in sodium handling in more proximal parts of the nephron allow compensatory mechanisms to maintain sodium balance, dysregulation of sodium transport in the distal nephron may not allow counterregulatory mechanisms to operate.

It has been hypothesized that defective sodium excretion in hypertension could be caused by vasoconstriction of the afferent arteriole.[9] This vasoconstriction could be mediated by mechanisms involving vasoactive substances, that is, either excessive production of vasoconstrictors, such as endothelin, or impaired vasodilation, for example, due to impaired release of nitric oxide (NO).[10] Alternatively, the vasoconstriction could result from increased sympathetic tone[11] or activation of the renin-angiotensin system (RAS).[12] This mechanism is not specific to patients with kidney disease but could also be operative in patients with primary hypertension.

RAAS

The RAAS directly controls peripheral vascular resistance and renal reabsorption of sodium and water. Renin is secreted from juxtaglomerular cells in response to reduction in effective circulating fluid volume. This condition is detected by reduction in arterial pressure, renal perfusion pressure, or chloride delivery to the macula densa. Adenosine, acting via adenosine 1 receptors, mediates the inhibition of renin secretion in response to both increased chloride delivery to the macula densa and increased renal perfusion pressure as detected by baroreceptors in the afferent arterioles. Both cyclooxygenase 2 and neuronal NO synthase mediate increases in renin release in response to low blood pressure. Renin is also released in response to increased sympathetic nerve stimulation via β_1-adrenoceptors. Renin release can be inhibited by the action of angiotensin II on juxtaglomerular cells.

Renin is an aspartyl protease that is synthesized in the juxtaglomerular cell as a proenzyme, prorenin. Prorenin is converted to renin exclusively within the juxtaglomerular cell, so plasma renin activity (PRA) is undetectable following bilateral nephrectomy. Renin cleaves angiotensinogen, produced by the liver, to yield a decapeptide angiotensin I. Then, angiotensin I is converted to the octapeptide angiotensin II by the angiotensin-converting enzyme (ACE), which is located on endothelial surfaces and in the circulation. Other metabolites of angiotensin I and II can be formed by ACE-2, a homolog of ACE.[13] Some of these metabolites have effects that oppose those of angiotensin II, resulting in vasodilation and antiproliferative effects. Inhibition of ACE-2 worsens glomerular injury and promotes proteinuria in mouse models of diabetic nephropathy.[14]

Prorenin is secreted constitutively by juxtaglomerular cells, resulting in plasma levels that are about 10 times higher than those of renin. Although this proenzyme was previously considered to have no physiologic role, a receptor, located on mesangial and smooth muscle cells, has now been identified that binds both prorenin and renin with equal affinity.[15] Once bound to the receptor, prorenin exhibits catalytic activity, enabling conversion of angiotensinogen to angiotensin I. Receptor binding also activates intracellular signaling pathways (eg, ERK and transforming growth factor β). Prorenin may be of particular importance in the pathogenesis of diabetic nephropathy.[16]

Angiotensin II acts on at least 2 different receptor subtypes: type 1 (AT1) and type 2 (AT2) receptors. The AT1 receptor mediates all the classical physiologic effects of angiotensin II. The functions of the AT2 receptor are less well understood, but in general, AT2 receptors seem to oppose the effects mediated by AT1. Angiotensin II increases blood pressure in several different ways, each of which is mediated by binding to the AT1 receptor. It causes immediate and powerful vasoconstriction, thereby increasing peripheral vascular resistance. It stimulates sodium reabsorption in the proximal tubule (via the sodium hydrogen exchanger isoform 3) and also possibly in other nephron segments. Angiotensin II also stimulates aldosterone synthesis and secretion by the zona glomerulosa of the adrenal gland. Aldosterone in turn stimulates reabsorption of sodium by the principal cells of the collecting duct.

Although the effects of RAAS stimulation in mediating hypertension and kidney injury have been generally ascribed to the actions of angiotensin II, there is increasingly substantial evidence that aldosterone may also play a key role.[17] It has been shown that administration of exogenous aldosterone to rats results in hypertension and kidney injury.[18] Many of the pathologic changes in the rodent remnant kidney model (eg, hypertension, glomerulosclerosis, and proteinuria) can be replicated by infusion of aldosterone, even when the actions of angiotensin II are pharmacologically inhibited.[19] Conversely, in partially nephrectomized rodents, concurrent adrenalectomy ameliorates the attendant hypertension.[20]

In addition to the circulating RAS, many tissues, including those of the kidney, can generate angiotensin II (and other components of RAS) locally. This tissue-based system can function independently of the circulating hormones and is thought to act in a paracrine manner.[21] Upregulation of the intrarenal RAS may play a pathologic role in progression of some forms of kidney disease. This system may explain the apparent paradox that in some disease states, notably, diabetic nephropathy, there can be an exaggerated hemodynamic response to treatment with ACE inhibitors in spite of low PRA.[22]

Sympathetic Nervous System

Inappropriate sympathetic drive may contribute to the development of hypertension. Excessive sympathetic drive results in sodium retention, renin stimulation, and diminished kidney function. The kidney itself plays a role in the generation of increased sympathetic activity by way of renal somatic afferent nerves directly linked to neural cardiovascular control centers in the midbrain. The kidney is therefore both a target and a contributor to increased sympathetic nerve activity.[23]

Increased sympathetic nerve activity is evident even in mild compensated CKD. It is present in models of mild acute kidney damage and in individuals with polycystic kidney disease (PKD) with normal GFR.[24] These observations suggest that sympathetic activation rather than being a consequence of uremia is an early event in the pathophysiology of CKD and that various forms of kidney damage activate the sympathetic nervous system via the afferents of renal sensory nerves.

Kidney transplant recipients with excellent graft function display increased sympathetic nerve activity similar to that of patients undergoing hemodialysis, whereas transplant recipients who undergo bilateral nephrectomy have normalized sympathetic nerve activity not different from healthy control subjects.[25] Sympathetic hyperactivity in human patients with CKD has been associated with an increased risk of adverse cardiovascular events.[26] In the 1950s (before the advent of effective pharmaceutics), it was shown that lumbar sympathectomy could be an effective treatment for malignant hypertension.[27] Because of the recent development of less-invasive techniques for sympathectomy, there is now a recrudescence in interest in this treatment for human patients with resistant hypertension.[28,29]

Renalase is a soluble monoamine oxidase that may be relatively deficient in patients with CKD, resulting in increased norepinephrine levels and consequently hypertension.[30] Renalase is predominantly expressed in glomeruli and proximal tubules, although it is also expressed in cardiac and skeletal muscles. Under basal conditions, it lacks enzymatic activity; however, physiologic stimuli, such as increases in blood pressure, increase its amine oxidase activity. Renalase is readily detectable in the plasma of normal humans but not in patients with uremia. Single nucleotide polymorphisms in the renalase gene have recently been associated with essential hypertension in man.[31]

Other Mechanisms

Concentrations of parathyroid hormone correlate with blood pressure in human patients with kidney disease.[32] Chronic hyperparathyroidism may lead to accumulation of calcium inside vascular smooth muscle cells, enhancing their sensitivity to norepinephrine.[33] This effect can be blocked by treatment with calcium-channel blockers.[32] However, in one study, parathyroidectomy did not alter blood pressure in patients who underwent kidney dialysis, thus arguing against an important role for this mechanism in the pathogenesis of hypertension in patients with kidney disease.[34]

Administration of erythropoietin may increase blood pressure.[35] This finding may be the reason why the use of this drug to achieve a relatively high packed-cell volume target in human patients with kidney disease was associated with an increased risk of adverse cardiovascular events in recent clinical trials.[36] These effects may occur independent of any viscosity changes that result from increasing hematocrit; it has been suggested that a direct effect on arteriolar constriction may be responsible,[37] although increased sensitivity to norepinephrine has also been demonstrated.[38]

PATHOGENESIS OF HYPERTENSION IN RENAL DISEASE

In humans, hypertension is considered to be both a cause and a consequence of CKD. The prevalence of hypertension is reciprocally related to GFR; the worse the kidney disease, the more likely that hypertension will be present.[39] It is important to recognize that no single mechanism is preeminent in the pathogenesis of hypertension in human patients with CKD but that the relative importance of the myriad mechanisms described earlier varies according to the particular form of kidney disease that is present. A few of the diseases that are of comparative interest in companion animals are discussed in more detail.

Patients who Undergo Dialysis

More than 90% of human patients with end-stage renal disease are hypertensive before the initiation of dialysis. In most human patients receiving maintenance hemodialysis, hypertension is caused by extracellular fluid expansion. Blood pressure can be controlled by adjusting the rates of ultrafiltration during dialysis and by restriction of dietary sodium intake. The importance of volume homeostasis in these patients is illustrated by results from the Tassin hemodialysis unit where long slow dialysis treatments are performed, and within a few months of starting dialysis, fewer than 5% of patients require antihypertensive medications for control of blood pressure. Dry weight (in which blood pressure remains normal both before and after dialysis sessions) is more often achieved in this system because the ultrafiltration rate is relatively low, blood-volume changes are relatively small, and intradialysis symptoms are in frequent.[40] This contrasts with results from most dialysis centers, where the prevalence of hypertension remains high in spite of treatment.

In a minority of patients who undergo hemodialysis, blood pressure is refractory to maneuvers directed at volume homeostasis. In these patients, excessive stimulation of RAAS seems to be the mechanism underlying the persistent hypertension. In a seminal study performed in the 1960s, Vertes and colleagues[41] found that maintaining dry weight helped control hypertension without medication in 35 of 40 (87.5%) hypertensive patients who underwent dialysis. In the remaining 5 patients (12.5%) in whom blood pressure remained elevated, PRA was significantly increased and they were designated as having renin-dependent hypertension. These patients were successfully treated (without antihypertensive medication) by bilateral nephrectomy that reduced PRA to undetectable levels.

Hypertension is common in dogs with severe acute kidney failure requiring dialysis. In a study of 153 dogs receiving dialysis treatment at the University of California, Davis, California, 78% had systolic hypertension (>150 mm Hg), 84% had diastolic hypertension (>95 mm Hg), and 87% had either systolic or diastolic hypertension.[42] In that study, hypertension was not significantly related to the cause of kidney failure or to urine output and did not alter survival. Another study also found that the blood pressure before initiating treatment was not related to survival in dogs receiving dialysis.[43]

In a study of 119 cats receiving hemodialysis at the same center, 40% were hypertensive (systolic blood pressure [SBP]>150 mm Hg) before the initiation of dialysis.[44] Blood pressure was not related to the cause of the kidney failure.

Renal Transplant Recipients

Several factors are known to contribute to the development of hypertension in human kidney transplant recipients; among the most important factors are immunosuppressive therapy, renin secretion from the native kidneys, transplant renal artery stenosis, allograft dysfunction, and hypertension in the donor. Cyclosporine is commonly incriminated in the pathogenesis of posttransplant hypertension. Cyclosporine (and other calcineurin inhibitors) causes constriction of the preglomerular afferent arterioles, resulting in a decrease in renal blood flow and GFR.[45] Several mediators have been implicated in this process, including endothelin, prostaglandins, inhibition of NO synthase, and activation of RAS.[46] Chronic cyclosporine nephrotoxicity is characterized by the presence of structural lesions in the kidney, predominantly interstitial fibrosis and tubular atrophy.[47] This condition is accompanied by reduction in GFR and systemic hypertension.[48] Development of structural lesions may be prevented by treatment with calcium channel blockers, suggesting that vasodilation of the afferent arterioles may ameliorate the chronic nephrotoxicity of cyclosporine.[49] Glucocorticoids may also contribute to the development of hypertension in transplant recipients.

Renal artery stenosis is a relatively frequent cause of hypertension and allograft dysfunction in humans, occurring in 5% to 10% of kidney transplant recipients.[50] It may present at any time but is most common between 3 months and 2 years following transplant. It may develop due to trauma to the donor or recipient vessels during the transplant, immune-mediated endothelial injury of the donor renal artery, or extension of atherosclerosis from the recipient's iliac artery. Renovascular hypertension in renal transplant recipients is the clinical correlate of the Goldblatt one-kidney one-clip model of hypertension that was first described in experimental dogs; hypoperfusion of the single functioning kidney causes stimulation of RAS that in turn causes sodium retention and extracellular volume expansion. These changes improve renal perfusion and reduces RAS activation to levels that are normal or low but inappropriate in relation to the degree of plasma volume expansion. Postglomerular arteriolar constriction maintains GFR at near-normal levels in spite of reduced renal blood flow caused by an increase in filtration fraction.[50]

In humans, transplanting a kidney from a donor with a familial history of hypertension results in a greater increase in blood pressure in the recipient than when the donor's family is normotensive.[51] The importance of the donor kidney has long been studied in experimental models. Kidney transplant from genetically hypertensive rats causes hypertension in the recipients, whereas renal grafts from genetically normotensive donors lower blood pressure in genetically hypertensive recipients.[52] Results of these studies reinforce the primacy of the kidney in the pathogenesis of hypertension.

Severe acute hypertension is common in the immediate perioperative period following a kidney transplant in cats.[53] Before the advent of perioperative blood pressure monitoring, many cats that underwent kidney transplant developed postoperative neurologic complications, most often seizures, and these cats often died as a result.[54,55] Stupor, ataxia, and blindness have also been reported. Treatment of hypertensive cats with hydralazine reduces the incidence of postoperative neurologic complications.[53] In 2 case series, severe hypertension reportedly developed in 21 of 34 (64%) and 9 of 30 (30%) cats that underwent kidney transplant, with blood pressure cutoffs of more than 170 and 160 mm Hg, respectively, to signify severe hypertension in each of the studies.[53,56] The reason for the apparent difference in the incidence of postoperative hypertension in the 2 case series is not clear. Schmiedt and colleagues[56] postulated that this difference may be related to the cold-organ storage techniques for preservation of the grafts before being transplanted because stimulation of the intrarenal RAS has been documented in rat kidneys subjected to ischemia-reperfusion[57] and production of such vasoactive mediators might be reduced at lower temperatures. However, in an experimental study, 10 cats were subjected to kidney autotransplant and contralateral nephrectomy, and none of the cats developed significant postoperative hypertension.[58] Renin activity was not increased in these cats following ischemia-reperfusion.[59] It therefore seems unlikely that ischemia and reperfusion injury is responsible for the development of hypertension following kidney transplant in cats.

The long-term prevalence of hypertension in cats that have received renal allografts and survived the perioperative period has not been reported. Histopathologic evaluations of donor kidneys from cats dying following kidney transplant have shown minimal arteriolar changes suggesting that hypertension may not be a frequent problem.[60] However, in the same study, changes consistent with cyclosporine nephropathy were documented. Cyclosporine concentration has been positively associated with resistive index in cats following kidney transplant, although this change was not associated with an increase in systemic blood pressure.[56]

Kidney transplant is infrequently performed in dogs, except as an experimental model for transplantation in humans. In one report of 15 clinical cases that underwent a kidney transplant, it was reported that the majority had intraoperative hypertension that was managed with opioids, although one dog also required treatment with nitroprusside.[61] One dog developed hypertension following surgery and was treated by removing the remaining native kidney 2 months after it was transplanted; however, whether or not there was resolution of the hypertension was not reported. It is not stated explicitly but seems that the remaining dogs were normotensive.

Diabetic Nephropathy

Diabetes is the most common cause of CKD in humans, accounting for approximately one-third of all cases. Hypertension often develops before any detectable reduction in GFR. Once diabetic nephropathy is established, there is a reduced ability of the kidney to excrete sodium and the systemic RAS is suppressed, although the intrarenal RAS may be simultaneously activated.[62] Many humans with type 2 diabetes are characterized as having the metabolic syndrome comprising insulin resistance, hypertension, hyperlipidemia, and obesity. Development of this syndrome is multifactorial, with both genetic and environmental influences playing a role. Hypertension may be caused or exacerbated by the accumulation of glycosylated end products within the endothelium, altered vasomotor activity, increased oxidative stress, and sympathetic overactivity.

Hypertension (SBP>160 mm Hg, mean BP>120 mm Hg or diastolic blood pressure >100 mm Hg) was reported in 23 of 50 (46%) dogs with diabetes mellitus in one study.[63] Several of these dogs were also proteinuric. In another report blood pressure of 31 dogs with diabetes mellitus was reportedly greater than that of healthy dogs, although the difference was small.[64] Mean (SE) SBP of the diabetic dogs was 142.6 (3.89) mm Hg, so it seems unlikely that many of the dogs were overtly hypertensive, although those data were not reported directly. The kidney function of the dogs was not assessed. There are isolated case reports in the veterinary literature of diabetic cats presenting with signs of hypertensive retinopathy.[65,66] However, there is currently no convincing evidence that diabetic cats are at increased risk for developing systemic hypertension. Blood pressure measurements have been reported in 2 small case series including, in total, 24 cats.[67,68] None of the cats had an SBP more than 180 mm Hg or were reported to have kidney dysfunction.

Hypertensive Nephrosclerosis

Hypertensive nephrosclerosis is reported to be the second most common cause of CKD in humans, accounting for 21% of adult CKD cases. The diagnosis of hypertensive nephrosclerosis implies that hypertension is the cause of the kidney disease, although this remains controversial. One problem is that hypertensive nephrosclerosis refers to a histologic diagnosis (with features including glomerulosclerosis, medial thickening of the arteriolar wall, and intimal fibrosis), but, in fact, biopsy specimens are rarely obtained in this patient subgroup and the pathologic features are, anyway, not specific to hypertensive injury. In addition, although the fact that malignant hypertension causes kidney failure in humans has been accepted for decades, the importance of mild-to-moderate or benign hypertension as a cause of kidney failure is still debated. Although some epidemiologic studies have indicated that hypertension is associated with subsequent development of kidney failure,[7] these studies have been criticized for the fact that preexisting renal disease was not tested for at study entry.[69] This fact essentially means that the hypertension could accelerate the progression of undetected kidney disease in the study participants rather than actually initiating a disease process in otherwise healthy kidneys.

Two seemingly contradictory pathophysiologic mechanisms have been proposed for the development of hypertensive nephrosclerosis.[69] The first putative mechanism is glomerular ischemia. This mechanism occurs as a consequence of chronic hypertension, causing narrowing of preglomerular arteries and arterioles, with a consequent reduction in glomerular blood flow. The second mechanism is glomerular hypertension and glomerular hyperfiltration. It is proposed that hypertension causes some glomeruli to become sclerotic. As an attempt to compensate for the resultant loss of renal function, the remaining nephrons undergo vasodilation of the preglomerular arterioles and experience an increase in renal blood flow and glomerular filtration. The result is glomerular hypertension, glomerular hyperfiltration, and progressive glomerulosclerosis. These mechanisms are not mutually exclusive and may operate simultaneously in the kidney.

There have been infrequent reports in which histologic features of hypertensive arteriosclerosis have been described in cats with antemortem clinical signs relating to hypertension.[66,70] However, because kidney disease and hypertension are usually discovered simultaneously in feline patients, it is impossible to determine whether the hypertension could, in some cases, be the cause of the kidney disease rather than vice versa. Although kidney failure is common in cats, there are very few systematic histopathologic descriptions of this condition. Lucke[71] examined 93 cats with gross kidney morphometric changes, only some of which had evidence of functional kidney impairment, and found fibrous arteriosclerotic plaques of the intima and media of interlobar and arcuate arteries. A comparative study of species differences in the development of arteriosclerosis with age also demonstrated a small, but measurable, degree of intimal hyperplasia in older cats.[72] In another small study of cats with kidney failure, medial hypertrophy of the renal arteries was present in 9 of 10 cats examined.[73] These results conflict with those of a study by DiBartola and colleagues[74] on 74 cats with an antemortem diagnosis of chronic kidney failure. No vascular lesions were described in the study, even though 3 cats had retinal detachment, and the investigators concluded that systemic hypertension was the likely cause. The most common histopathologic diagnosis in that study was chronic tubulointerstitial nephritis; the investigators did not comment on whether vascular lesions were not found or simply not considered significant. Blood pressure measurements were not reported in any of these studies. Further advancement of the understanding of the role that systemic hypertension plays in the development or progression of kidney failure in cats requires systematic histopathologic studies. In a preliminary study of kidney specimens obtained at post mortem examination from cats with naturally occurring systemic hypertension histopathologic changes, including glomerulosclerosis, were more marked than in the control group of normotensive cats with CKD.[75] This was in spite of the fact that the hypertensive cats had been treated with amlodipine for months or even years before death. However, whether these changes are the cause or the result of the hypertension (or its treatment) is impossible to determine.

PKD

Hypertension is common in humans with PKD, often developing before any detectable decline in kidney function. Blood pressure is related to renal volume in children[76] and adults.[77] Hypertension may actually accelerate growth of the cysts because effective control of blood pressure with ACE inhibitors seems to retard cyst enlargement.[78] Hypertension is thought to occur in PKD because the enlarging cysts attenuate flow in the renal blood vessels, resulting in areas of local hypoxia. Accordingly, erythropoietin concentrations are relatively increased in hypertensive patients. Although initial studies failed to demonstrate an absolute increase in PRA or angiotensin II levels in patients with PKD, it has subsequently been demonstrated that activation of RAS is increased relative to patients with essential hypertension.[79] It is proposed that because the disease is bilateral, initial activation of RAS is accompanied by sodium retention, which in turn reduces RAS to normal levels, although inappropriate, relative to the degree of extracellular volume expansion.[80] Intrarenal RAS activation has been demonstrated by immunohistochemistry in kidneys that were surgically removed from kidney transplant recipients.[81] Activation of the sympathetic nervous system[82] and increased production of endothelin 1[83] have also been implicated in the pathogenesis of hypertension in patients with PKD.

Autosomal dominant PKD in cats is the direct clinical correlate of the disease in humans. The underlying mutation in cats is located in the feline PKD1 gene, the homolog of the gene that is affected in 85% of humans with the disease.[84] PKD is not common amongst cats presenting with ocular lesions caused by severe hypertension, although isolated cases may occur. In one small study of 6 cats with PKD and 6 control cats monitored with a directly implanted arterial catheter and a radiotelemetric recording system, no difference in blood pressure was identified.[85] Enalapril was administered to both groups of cats, and an equivalent decrease in blood pressure and increase in PRA was observed in both groups. However, a second study demonstrated that cats with PKD (n = 14) had higher mean blood pressure than gender- and age-matched Persian cats (n = 7), although the SBP and diastolic blood pressure did not differ significantly between the groups and none of the cats were overtly hypertensive.[86] There was a tendency for PRA to be lower in the cats with PKD, and this tendency was reflected by a decrease in the aldosterone to renin ratio compared with the control cats. By analogy with what is found in humans (as described earlier), reduction in PRA does not necessarily indicate that RAS is not implicated in the pathogenesis of any observed increase in blood pressure because RAS should be considered in conjunction with extracellular volume status and PRA should be suppressed if blood pressure is elevated and renal perfusion pressures are increased. It has therefore yet to be conclusively established whether cats with PKD develop hypertension in the same manner as humans.

PKD is infrequently described in dogs but does occur in a population of bull terriers in Australia.[87] Hypertension has not been reported in these dogs, although interpretation of their blood pressure measurements is complicated because many of them have concurrent valvular heart disease.[88]

Glomerular Diseases and the Nephrotic Syndrome

In humans, hypertension is reported to be more common in patients with glomerular than tubulointerstitial diseases and this association is independent of GFR.[39] In patients with nephrotic syndrome, hypertension is common but is usually relatively mild because much of the retained fluid is distributed to the interstitial rather than the vascular space. Historically, it was considered that reduced plasma oncotic pressure caused hypovolemia and sodium retention in the nephrotic syndrome. However, blood volume measurements are generally normal or mildly increased in patients with nephrotic syndrome,[89] and at present it is thought that sodium retention is a primary feature of glomerular disease.[90] Micropuncture studies using experimental models of nephrotic syndrome have localized defective sodium excretion to the connecting tubule and collecting duct.[91] This finding has in turn been linked to aldosterone-independent activation of the epithelial sodium channel and concomitant upregulation of Na^+, K^+-ATPase in the basolateral cell membrane.[92] Renal resistance to the actions of atrial natriuretic peptide has also been proposed as an underlying mechanism for the sodium retention that occurs in proteinuric kidney diseases.[93]

Substantial differences have been reported in the prevalence of hypertension in dogs with naturally occurring kidney disease. This disparity is probably in the main because of methodological differences in blood pressure measurement between the studies; however, it has been suggested that, in general, the prevalence of hypertension is higher in the studies in which glomerular diseases predominate.[94,95] In some cross-sectional studies of dogs with CKD (in which in general, nonproteinuric kidney diseases predominate), correlation between blood pressure and urine protein/creatinine (UPC) ratio has been observed,[96,97] although in other studies a relationship was not evident.[98] A recent study found that blood pressure in dogs with nephrotic syndrome was slightly, but significantly, higher than that in the control group with protein-losing nephropathy but without edema or ascites.[99]

Leishmaniasis is a common cause of glomerular disease in dogs living in endemic areas, notably the Mediterranean basin. In a prospective study of 105 dogs with leishmaniasis, almost half (49.5%) were found to have kidney disease as evidenced by azotemia (creatinine>1.4 mg/dL) and/or proteinuria (UPC ratio >0.5). Of the dogs with kidney disease, 61.5% (n = 32) were reported to be hypertensive with an SBP more than 180 mm Hg (n = 25) or more than 150 mm Hg in conjunction with left ventricular hypertrophy (n = 7).[95] Interestingly, the prevalence of hypertension in the dogs that were proteinuric but not azotemic was 70.6% (12 of 17 dogs). Leishmaniasis may serve as a useful naturally occurring model for the further study of systemic hypertension in dogs with glomerular disease.

There are only limited reports of blood pressure measurements from other spontaneously occurring glomerular diseases in dogs. Hypertension (SBP>180 mm Hg) was present in 22 of 69 (31.9%) dogs in which blood pressure was measured before obtaining a kidney biopsy sample; many but not all of these dogs were suspected to have glomerular disease.[100] A juvenile glomerulopathy has recently been described in French mastiffs; blood pressure was only measured in 4 dogs, and none were reported to be hypertensive.[101] One study reported that only 12 of 146 (8.2%) soft-coated wheaten terriers with protein-losing nephropathy were hypertensive, with 5 of the dogs having retinal lesions; however, it is not clear in how many dogs blood pressure measurements were actually obtained, so the true prevalence of hypertension in this disease remains uncertain.[102] Hypertension has been reported in dogs with Lyme nephropathy but again its frequency is uncertain.[103]

Hypertension has not been reported in association with the membranous glomerulonephritis that is sometimes seen in young, predominantly male, cats.[104]

CKD of Undetermined Cause

In many veterinary patients in whom CKD is diagnosed, proteinuria is mild and no specific underlying cause for the kidney disease is identified. In many of these patients, the kidneys are small and it is presumed that were a biopsy to be performed (although this is rarely clinically indicated), tubulointerstitial nephritis and fibrosis would be identified. It is in this group of relatively poorly characterized patients, in particular elderly cats, that hypertension is most frequently recognized. In most studies, about two-thirds of cats presenting with signs of hypertension-induced ocular damage are azotemic.[65,66,70] However, estimates of the proportion of azotemic cats that are hypertensive are much less consistent, ranging from 19% to 65%.[105–107] These widely differing estimates of the proportion of azotemic cats that are hypertensive are probably in large part because of differences in the populations studied and differences in the cutoff points used to define hypertension. An interesting observation is that cats presenting with signs of hypertensive end-organ damage tend to be mildly azotemic.[105,106] Similarly, it is relatively uncommon for normotensive cats diagnosed with CKD to subsequently develop hypertension, even if their kidney disease is progressive. This finding is in contrast to the observation in humans that blood pressure is inversely related to GFR.

Ocular lesions caused by systemic hypertension are less frequently encountered in dogs than in cats. Nonetheless, a small number of case reports exist.[108] Dogs may be relatively resistant to the development of ocular lesions, even when relatively severe increases in blood pressure occur, so substantiating a diagnosis of hypertension is more difficult in dogs than in cats.[95] In studies in which blood pressure measurement has been performed systematically in dogs with azotemic CKD, the prevalence of hypertension has been reported as 31% and 54% using blood pressure cutoffs of 160 and 140 mm Hg, respectively.[96,97] In another study, although blood pressure was higher in dogs with kidney disease than clinically healthy dogs, the difference was small[64] and hypertension was reported to be uncommon[109]; however, estimates of prevalence were not reported.

Hypertensive cats tend to have slightly lower serum or plasma potassium concentrations than normotensive cats, although in the majority the potassium concentration remains within, or only just less than, the laboratory reference range.[70,106] A potential explanation for this difference is relative or absolute hyperaldosteronism in the hypertensive cats—a hypothesis that has been tested in several different studies. Jensen and colleagues[110] showed that aldosterone concentration was significantly higher in hypertensive cats with kidney disease than in a control population of young normal cats. A limitation of the study is that it is not possible to tell whether the differences observed were because of the study group being hypertensive or other differences between the groups (eg, in kidney function, diet, or age). However, a subsequent study comparing hypertensive and normotensive cats with CKD also indicated that aldosterone concentrations were slightly higher in cats with hypertension, although there was considerable overlap between groups, and in most instances, aldosterone concentration remained within the laboratory reference range.[111] Taken together, these observations seem to support a role for hyperaldosteronism in the pathogenesis of hypertension in cats with CKD, although the relative importance of this mechanism, given the very small observed differences, is unknown.

The cause of hyperaldosteronism in patients with CKD is presumed to be increased renin production caused by a subpopulation of underperfused nephrons. However, in the small number of cats with CKD and hypertension in which PRA has been measured, it has been normal or low.[110,111] This result suggests that the relative hyperaldosteronism observed in cats with CKD is independent of RAS stimulation. This suggestion is supported by the clinical observation that there is minimal change in blood pressure when hypertensive cats are treated with ACE inhibitors.[110] Accordingly, in a study that measured PRA and aldosterone in hypertensive cats before and after treatment with ACE inhibitors, concentrations of these hormones did not change with treatment.[112]

The idea that hyperaldosteronism plays a role in the development of hypertension in cats with CKD is also supported by the observation that in a small group of cats presented with signs of hypertension, histologic examination of their adrenal glands revealed extensive micronodular hyperplasia of the zona glomerulosa.[113] However, a study that compared adrenocortical histopathologic findings in hypertensive (n = 37) and normotensive cats (n = 30) found no difference between the 2 groups, although adrenocortical hyperplasia was common (present in 65 of 67 cats). In addition, 2 cats, both in the hypertensive group, had adrenocortical adenomas.[114] Thus, although adrenocortical pathology is common in old cats, it does not, in isolation, explain the development of hypertension; although relative nonsuppressible hyperaldosteronism could be one contribution to a multifactorial cause.

Several other potential mechanisms for the development of hypertension in cats with CKD have been investigated. The syndrome of apparent mineralocorticoid excess occurs when there is decreased conversion of hormonally active cortisol to inactive cortisone within mineralocorticoid-target tissues, such as those of the kidney. This conversion is catalyzed by the enzyme 11β-hydroxysteroid dehydrogenase type 2, and activity of this enzyme is impaired in human patients with CKD.[115] Cortisol has great affinity for mineralocorticoid receptors and its concentration is much higher than that of aldosterone; therefore, if conversion of cortisol to cortisone is reduced, signs of mineralocorticoid excess (hypokalemia and hypertension) develop. To determine whether reduced conversion of cortisol to cortisone could play a role in development of hypertension in cats with CKD, cortisol/cortisone ratios were compared in hypertensive and normotensive cats, but no difference was found. In fact, the cortisol to cortisone shuttle seems to be more effective in cats with CKD than in clinically normal cats.[116] The reason for this potentially adaptive response to kidney disease is unclear.

NO is a vasodilator with an important physiologic role in the regulation of renal blood flow and control of vascular tone. As might be expected, chronic administration of L-NAME ($N\omega$-nitro-L-arginine methyl ester), an inhibitor of NO production, to clinically normal cats causes a significant increase in blood pressure.[117] Reduced availability of NO resulting in endothelial dysfunction has been implicated in the pathogenesis of hypertension and progression of kidney disease.[118] Two proposed causes of NO deficiency in human patients with CKD are L-arginine deficiency (because the kidney is a primary site for its synthesis) and accumulation of endogenous inhibitors of NO synthase, most notably asymmetric dimethylarginine (ADMA).[119] Studies in cats with CKD did not find any evidence for L-arginine deficiency in this species, but ADMA and creatinine concentrations were positively correlated.[120] However, ADMA concentrations did not differ between hypertensive and normotensive cats and there was no correlation between ADMA measurements and SBP. Therefore, although the possibility exists that the accumulation of ADMA in cats with CKD results in endothelial dysfunction, this does not seem to be associated with the development of systemic hypertension.

The observation that PRA tends to be normal or low in cats with hypertension (see earlier discussion) points to a role for sodium retention and plasma volume expansion in the pathogenesis of renal hypertension in this species. The volume status of cats with CKD has not been systematically studied. In one very small study, plasma volume in 4 hypertensive cats with CKD (33.1 mL/kg) was not significantly different from that of the young normal controls (29.3 mL/kg).[121] No normotensive cats with CKD were included for comparison in the study. Further characterization of plasma volume in larger numbers of cats with CKD is required before conclusions can be drawn. However, consideration of volume in isolation is inherently flawed because blood pressure is essentially a function of the degree of vasoconstriction of the vascular bed relative to its degree of filling (the so-called vasoconstriction-volume hypothesis); simultaneous measurement of both volume and vascular tone is required, although difficult in practice.[122] Increased vascular tone may be particularly important in the pathogenesis of hypertension in cats because they show a profound response to treatment with calcium-channel blockers and other arteriolar dilators. This response is much more dramatic than the typical responses observed in dogs or humans.[96,123]

Changes in sodium intake have a direct influence on blood pressure in human patients with CKD, and this relationship seems to be stronger at low levels of kidney function.[6] The limited studies performed to date in cats do not indicate that blood pressure in this species is generally salt sensitive.[124–126] However, only small numbers of cats with either naturally occurring[126] or induced[125] renal dysfunction have been included. The salt sensitivity of blood pressure in hypertensive cats with naturally occurring CKD has not been reported and would be an interesting area for study in the future. In clinically normal dogs, increasing salt intake increases total body water with no change in blood pressure.[127] Varying dietary salt intake also does not alter blood pressure in dogs with experimentally reduced renal mass.[128] No studies have been performed in dogs with naturally occurring CKD.

Nonazotemic CKD

As discussed earlier, contrary to expectation, cats are usually only mildly azotemic when hypertension is diagnosed. In all the larger series of hypertensive cats published to date, about 20% of the cats have been nonazotemic and nonhyperthyroid.[65,129] Although some of these cats may have had less common causes of hypertension, such as primary hyperaldosteronism or pheochromocytoma, it seems unlikely that this would account for all of these patients. These cats have been described as having idiopathic hypertension. In these cats, the hypertension may be actually primary, unassociated with any underlying disease process, or may be related to underlying CKD that is not severe enough to result in azotemia. It is well documented in human medicine that the prevalence of hypertension increases in patients with kidney disease, even when GFR is normal.[39]

TREATMENT

Although a reduction in dietary sodium intake is often recommended as an initial step in the management of systemic hypertension in humans, there is no evidence that this intervention is of any benefit in the management of hypertension in cats or dogs because blood pressure does not seem to change in response to sodium restriction/loading. Reduction in sodium intake does, however, result in potentially deleterious effects including activation of RAS and kaliuresis.[125] At present, the recommendation for cats and dogs with spontaneous hypertension is to avoid unusually high salt intake without making a specific effort to restrict it.[3] It is currently unknown whether administering subcutaneous fluids to patients with CKD will alter blood pressure in hypertension-susceptible individuals. Until more information is available, it seems prudent to reserve this treatment for specific patients with a tendency to become dehydrated without fluid therapy.

Pharmacologic management is the mainstay of treatment of hypertension in both dogs and cats. In human medicine, it has been proposed that the relative activation of RAS should be an important consideration in the selection of initial treatment.[130] Drugs that interrupt RAS are likely to be most effective in the treatment of the high-renin forms of hypertension (**Box 1**). In low-renin forms of hypertension, treatment with drugs that target the sodium volume–mediated mechanisms of hypertension is

---

Box 1
Classification of antihypertensive agents based on whether their predominant effect is through renin- or volume-dependent mechanisms

Renin-dependent hypertension

ACE inhibitors

Angiotensin receptor blockers

Renin inhibitors

Centrally acting α_2-receptor agonists

β-Blockers

Volume-dependent hypertension

Diuretics

Calcium-channel blockers

α_1-Receptor blockers

most logical. Moreover, when combining multiple agents to increase efficacy, selecting the combination of a drug that interrupts RAS and a drug with a predominant effect on sodium volume may be more effective than selecting 2 drugs from the same group. For example, treatment of hypertensive humans with thiazide diuretics is commonplace, but this drug results in stimulation of RAS, which blunts the drugs' efficacy. Combined therapy with an ACE inhibitor improves blood pressure control.

Treatment of Hypertension in Cats

The choice of an antihypertensive agent for cats with systemic hypertension is largely governed by the requirement for a dramatic sustained reduction in blood pressure without the development of unwanted side effects and, in general, without the necessity to administer multiple medications. This situation is in contrast to human medicine in which administration of 2 or more drugs is generally accepted, particularly in patients with kidney disease.[123]

A marked decrease in blood pressure, typically of the order of 30 to 60 mm Hg, can be achieved by treating hypertensive cats with the second-generation dihydropyridine calcium-channel blocker amlodipine.[65,131–134] This drug is well tolerated. Although the half-life of the drug in cats has not been measured, its duration of effect seems to be maintained for more than 24 hours, making it suitable for once-daily dosing and meaning that the lack of precision in daily dosing (due to administering fractions of tablets) is not an issue.[133,135] The use of a transdermal formulation of amlodipine in hypertensive cats has been reported.[136] Bioavailability of the transdermal formulation was only reported to be about 30% of the oral formulation, and it is possible that even this availability was because of the cats' grooming and ingesting the product from the pinnae. Given the ease with which amlodipine can be administered orally, the requirement for a transdermal formulation seems debatable.

In an experimental model of induced kidney insufficiency and hypertension in cats, diltiazem was shown to decrease blood pressure but the effect was not maintained for 24 hours, indicating that the drug would need to be given at least twice daily for effective blood pressure control.[135] Diltiazem is a member of the benzothiazepine class of calcium-channel blockers and would be anticipated to have more cardiac effects than the drugs of the dihydropyridine class, such as amlodipine. Use of diltiazem has been reported in a small number of cats with spontaneous disease, and although some improvement in blood pressure was noted, amlodipine was found to be more efficacious.[65]

Another vasodilator drug, hydralazine, has also shown efficacy in the treatment of renal hypertension in cats. Use of this drug may be considered in the emergency setting because with parenteral administration, a response may be demonstrated within 15 minutes of administration.[53] It has been used to treat hypertension when it develops acutely following kidney transplant. However, in most clinical situations, the time taken to respond to orally administered amlodipine is perfectly adequate, so in view of the increased potential for side effects when treating with hydralazine (most notably, symptomatic hypotension and tachycardia), treatment with amlodipine is generally preferred.

A potential disadvantage of treating cats with kidney disease with amlodipine is that it causes dilation of the afferent renal arteriole. If sufficient reduction in systemic blood pressure is not achieved, intraglomerular pressure could increase. This disadvantage has led to suggestion that drugs with preferential effect on the efferent arteriole be used instead. In this regard, ACE inhibitors and/or angiotensin receptor blockers (ARBs) are considered to be the first line agents of antihypertensive therapy in humans with CKD,[137] although evidence exists that the benefit of specific types of drug is not as important as the magnitude of their antihypertensive effect.[138] ACE inhibitors have not been demonstrated to be sufficiently effective antihypertensive agents in cats with naturally occurring systemic hypertension to recommend their use, at least as sole therapy.[66,110,131] Studies of cats with induced kidney insufficiency have demonstrated that ACE inhibitors decrease systemic blood pressure, but the magnitude of the measured effect is very small.[85,117,139] It is notable, however, that in these experimental settings, hypertension was either absent or mild, and there was no evidence that RAAS was stimulated, which may explain the apparent lack of efficacy of the ACE inhibitor. An alternative explanation is suggested by the observation that a conventional dose of enalapril (0.5 mg/kg every 24 hours) was insufficient to completely block the pressor effect of angiotensin I infusion in experimental cats, indicating that additional pathways for conversion of angiotensin I to angiotensin II may exist in this species.[140] ARBs have not been used to any great extent in feline medicine. Losartan was ineffective as an antihypertensive agent in cats with experimentally induced renal hypertension.[135,140]

A variety of drugs were used to treat systemic hypertension in cats before the effectiveness of amlodipine was established. Thus, some limited clinical experience of treating cats with β-blockers, diuretics, and spironolactone exists, but none is currently recommended as first line therapy. β-Blockers have the potential to reduce blood pressure in renal hypertension not only by decreasing heart rate and stroke volume but also by inhibiting the release of renin. However, β-blockers are not very effective in the treatment of hypertension in cats.[110,141] Although diuretics are frequently administered to hypertensive people, even those with kidney disease, these agents are not recommended in cats with CKD due to the risk of volume depletion and hypokalemia. Given that mild relative hyperaldosteronism has been demonstrated in cats with hypertensive renal disease, treatment with spironolactone is an attractive option. However, the effectiveness of this therapy has been marginal when used as a sole therapy for the management of hypertension, even in cats with aldosterone-secreting tumors.[142] When spironolactone was used for treatment of heart disease, 4 of 13 cats developed a cutaneous drug reaction; this reaction may also limit its use in patients with hypertension.[143] In addition to their effects on vascular smooth muscle, it has been proposed that calcium-channel blockers could act directly to reduce secretion of aldosterone by the adrenal gland, so this may be an additional reason to favor this class of drugs.[144]

The desired end point of antihypertensive therapy in cats with CKD is to minimize the risk of end-organ damage and to maximize the quantity and the quality of life after implementing therapy. Treatment with amlodipine in cats is sufficient to prevent the development of hypertensive encephalopathy and ongoing ocular damage and to stabilize, or reverse, cardiac hypertrophy.[53,65,134] However, although kidney disease is reportedly the most common cause of death in cats with hypertension,[131,145] whether treatment of cats with a particular class of drug has additional benefits in terms of slowing the progression of CKD remains to be determined.

In one study of 136 cats with naturally occurring CKD, blood pressure was not independently related to survival, although all the hypertensive cats were treated, which may have affected patient outcome.[146] However, in an earlier case series in which blood pressure was not controlled (the report predated the discovery that amlodipine was effective), it is notable that many of the cats lived for long periods in spite of the evidence of ongoing ocular injury.[66] In a further study, 141 hypertensive cats (most of them azotemic) were treated with amlodipine. A composite measure of the cats' blood pressure while on treatment was calculated over the entire period of follow-up and used to evaluate for an association between the degree of blood pressure control and survival.[129] No independent association of blood pressure with survival was found. However, the cats with the highest blood pressure (both before and during treatment) tended to be the most proteinuric, and proteinuria was associated with survival. It remains to be determined whether this association between proteinuria and survival is causative. It remains possible that proteinuria is merely a marker for a more rapidly progressive form of kidney disease.

Treatment with amlodipine in hypertensive cats could in theory cause or exacerbate proteinuria because this drug causes greater dilation of the afferent than the efferent renal arterioles, potentially allowing the transmission of high systemic pressures to the glomerular capillaries. However, treatment of hypertensive cats with amlodipine causes a reduction in proteinuria. This change is presumably because of the profound decrease in blood pressure that occurs.

Treatment with ACE inhibitors has been demonstrated to reduce proteinuria in cats with normotensive CKD.[147,148] As might be expected, reduction in proteinuria is greatest in those cats that are the most proteinuric before treatment. Unfortunately, despite reducing proteinuria, ACE inhibitors have not shown demonstrable benefit in terms of increased survival times[147] or retarded disease progression[148] in normotensive cats with CKD. It is, however, possible that a similar study of hypertensive cats with CKD would yield more favorable results, particularly because hypertensive cats tend to be more proteinuric than their normotensive counterparts.[146] A small pilot study has demonstrated that combination therapy with benazepril and amlodipine is well tolerated by cats but the UPC ratios were not significantly different from those of cats receiving sole therapy with amlodipine.[149]

Treatment of Hypertension in Dogs

In dogs the optimal treatment of hypertension has yet to be established. Although there are published studies of the use of antihypertensive agents in normal dogs[150] and in dogs with experimentally induced kidney disease,[151,152] there are few systematic studies of dogs with naturally occurring renal hypertension. Anecdotally, it is reported that hypertension is difficult to control in dogs. In one study in which 14 dogs with renal hypertension were treated with a variety of antihypertensive agents, blood pressure was controlled (<160 mm Hg) in only 1 dog.[96]

Use of ACE inhibitors is generally considered to be the first line treatment of hypertension in dogs.[3] This is not because these drugs have been found to be particularly effective in reducing blood pressure, but because they are indicated in the management of proteinuric kidney disease. Treatment with ACE inhibitors has been shown to reduce proteinuria and improve patient outcome in dogs with glomerulonephritis,[153] hereditary nephropathy,[154] and CKD.[155] ACE inhibitors slightly reduced blood pressure in a study of dogs with experimentally induced kidney disease.[151] In the same study, glomerular capillary pressure and histologic scores for glomerular and tubular injury were reduced in dogs treated with enalapril.

In general, except in the emergency setting, treatment of hypertension in dogs is staged: an ACE inhibitor is introduced first, and if the response is inadequate, a second agent, usually amlodipine, is added. Amlodipine is generally preferred to other arteriolar dilators because its use is associated with minimal reflex tachycardia. Combination therapy with an ACE inhibitor and amlodipine may be rational because the former blunts the stimulation of RAS caused by amlodipine.[150] However, even when used in combination, the change in blood pressure (at least in normal dogs) is small.[150] The dose of amlodipine is typically sequentially increased to the maximum recommended dose (**Table 1**), with adjustments made on a weekly to fortnightly basis. The half-life of amlodipine in dogs is reported to be 30 hours, so it is inadvisable to make more rapid

Table 1
Recommended dosages for different antihypertensive agents in dogs and cats

Drug	Action	Dose in Cats	Dose in Dogs
Amlodipine	Calcium-channel blocker	0.625–1.25 mg/cat q 24 h	0.1–0.4 mg/kg q 24 h
Diltiazem	Calcium-channel blocker	10 mg/cat q 8 h (regular formulation) 10 mg/kg q 12 h (sustained release)	0.5–2.0 mg/kg q 8 h (regular formulation)
Enalapril	ACE inhibitor	0.25–0.5 mg/kg q 12–24 h	0.5–1.0 mg/kg q 12–24 h
Benazepril	ACE inhibitor	0.5–1.0 mg/kg q 12–24 h	0.25–0.5 mg/kg q 12–24 h
Ramipril	ACE inhibitor	0.125 mg/kg q 24 h	0.125 mg/kg q 24 h
Atenolol	β_1-Adrenergic blocker	6.25–12.5 mg/cat q 12–24 h	0.25–1.0 mg/kg q 12–24 h
Hydralazine	Direct arteriolar dilator	1.0–2.5 mg/cat subcutaneously	0.5–3.0 mg/kg q 8–12 h
Phenoxybenzamine	α-Adrenergic blocker	Not recommended	0.25–2.5 mg/kg q 12 h
Prazosin	α-Adrenergic blocker	Not recommended	0.5–2.0 mg/dog q 12 h
Spironolactone	Aldosterone antagonist	1–2 mg/kg q 12 h	1–2 mg/kg q 12 h

With the exception of the dose for hydralazine in the cat, all other drugs are administered orally. If a dose range is given, treatment is usually initiated at the low end of the range and titrated upward to effect. Once the maximum dose is reached, an additional agent may be added in some instances (see text for details).

adjustments to the administered dose[156] and also unnecessary to administer it more than once daily. Gingival hyperplasia has been reported in a small percentage of dogs treated chronically with amlodipine.[157] Otherwise, the drug is generally well tolerated.

A significant proportion of hypertensive dogs seem to be relatively refractory to treatment. In these cases, it is difficult to know what therapeutic regimen should be followed; certainly there is no evidence base to guide therapy. If the patient is tachycardic, then administration of a low dose of atenolol may be logical. Otherwise, a different vasodilator (hydralazine or phenoxybenzamine) can be substituted for the amlodipine to see if it is more effective. The impetus to reduce blood pressure in these refractory cases tends to be the evidence of nonrenal end-organ damage, such as ventricular hypertrophy, or retinal changes. In some cases without end-organ damage, at least in the author's opinion, the risks of further therapy are difficult to justify. However, there is a risk that uncontrolled hypertension will accelerate progression of the patient's kidney disease.

In a remnant kidney model of kidney failure in dogs, blood pressure was related to both proteinuria and severity of renal morphologic lesions (mesangial matrix accumulation, tubular lesions, and fibrosis) at the termination of the study.[158] GFR tended to increase over time following the kidney insult; however, this increase was less evident in the dogs that had the highest blood pressure.[158] In dogs with naturally occurring CKD, hypertension has also been related to progression of kidney disease. In one study of 45 dogs, the median survival times of dogs in the high–blood-pressure (>161 mm Hg), medium–blood-pressure (144–160 mm Hg), and low–blood-pressure

(<144 mm Hg) groups were 425, 348, and 154 days, respectively.[96] There was a statistically significant difference in survival between the high– and low–blood-pressure groups. Differences in survival were mainly attributable to progression of kidney disease in the dogs with the highest blood pressure. It is notable, however, that the dogs with the highest blood pressure also tended to be those that were the most proteinuric.[159] Another study has also reported an association between hypertension and/or proteinuria and shortened survival times.[97] Thus, in dogs, as with cats, it is difficult to differentiate the effect of blood pressure and proteinuria on survival; it is possible that the dogs that are the most hypertensive (and proteinuric) have a type of kidney disease that is inherently more rapidly progressive. In humans with kidney disease, the importance of blood pressure control depends on the severity of proteinuria.

SUMMARY

The pathogenesis of hypertension is multifactorial. Uncontrolled hypertension leads to end-organ damage in both dogs and cats. Early recognition and treatment are the keys to preventing end-organ damage.

REFERENCES

1. Crispin SM, Mould JR. Systemic hypertensive disease and the feline fundus. Vet Ophthalmol 2001;4(2):131–40.
2. Acierno MJ, Labato MA. Hypertension in renal disease: diagnosis and treatment. Clin Tech Small Anim Pract 2005;20(1):23–30.
3. Brown S, Atkins C, Bagley R, et al. Guidelines for the identification, evaluation, and management of systemic hypertension in dogs and cats. J Vet Intern Med 2007;21(3):542–58.
4. Henik RA, Stepien RL, Bortnowski HB. Spectrum of M-Mode echocardiographic abnormalities in 75 cats with systemic hypertension. J Am Anim Hosp Assoc 2004;40(5):359–63.
5. Olsen ME, Hall JE, Montani JP, et al. Mechanisms of angiotensin II natriuresis and antinatriuresis. Am J Physiol 1985;249(2 Pt 2):F299–307.
6. Koomans HA, Roos JC, Boer P, et al. Salt sensitivity of blood pressure in chronic renal failure. Evidence for renal control of body fluid distribution in man. Hypertension 1982;4(2):190–7.
7. Klag MJ, Whelton PK, Randall BL, et al. Blood pressure and end-stage renal disease in men. N Engl J Med 1996;334(1):13–8.
8. Lifton RP, Gharavi AG, Geller DS. Molecular mechanisms of human hypertension. Cell 2001;104(4):545–56.
9. Johnson RJ, Rodriguez-Iturbe B, Nakagawa T, et al. Subtle renal injury is likely a common mechanism for salt-sensitive essential hypertension. Hypertension 2005;45(3):326–30.
10. Quiroz Y, Pons H, Gordon KL, et al. Mycophenolate mofetil prevents salt-sensitive hypertension resulting from nitric oxide synthesis inhibition. Am J Physiol Renal Physiol 2001;281(1):F38–47.
11. Johnson RJ, Gordon KL, Suga S, et al. Renal injury and salt-sensitive hypertension after exposure to catecholamines. Hypertension 1999;34(1):151–9.
12. Lombardi D, Gordon KL, Polinsky P, et al. Salt-sensitive hypertension develops after short-term exposure to angiotensin II. Hypertension 1999;33(4):1013–9.
13. Ribeiro-Oliveira A Jr, Nogueira AI, Pereira RM, et al. The renin-angiotensin system and diabetes: an update. Vasc Health Risk Manag 2008;4(4):787–803.

14. Wong DW, Oudit GY, Reich H, et al. Loss of angiotensin-converting enzyme-2 (Ace2) accelerates diabetic kidney injury. Am J Pathol 2007;171(2):438–51.
15. Nguyen G, Delarue F, Burckle C, et al. Pivotal role of the renin/prorenin receptor in angiotensin II production and cellular responses to renin. J Clin Invest 2002; 109(11):1417–27.
16. Hollenberg NK. Direct renin inhibition and the kidney. Nat Rev Nephrol 2010; 6(1):49–55.
17. Epstein M. Aldosterone as a mediator of progressive renal disease: pathogenetic and clinical implications. Am J Kidney Dis 2001;37(4):677–88.
18. Gomez-Sanchez EP, Zhou M, Gomez-Sanchez CE. Mineralocorticoids, salt and high blood pressure. Steroids 1996;61(4):184–8.
19. Greene EL, Kren S, Hostetter TH. Role of aldosterone in the remnant kidney model in the rat. J Clin Invest 1996;98(4):1063–8.
20. Quan ZY, Walser M, Hill GS. Adrenalectomy ameliorates ablative nephropathy in the rat independently of corticosterone maintenance level. Kidney Int 1992; 41(2):326–33.
21. Kobori H, Nangaku M, Navar LG, et al. The intrarenal renin-angiotensin system: from physiology to the pathobiology of hypertension and kidney disease. Pharmacol Rev 2007;59(3):251–87.
22. Hollenberg NK, Price DA, Fisher ND, et al. Glomerular hemodynamics and the renin-angiotensin system in patients with type 1 diabetes mellitus. Kidney Int 2003;63(1):172–8.
23. Schlaich MP, Socratous F, Hennebry S, et al. Sympathetic activation in chronic renal failure. J Am Soc Nephrol 2009;20(5):933–9.
24. Klein IH, Ligtenberg G, Oey PL, et al. Sympathetic activity is increased in polycystic kidney disease and is associated with hypertension. J Am Soc Nephrol 2001;12(11):2427–33.
25. Hausberg M, Kosch M, Harmelink P, et al. Sympathetic nerve activity in end-stage renal disease. Circulation 2002;106(15):1974–9.
26. Penne EL, Neumann J, Klein IH, et al. Sympathetic hyperactivity and clinical outcome in chronic kidney disease patients during standard treatment. J Nephrol 2009;22(2):208–15.
27. Smithwick RH, Thompson JE. Splanchnicectomy for essential hypertension; results in 1,266 cases. J Am Med Assoc 1953;152(16):1501–4.
28. Schlaich MP, Sobotka PA, Krum H, et al. Renal sympathetic-nerve ablation for uncontrolled hypertension. N Engl J Med 2009;361(9):932–4.
29. Krum H, Schlaich M, Whitbourn R, et al. Catheter-based renal sympathetic denervation for resistant hypertension: a multicentre safety and proof-of-principle cohort study. Lancet 2009;373(9671):1275–81.
30. Desir GV. Regulation of blood pressure and cardiovascular function by renalase. Kidney Int 2009;76(4):366–70.
31. Zhao Q, Fan Z, He J, et al. Renalase gene is a novel susceptibility gene for essential hypertension: a two-stage association study in northern Han Chinese population. J Mol Med 2007;85(8):877–85.
32. Raine AE, Bedford L, Simpson AW, et al. Hyperparathyroidism, platelet intracellular free calcium and hypertension in chronic renal failure. Kidney Int 1993; 43(3):700–5.
33. Schiffl H, Fricke H, Sitter T. Hypertension secondary to early-stage kidney disease: the pathogenetic role of altered cytosolic calcium (Ca2+) homeostasis of vascular smooth muscle cells. Am J Kidney Dis 1993;21(5 Suppl 2): 51–7.

34. Ifudu O, Matthew JJ, Macey LJ, et al. Parathyroidectomy does not correct hypertension in patients on maintenance hemodialysis. Am J Nephrol 1998; 18(1):28–34.
35. Krapf R, Hulter HN. Arterial hypertension induced by erythropoietin and erythro-poiesis-stimulating agents (ESA). Clin J Am Soc Nephrol 2009;4(2):470–80.
36. Singh AK, Szczech L, Tang KL, et al. Correction of anemia with epoetin alfa in chronic kidney disease. N Engl J Med 2006;355(20):2085–98.
37. Heidenreich S, Rahn KH, Zidek W. Direct vasopressor effect of recombinant human erythropoietin on renal resistance vessels. Kidney Int 1991;39(2): 259–65.
38. Hand MF, Haynes WG, Johnstone HA, et al. Erythropoietin enhances vascular responsiveness to norepinephrine in renal failure. Kidney Int 1995;48(3):806–13.
39. Buckalew VM Jr, Berg RL, Wang SR, et al. Prevalence of hypertension in 1,795 subjects with chronic renal disease: the modification of diet in renal disease study baseline cohort. Modification of Diet in Renal Disease Study Group. Am J Kidney Dis 1996;28(6):811–21.
40. Charra B. Fluid balance, dry weight, and blood pressure in dialysis. Hemodial Int 2007;11(1):21–31.
41. Vertes V, Cangiano JL, Berman LB, et al. Hypertension in end-stage renal disease. N Engl J Med 1969;280(18):978–81.
42. Francey T, Cowgill LD. Hypertension in dogs with severe acute renal failure. J Vet Intern Med 2004;18(3):418.
43. Segev G, Kass PH, Francey T, et al. A novel clinical scoring system for outcome prediction in dogs with acute kidney injury managed by hemodialysis. J Vet Intern Med 2008;22(2):301–8.
44. Pantaleo V, Francey T, Fischer JR, et al. Application of hemodialysis for the management of acute uremia in cats: 119 cases (1993–2003). J Vet Intern Med 2004;18(3):418.
45. Morales JM, Andres A, Rengel M, et al. Influence of cyclosporin, tacrolimus and rapamycin on renal function and arterial hypertension after renal transplantation. Nephrol Dial Transplant 2001;16(Suppl 1):121–4.
46. Bobadilla NA, Gamba G. New insights into the pathophysiology of cyclosporine nephrotoxicity: a role of aldosterone. Am J Physiol Renal Physiol 2007;293(1):F2–9.
47. Naesens M, Kuypers DR, Sarwal M. Calcineurin inhibitor nephrotoxicity. Clin J Am Soc Nephrol 2009;4(2):481–508.
48. First MR, Neylan JF, Rocher LL, et al. Hypertension after renal transplantation. J Am Soc Nephrol 1994;4(Suppl 8):S30–6.
49. McCulloch TA, Harper SJ, Donnelly PK, et al. Influence of nifedipine on intersti-tial fibrosis in renal transplant allografts treated with cyclosporin A. J Clin Pathol 1994;47(9):839–42.
50. Bruno S, Remuzzi G, Ruggenenti P. Transplant renal artery stenosis. J Am Soc Nephrol 2004;15(1):134–41.
51. Guidi E, Menghetti D, Milani S, et al. Hypertension may be transplanted with the kidney in humans: a long-term historical prospective follow-up of recipients grafted with kidneys coming from donors with or without hypertension in their families. J Am Soc Nephrol 1996;7(8):1131–8.
52. Rettig R, Grisk O. The kidney as a determinant of genetic hypertension: evidence from renal transplantation studies. Hypertension 2005;46(3):463–8.
53. Kyles AE, Gregory CR, Wooldridge JD, et al. Management of hypertension controls postoperative neurologic disorders after renal transplantation in cats. Vet Surg 1999;28(6):436–41.

54. Mathews KG, Gregory CR. Renal transplants in cats: 66 cases (1987–1996). J Am Vet Med Assoc 1997;211(11):1432–6.
55. Gregory CR, Mathews KG, Aronson LR, et al. Central nervous system disorders after renal transplantation in cats. Vet Surg 1997;26(5):386–92.
56. Schmiedt CW, Holzman G, Schwarz T, et al. Survival, complications, and analysis of risk factors after renal transplantation in cats. Vet Surg 2008;37(7):683–95.
57. Allred AJ, Chappell MC, Ferrario CM, et al. Differential actions of renal ischemic injury on the intrarenal angiotensin system. Am J Physiol Renal Physiol 2000; 279(4):F636–45.
58. Schmiedt CW, Mercurio AD, Glassman MM, et al. Effects of renal autograft ischemia and reperfusion associated with renal transplantation on arterial blood pressure variables in clinically normal cats. Am J Vet Res 2009;70(11): 1426–32.
59. Schmiedt CW, Hurley KAE, Tong X, et al. Measurement of plasma renin concentration in cats by use of a fluorescence resonance energy transfer peptide substrate of renin. Am J Vet Res 2009;70(11):1315–22.
60. De Cock HE, Kyles AE, Griffey SM, et al. Histopathologic findings and classification of feline renal transplants. Vet Pathol 2004;41(3):244–56.
61. Mathews KA, Holmberg DL, Miller CW. Kidney transplantation in dogs with naturally occurring end-stage renal disease. J Am Anim Hosp Assoc 2000;36(4): 294–301.
62. Price DA, Porter LE, Gordon M, et al. The paradox of the low-renin state in diabetic nephropathy. J Am Soc Nephrol 1999;10(11):2382–91.
63. Struble AL, Feldman EC, Nelson RW, et al. Systemic hypertension and proteinuria in dogs with diabetes mellitus. J Am Vet Med Assoc 1998;213(6):822–5.
64. Bodey AR, Michell AR. Epidemiological study of blood pressure in domestic dogs. J Small Anim Pract 1996;37(3):116–25.
65. Maggio F, DeFrancesco TC, Atkins CE, et al. Ocular lesions associated with systemic hypertension in cats: 69 cases (1985–1998). J Am Vet Med Assoc 2000;217(5):695–702.
66. Littman MP. Spontaneous systemic hypertension in 24 cats. J Vet Intern Med 1994;8(2):79–86.
67. Norris CR, Nelson RW, Christopher MM. Serum total and ionized magnesium concentrations and urinary fractional excretion of magnesium in cats with diabetes mellitus and diabetic ketoacidosis. J Am Vet Med Assoc 1999;215(10):1455–9.
68. Sennello KA, Schulman RL, Prosek R, et al. Systolic blood pressure in cats with diabetes mellitus. J Am Vet Med Assoc 2003;223(2):198–201.
69. Luke RG. Hypertensive nephrosclerosis: pathogenesis and prevalence. Essential hypertension is an important cause of end-stage renal disease. Nephrol Dial Transplant 1999;14(10):2271–8.
70. Sansom J, Rogers K, Wood JL. Blood pressure assessment in healthy cats and cats with hypertensive retinopathy. Am J Vet Res 2004;65(2):245–52.
71. Lucke VM. Renal disease in the domestic cat. J Pathol Bacteriol 1968;95(1): 67–91.
72. Tracy RE, Johnson LK. Aging of a class of arteries in various mammalian species in relation to the life span. Gerontology 1994;40(6):291–7.
73. Taugner F, Baatz G, Nobiling R. The renin-angiotensin system in cats with chronic renal failure. J Comp Pathol 1996;115(3):239–52.
74. DiBartola SP, Rutgers HC, Zack PM, et al. Clinicopathologic findings associated with chronic renal disease in cats: 74 cases (1973–1984). J Am Vet Med Assoc 1987;190(9):1196–202.

75. Fletcher M, Syme H, Brown SA, et al. Histological assessment of renal pathology in treated hypertensive and normotensive azotaemic cats. ACVIM. J Vet Intern Med 2004;18(5):788.

76. Cadnapaphornchai MA, McFann K, Strain JD, et al. Increased left ventricular mass in children with autosomal dominant polycystic kidney disease and borderline hypertension. Kidney Int 2008;74(9):1192–6.

77. Gabow PA, Chapman AB, Johnson AM, et al. Renal structure and hypertension in autosomal dominant polycystic kidney disease. Kidney Int 1990;38(6):1177–80.

78. Cadnapaphornchai MA, McFann K, Strain JD, et al. Prospective change in renal volume and function in children with ADPKD. Clin J Am Soc Nephrol 2009;4(4): 820–9.

79. Chapman AB, Johnson A, Gabow PA, et al. The renin-angiotensin-aldosterone system and autosomal dominant polycystic kidney disease. N Engl J Med 1990;323(16):1091–6.

80. Schrier RW. Renal volume, renin-angiotensin-aldosterone system, hypertension, and left ventricular hypertrophy in patients with autosomal dominant polycystic kidney disease. J Am Soc Nephrol 2009;20(9):1888–93.

81. Loghman-Adham M, Soto CE, Inagami T, et al. The intrarenal renin-angiotensin system in autosomal dominant polycystic kidney disease. Am J Physiol Renal Physiol 2004;287(4):F775–88.

82. Cerasola G, Vecchi M, Mule G, et al. Sympathetic activity and blood pressure pattern in autosomal dominant polycystic kidney disease hypertensives. Am J Nephrol 1998;18(5):391–8.

83. Hocher B, Zart R, Schwarz A, et al. Renal endothelin system in polycystic kidney disease. J Am Soc Nephrol 1998;9(7):1169–77.

84. Lyons LA, Biller DS, Erdman CA, et al. Feline polycystic kidney disease mutation identified in PKD1. J Am Soc Nephrol 2004;15(10):2548–55.

85. Miller RH, Lehmkuhl LB, Smeak DD, et al. Effect of enalapril on blood pressure, renal function, and the renin-angiotensin-aldosterone system in cats with autosomal dominant polycystic kidney disease. Am J Vet Res 1999;60(12): 1516–25.

86. Pedersen KM, Pedersen HD, Haggstrom J, et al. Increased mean arterial pressure and aldosterone-to-renin ratio in Persian cats with polycystic kidney disease. J Vet Intern Med 2003;17(1):21–7.

87. Burrows AK, Malikt R, HuntS GB, et al. Familial polycystic kidney disease in bull terriers. J Small Anim Pract 1994;35(7):364–9.

88. O'Leary CA, Mackay BM, Taplin RH, et al. Auscultation and echocardiographic findings in Bull Terriers with and without polycystic kidney disease. Aust Vet J 2005;83(5):270–5.

89. Geers AB, Koomans HA, Boer P, et al. Plasma and blood volumes in patients with the nephrotic syndrome. Nephron 1984;38(3):170–3.

90. Orth SR, Ritz E. The nephrotic syndrome. N Engl J Med 1998;338(17):1202–11.

91. Buerkert J, Martin DR, Trigg D, et al. Sodium handling by deep nephrons and the terminal collecting duct in glomerulonephritis. Kidney Int 1991;39(5):850–7.

92. Gadau J, Peters H, Kastner C, et al. Mechanisms of tubular volume retention in immune-mediated glomerulonephritis. Kidney Int 2009;75(7):699–710.

93. Perico N, Delaini F, Lupini C, et al. Blunted excretory response to atrial natriuretic peptide in experimental nephrosis. Kidney Int 1989;36(1):57–64.

94. Cook AK, Cowgill LD. Clinical and pathological features of protein-losing glomerular disease in the dog: a review of 137 cases (1985–1992). J Am Anim Hosp Assoc 1996;32(4):313–22.

95. Cortadellas O, del Palacio MJ, Bayon A, et al. Systemic hypertension in dogs with leishmaniasis: prevalence and clinical consequences. J Vet Intern Med 2006;20(4):941–7.

96. Jacob F, Polzin DJ, Osborne CA, et al. Association between initial systolic blood pressure and risk of developing a uremic crisis or of dying in dogs with chronic renal failure. J Am Vet Med Assoc 2003;222(3):322–9.

97. Wehner A, Hartmann K, Hirschberger J. Associations between proteinuria, systemic hypertension and glomerular filtration rate in dogs with renal and non-renal diseases. Vet Rec 2008;162(5):141–7.

98. Buranakarl C, Ankanaporn K, Thammacharoen S, et al. Relationships between degree of azotaemia and blood pressure, urinary protein:creatinine ratio and fractional excretion of electrolytes in dogs with renal azotaemia. Vet Res Commun 2007;31(3):245–57.

99. Klosterman ES, Moore GE, De Brito Galvao JF, et al. A case-control study of nephrotic syndrome in dogs: 78 cases. J Vet Intern Med 2010;24(3):678.

100. Vaden SL. Renal biopsy of dogs and cats. Clin Tech Small Anim Pract 2005;20(1):11–22.

101. Lavoué R, van der Lugt JJ, Day MJ, et al. Progressive juvenile glomerulonephropathy in 16 related French Mastiff (Bordeaux) dogs. J Vet Intern Med 2010;24(2):314–22.

102. Littman MP, Dambach DM, Vaden SL, et al. Familial protein-losing enteropathy and protein-losing nephropathy in soft coated Wheaten Terriers: 222 cases (1983–1997). J Vet Intern Med 2000;14(1):68–80.

103. Littman MP, Goldstein RE, Labato MA, et al. ACVIM small animal consensus statement on Lyme disease in dogs: diagnosis, treatment, and prevention. J Vet Intern Med 2006;20(2):422–34.

104. Nash AS, Wright NG, Spencer AJ, et al. Membranous nephropathy in the cat: a clinical and pathological study. Vet Rec 1979;105(4):71–7.

105. Stiles J, Polzin DJ, Bistner DI. The prevalence of retinopathy in cats with systemic hypertension and chronic renal failure or hyperthyroidism. J Am Anim Hosp Assoc 1994;30:564–72.

106. Syme HM, Barber PJ, Markwell PJ, et al. Prevalence of systolic hypertension in cats with chronic renal failure at initial evaluation. J Am Vet Med Assoc 2002;220(12):1799–804.

107. Kobayashi DL, Peterson ME, Graves TK, et al. Hypertension in cats with chronic renal failure or hyperthyroidism. J Vet Intern Med 1990;4(2):58–62.

108. Littman MP, Robertson JL, Bovee KC. Spontaneous systemic hypertension in dogs: five cases (1981–1983). J Am Vet Med Assoc 1988;193(4):486–94.

109. Michell AR, Bodey AR, Gleadhill A. Absence of hypertension in dogs with renal insufficiency. Ren Fail 1997;19(1):61–8.

110. Jensen J, Henik RA, Brownfield M, et al. Plasma renin activity and angiotensin I and aldosterone concentrations in cats with hypertension associated with chronic renal disease. Am J Vet Res 1997;58(5):535–40.

111. Syme HM, Markwell PJ, Elliott J. Aldosterone and plasma renin activity in cats with hypertension and/or chronic renal failure. J Vet Intern Med 2002;16(3):354.

112. Steele JL, Henik RA, Stepien RL. Effects of angiotensin-converting enzyme inhibition on plasma aldosterone concentration, plasma renin activity, and blood pressure in spontaneously hypertensive cats with chronic renal disease. Vet Ther 2002;3(2):157–66.

113. Javadi S, Djajadiningrat-Laanen SC, Kooistra HS, et al. Primary hyperaldosteronism, a mediator of progressive renal disease in cats. Domest Anim Endocrinol 2005;28(1):85–104.

114. Keele SJ, Smith KC, Elliott J, et al. Adrenocortical morphology in cats with chronic kidney disease (CKD) and systemic hypertension. J Vet Intern Med 2009;23(6):1319–50.

115. Homma M, Tanaka A, Hino K, et al. Assessing systemic 11beta-hydroxysteroid dehydrogenase with serum cortisone/cortisol ratios in healthy subjects and patients with diabetes mellitus and chronic renal failure. Metabolism 2001; 50(7):801–4.

116. Walker DJ, Elliott J, Syme HM. Urinary cortisol/cortisone ratios in hypertensive and normotensive cats. J Feline Med Surg 2009;11(6):442–8.

117. Brown SA, Langford K, Tarver S. Effects of certain vasoactive agents on the long-term pattern of blood pressure, heart rate, and motor activity in cats. Am J Vet Res 1997;58(6):647–52.

118. Baylis C, Mitruka B, Deng A. Chronic blockade of nitric oxide synthesis in the rat produces systemic hypertension and glomerular damage. J Clin Invest 1992; 90(1):278–81.

119. Baylis C. Arginine, arginine analogs and nitric oxide production in chronic kidney disease. Nat Clin Pract Nephrol 2006;2(4):209–20.

120. Jepson RE, Syme HM, Vallance C, et al. Plasma asymmetric dimethylarginine, symmetric dimethylarginine, l-arginine, and nitrite/nitrate concentrations in cats with chronic kidney disease and hypertension. J Vet Intern Med 2008;22(2):317–24.

121. Hogan DF, Sisson DD, Solter P. Characterisation of plasma volume and neuroendocrine status in renal hypertensive cats. J Vet Intern Med 1999;13(3):249.

122. Salem MM. Pathophysiology of hypertension in renal failure. Semin Nephrol 2002;22(1):17–26.

123. Cushman WC, Ford CE, Einhorn PT, et al. Blood pressure control by drug group in the Antihypertensive and Lipid-Lowering Treatment to Prevent Heart Attack Trial (ALLHAT). J Clin Hypertens (Greenwich) 2008;10(10):751–60.

124. Luckschander N, Iben C, Hosgood G, et al. Dietary NaCl does not affect blood pressure in healthy cats. J Vet Intern Med 2004;18(4):463–7.

125. Buranakarl C, Mathur S, Brown SA. Effects of dietary sodium chloride intake on renal function and blood pressure in cats with normal and reduced renal function. Am J Vet Res 2004;65(5):620–7.

126. Kirk CA, Jewell DE, Lowry SR. Effects of sodium chloride on selected parameters in cats. Vet Ther 2006;7(4):333–46.

127. Krieger JE, Liard JF, Cowley AW Jr. Hemodynamics, fluid volume, and hormonal responses to chronic high-salt intake in dogs. Am J Physiol 1990;259(6 Pt 2): H1629–36.

128. Greco DS, Lees GE, Dzendzel G, et al. Effects of dietary sodium intake on blood pressure measurements in partially nephrectomized dogs. Am J Vet Res 1994; 55(1):160–5.

129. Jepson RE, Elliott J, Brodbelt D, et al. Effect of control of systolic blood pressure on survival in cats with systemic hypertension. J Vet Intern Med 2007;21(3):402–9.

130. Laragh J. Laragh's lessons in pathophysiology and clinical pearls for treating hypertension. Am J Hypertens 2001;14(9 Pt 1):837–54.

131. Elliott J, Barber PJ, Syme HM, et al. Feline hypertension: clinical findings and response to antihypertensive treatment in 30 cases. J Small Anim Pract 2001; 42(3):122–9.

132. Henik RA, Snyder PS, Volk LM. Treatment of systemic hypertension in cats with amlodipine besylate. J Am Anim Hosp Assoc 1997;33(3):226–34.
133. Snyder PS. Amlodipine: a randomized, blinded clinical trial in 9 cats with systemic hypertension. J Vet Intern Med 1998;12(3):157–62.
134. Snyder PS, Sadek D, Jones GL. Effect of amlodipine on echocardiographic variables in cats with systemic hypertension. J Vet Intern Med 2001;15(1):52–6.
135. Mathur S, Brown CA, Dietrich UM, et al. Evaluation of a technique of inducing hypertensive renal insufficiency in cats. Am J Vet Res 2004;65(7):1006–13.
136. Helms SR. Treatment of feline hypertension with transdermal amlodipine: a pilot study. J Am Anim Hosp Assoc 2007;43(3):149–56.
137. Ferrari P. Prescribing angiotensin-converting enzyme inhibitors and angiotensin receptor blockers in chronic kidney disease. Nephrology (Carlton) 2007;12(1): 81–9.
138. Peterson JC, Adler S, Burkart JM, et al. Blood pressure control, proteinuria, and the progression of renal disease. The Modification of Diet in Renal Disease Study. Ann Intern Med 1995;123(10):754–62.
139. Brown SA, Brown CA, Jacobs G, et al. Effects of the angiotensin converting enzyme inhibitor benazepril in cats with induced renal insufficiency. Am J Vet Res 2001;62(3):375–83.
140. Reynolds V, Mathur S, Sheldon S, et al. Losartan fails to block angiotensin pressor response in cats. ACVIM forum. J Vet Intern Med 2002;16(3):341.
141. Henik RA, Stepien RL, Wenholz LJ, et al. Efficacy of atenolol as a single antihypertensive agent in hyperthyroid cats. J Feline Med Surg 2008;10(6): 577–82.
142. Ash RA, Harvey AM, Tasker S. Primary hyperaldosteronism in the cat: a series of 13 cases. J Feline Med Surg 2005;7(3):173–82.
143. MacDonald KA, Kittleson MD, Kass PH. Effect of spironolactone on diastolic function and left ventricular mass in Maine Coon cats with familial hypertrophic cardiomyopathy. J Vet Intern Med 2008;22(2):335–41.
144. Nadler JL, Hsueh W, Horton R. Therapeutic effect of calcium channel blockade in primary aldosteronism. J Clin Endocrinol Metab 1985;60(5):896–9.
145. Chetboul V, Lefebvre HP, Pinhas C, et al. Spontaneous feline hypertension: clinical and echocardiographic abnormalities, and survival rate. J Vet Intern Med 2003;17(1):89–95.
146. Syme HM, Markwell PJ, Pfeiffer D, et al. Survival of cats with naturally occurring chronic renal failure is related to severity of proteinuria. J Vet Intern Med 2006; 20(3):528–35.
147. King JN, Gunn-Moore DA, Tasker S, et al. Tolerability and efficacy of benazepril in cats with chronic kidney disease. J Vet Intern Med 2006;20(5):1054–64.
148. Mizutani H, Koyama H, Watanabe T, et al. Evaluation of the clinical efficacy of benazepril in the treatment of chronic renal insufficiency in cats. J Vet Intern Med 2006;20(5):1074–9.
149. Elliott J, Fletcher MG, Souttar K, et al. Effect of concomitant amlodipine and benazepril therapy in the management of feline hypertension. J Vet Intern Med 2004;18(5):788.
150. Atkins CE, Rausch WP, Gardner SY, et al. The effect of amlodipine and the combination of amlodipine and enalapril on the renin-angiotensin-aldosterone system in the dog. J Vet Pharmacol Ther 2007;30(5):394–400.
151. Brown SA, Finco DR, Brown CA, et al. Evaluation of the effects of inhibition of angiotensin converting enzyme with enalapril in dogs with induced chronic renal insufficiency. Am J Vet Res 2003;64(3):321–7.

152. Mishina M, Watanabe T. Development of hypertension and effects of benazepril hydrochloride in a canine remnant kidney model of chronic renal failure. J Vet Med Sci 2008;70(5):455–60.
153. Grauer GF, Greco DS, Getzy DM, et al. Effects of enalapril versus placebo as a treatment for canine idiopathic glomerulonephritis. J Vet Intern Med 2000; 14(5):526–33.
154. Grodecki KM, Gains MJ, Baumal R, et al. Treatment of X-linked hereditary nephritis in Samoyed dogs with angiotensin converting enzyme (ACE) inhibitor. J Comp Pathol 1997;117(3):209–25.
155. Tenhundfeld J, Wefstaedt P, Nolte IJ. A randomized controlled clinical trial of the use of benazepril and heparin for the treatment of chronic kidney disease in dogs. J Am Vet Med Assoc 2009;234(8):1031–7.
156. Stopher DA, Beresford AP, Macrae PV, et al. The metabolism and pharmacokinetics of amlodipine in humans and animals. J Cardiovasc Pharmacol 1988; 12(Suppl 7):S55–9.
157. Thomason JD, Fallaw TL, Carmichael KP, et al. Gingival hyperplasia associated with the administration of amlodipine to dogs with degenerative valvular disease (2004–2008). J Vet Intern Med 2009;23(1):39–42.
158. Finco DR. Association of systemic hypertension with renal injury in dogs with induced renal failure. J Vet Intern Med 2004;18(3):289–94.
159. Jacob F, Polzin DJ, Osborne CA, et al. Evaluation of the association between initial proteinuria and morbidity rate or death in dogs with naturally occurring chronic renal failure. J Am Vet Med Assoc 2005;226(3):393–400.

Peritoneal Dialysis in Veterinary Medicine

Rachel L. Cooper, DVM[a], Mary Anna Labato, DVM[b],*

KEYWORDS

- Peritoneal dialysis • Acute kidney injury • Anuria • Urea kinetic

Peritoneal dialysis is a modality of renal replacement therapy that is commonly used in human medicine for treatment of chronic kidney disease and end-stage kidney failure. Peritoneal dialysis employs the same principle as other forms of renal replacement therapy: the removal of uremic solutes by diffusion across a semipermeable membrane. In hemodialysis and continuous renal replacement therapy, blood is passed through straw-like semipermeable membranes, which are bathed in a dialysate. By contrast, peritoneal dialysis uses the peritoneum as a membrane across which fluids and uremic solutes are exchanged. In this process, dialysate is instilled into the peritoneal cavity and, through the process of diffusion and osmosis, water, toxins, electrolytes, and other small molecules are allowed to equilibrate. The dialysate is then removed and discarded, carrying with it uremic toxins and water. This process is repeated continuously as needed to achieve control of uremia.

Although peritoneal dialysis is used primarily for the treatment of chronic kidney disease in people, reports from as early as 1923 demonstrate its role in treating acute kidney injury.[1] Its use has also been described for removal of dialyzable toxins and to treat pancreatitis, electrolyte and acid base abnormalities, refractory congestive heart failure, and inborn errors of metabolism. In veterinary medicine, the most common use of peritoneal dialysis is to treat acute kidney injury, though it can be used for any of the aforementioned indications as well.

PHYSIOLOGY OF PERITONEAL DIALYSIS

The peritoneum is the serosal membrane that lines the abdominal cavity. The parietal peritoneum lines the abdominal cavity and is continuous with the visceral peritoneum, which lines the abdominal organs. The visceral peritoneum accounts for 80% of the peritoneal surface area; with the parietal peritoneum making up the remaining 20%.[2] The peritoneum has a surface area that is approximately the same as that of a normal

---

The authors have nothing to disclose.

[a] Department of Clinical Sciences, Matthew J. Ryan Veterinary Hospital, University of Pennsylvania, 3900 Delancey Street, Philadelphia, PA 19104, USA

[b] Small Animal Medicine, Department of Clinical Sciences, Cummings School of Veterinary Medicine, Tufts University, 200 Westboro Road, North Grafton, MA 01536, USA

* Corresponding author.

E-mail address: Mary.labato@tufts.edu

Vet Clin Small Anim 41 (2011) 91–113

doi:10.1016/j.cvsm.2010.10.002

0195-5616/11/$ – see front matter © 2011 Elsevier Inc. All rights reserved.

vetsmall.theclinics.com

body surface area; typically 1 to 2 m² in an adult.[2] Children have a disproportionately larger peritoneal surface area than adults.[2] Arterial circulation to the peritoneum is supplied by the cranial mesenteric artery for the visceral peritoneum and by the lumbar, intercostal, and epigastric arteries for the parietal peritoneum. The portal system provides drainage for the visceral peritoneum while the caudal vena cava drains the parietal peritoneum. One important clinical implication of this anatomic variant is that drugs that are absorbed via the visceral peritoneum undergo first-pass clearance by the liver. Lymphatic drainage is provided through stomata in the diaphragmatic peritoneum.

Microscopically, the peritoneum is made up of a single layer of mesothelial cells overlying an interstitial layer. The mesothelial cells are covered by microvilli, which contribute greatly to the large overall surface area of the peritoneum. These mesothelial cells are ultrastructurally similar to the type II pneumocytes of the lung, producing a film of glycosaminoglycans that function to lubricate and protect the abdominal viscera.[3] The interstitial layer is made of a mucopolysaccharide matrix with collagenous fibers, peritoneal capillaries, and lymphatics. A basement membrane composed of type IV collagen lies between the mesothelial cells and the interstitium. The interstitium has been described as a 2-phase system, consisting of a balance between a water-rich colloid-poor phase and a colloid-rich water-poor phase.[3] All of these structures act as barriers between fluid instilled into the peritoneal cavity and the endothelial surface of capillaries (**Fig. 1**).

The 3-pore model of peritoneal transport treats the capillary as the limiting factor in solute and water transport across the peritoneum (**Fig. 2**). This model proposes that pores of 3 different sizes mediate this transport. Large pores are present in small numbers, contributing less than 0.1% of total number of pores; they are significantly larger than the other pores, with a radius of 20 to 40 nm. These pores transport macromolecules such as proteins via convection. Small pores have a radius of 4 to 6 nm and are present in large numbers, accounting for 90% to 93% of total pore area.[4] These pores are thought to be involved in transport of small solutes such as urea, creatinine, sodium, and potassium in association with water.[2] The amount of transport is limited by the total number of small pores. Ultrasmall pores have a radius of less than 0.8 nm. These pores are involved in water transport only, and are thought to represent the same aquaporin-1 molecules that are present in the renal proximal tubules and red blood cells.[2] Ultrasmall pores account for 40% of total capillary ultrafiltration.[4] The rate of transport through the ultrasmall pores is determined

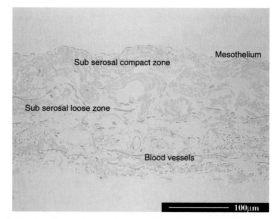

Fig. 1. Histology of the peritoneal membrane. (*Courtesy of* JD Williams, Cardiff University, Cardiff, Wales.)

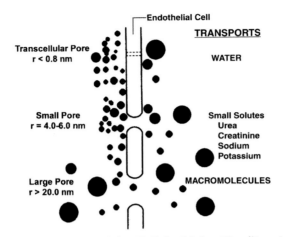

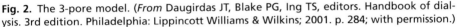

Fig. 2. The 3-pore model. (*From* Daugirdas JT, Blake PG, Ing TS, editors. Handbook of dialysis. 3rd edition. Philadelphia: Lippincott Williams & Wilkins; 2001. p. 284; with permission.)

primarily by osmotic gradient, in contrast to the small pores that are affected by mainly nonosmotic factors.

Diffusion is the most important mechanism responsible for solute transport in peritoneal dialysis. The dialysate, which contains high concentrations of glucose, encourages diffusion of these substances from dialysate into the bloodstream. Molecules in the blood that are not present in high concentrations in the dialysate such as uremic toxins and potassium diffuse from the peritoneal blood into the dialysate (**Fig. 3**) Acid-base disturbances are corrected by having higher concentrations of bicarbonate and lactate in the dialysate than in the plasma, which allows for diffusion of these substances from the dialysate into the body. The rate of diffusion of individual solutes is dependent on many factors, such as the concentration gradient, the molecular weight of solute, and the peritoneal surface area.

Ultrafiltration describes the movement of water across a semipermeable membrane, and can be driven by hydrostatic or osmotic forces. In peritoneal dialysis, a highly osmolar dialysate (the glucose rich solution) causes water to leave the body and enter the dialysate by osmosis. As the water crosses the peritoneal membrane, it carries small molecules into the dialysate (eg, urea, creatinine). This process is also known as convection. Ultrafiltration is an important clinical aspect of peritoneal dialysis that allows manipulation of fluid balance in the patient.

In humans, there is significant variation in the rate of solute transport among different peritoneal dialysis patients. High transporters diffuse substances well but have a low rate of ultrafiltration. Conversely, low transporters have high rates of

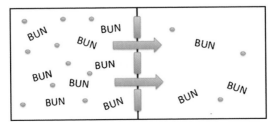

Fig. 3. The process of diffusion across the semipermeable peritoneal membrane.

ultrafiltration but take a longer time for substances to diffuse across the peritoneum. This transport is routinely determined using a peritoneal equilibration test. No studies on peritoneal transport have been performed in veterinary patients. It is not known whether cats or dogs have significant individual variation in their transport status, which may be a contributing factor to the effectiveness of peritoneal dialysis in individual veterinary patients.

INDICATIONS FOR PERITONEAL DIALYSIS

The first and foremost indication for peritoneal dialysis in dogs and cats is anuric acute kidney injury refractory to fluid therapy. Dialysis may also be indicated in nonanuric patients with severe acute uremia, in which the blood urea nitrogen (BUN) exceeds 100 mg/dL, or in which the creatinine exceeds 10 mg/dL.[5] Peritoneal dialysis can also be used to stabilize patients with a uroabdomen or urinary tract obstructions prior to surgery or anesthesia.

Peritoneal dialysis can also be used for a variety of intoxications and metabolic abnormalities. It can be used to remove dialyzable toxins such as ethylene glycol, ethanol, barbiturates, propoxyphene, and hydantoin, and correct electrolyte disturbances such as hyperkalemia.[6,7] However, peritoneal dialysis is limited in its ability to remove toxins from the blood and is about one-eighth to one-fourth as efficient as hemodialysis.[8] In situations where hemodialysis, hemofiltration, or charcoal hemoperfusion is unavailable, vascular access is difficult to obtain or the refractory hypotension makes hemodialysis a high-risk procedure, peritoneal dialysis may be indicated. When performing peritoneal dialysis for intoxications that have life-threatening side effects (hyperkalemia, ethylene glycol), very frequent exchanges should be made to promote a faster rate of clearance.[9] Electrolyte abnormalities such as hyperkalemia and hypercalcemia can also be effectively managed with peritoneal dialysis.

Life-threatening derangements in body temperature can also be corrected with peritoneal dialysis. The concentration of electrolytes in the dialysate solution should be similar to that in plasma to prevent extreme or rapid electrolyte fluctuations.[9] In cases of life-threatening hypothermia, dialysate at a temperature of 42°C to 43°C is instilled into the abdomen with a goal rewarming rate of 1°C to 2°C per hour.[7] In cases of life-threatening hyperthermia, dialysate should be administered at room temperature.[9]

Peritoneal dialysis has also been extensively used in human neonates with disorders of the urea cycle.[7] It is used as an emergency tool for correction of hyperammonemia along with additional medical management to stabilize this condition until liver transplant. It has recently been demonstrated that detoxification is more efficient with hemodialysis or continuous hemofiltration.[10] No studies have been done in veterinary patients to evaluate the utility of peritoneal dialysis to treat life-threatening hyperammonemia secondary to hepatic encephalopathy or urea cycle deficiencies.

Congestive heart failure refractory to medical management is another indication in human medicine for peritoneal dialysis. A recent study looked at patients with severe congestive heart failure, and found decreased mortality with use of hemofiltration followed by automated peritoneal dialysis as compared with patients with similar severities of heart disease.[11] This concept can also be applied to animals with severe volume overload. Exchanges should be performed hourly if the fluid overload is severe, and a markedly hyperosmotic (4.5%) dialysate should be used to encourage ultrafiltration.

CONTRAINDICATIONS FOR PERITONEAL DIALYSIS

Peritoneal dialysis is contraindicated in patients with peritoneal adhesions, fibrosis, or malignancies.[12] The presence of adhesions or fibrosis effectively decreases the surface area and the efficiency of peritoneal dialysis. Peritoneal dialysis is also contraindicated in patients with pleuroperitoneal leaks because of their predisposition to develop pleural effusion during dialysis.[12] Relative contraindications exist for patients with recent abdominal surgery, and inguinal or abdominal hernias because of the risk for herniation caused by increased intraperitoneal pressures. Patients in a severe hypercatabolic state such as burn victims or extremely malnourished states have a relative contraindication due to their propensity for protein loss through the peritoneum during dialysis.[6] Animals with recent abdominal surgery, especially gastrointestinal surgery, are at risk for dehiscence and infection during peritoneal dialysis because of the increased intraperitoneal pressure and potential fluid leakage through the incision site.[13]

CATHETERS AND CATHETER PLACEMENT

The ideal peritoneal dialysis catheter allows adequate inflow and outflow of dialysate, prevents subcutaneous leakage, and minimizes infection, in both the peritoneal cavity and the subcutaneous tissue.[14] Many of the common complications associated with peritoneal dialysis in veterinary medicine are catheter related, so it is important to consider different catheter types and placement techniques when choosing this modality.

Acute peritoneal dialysis catheters are designed to be placed percutaneously cage-side with a stylet in animals with sedation. These catheters are typically straight with holes at the distal end on the catheter tip. Acute catheters generally do not have cuffs to protect against bacterial infection and catheter migration, which is likely to lead to a high rate of peritonitis with prolonged use.[3] There is also an increased risk of bowel perforation during placement of these catheters.[14]

Chronic peritoneal dialysis catheters have specific designs in both the intraperitoneal and extraperitoneal portions of the catheters to reduce side effects and minimize clogging. Chronic peritoneal dialysis catheters are generally made from silicone rubber or polyurethane. The intraperitoneal portion of the catheters has numerous side holes at the distal tip to allow free flow of dialysate. The distal end of the peritoneal dialysis catheter may be straight or coiled. The coiled tip may help minimize outflow obstruction. The portion of the catheter that leaves the abdomen often has 1 or 2 Dacron cuffs. The most distal cuff is typically embedded in the abdominal rectus muscle. In humans the superficial cuff is placed subcutaneously 2 cm from the catheter exit site on the abdominal wall. The Dacron cuffs cause a local inflammatory response that causes fibrous and granulation tissue to form. This tissue fixes the catheter in position and prevents bacterial migration from the skin into the peritoneal cavity.[14] Some studies have shown that the single-cuff catheter is associated with a shorter time to peritonitis, a shorter catheter survival time, and a higher rate of exit site infections, although other studies have found no difference between numbers of cuffs.[15–17] The extraperitoneal portion of the catheter can be straight or can have a permanent bend between the 2 cuffs. The permanent bend or "Swan-neck" catheters are produced to have a subcutaneous tunnel that is directed downward to decrease the risk of catheter-related infections in humans.

Several different catheter types have been used to perform acute peritoneal dialysis in veterinary medicine. Simple tube catheters with trocars can be placed in conscious animals using local anesthetics in emergency situations.[6] A percutaneous cystotomy tube catheter (Stamey percutaneous suprapubic catheter set; Cook, Spencer, IN, USA) has also been reported as being used in veterinary medicine (**Fig. 4**).[12]

When placing a peritoneal dialysis catheter that is expected to function for longer than 3 days, a more permanent peritoneal dialysis catheter is recommended. A surgical omentectomy is also recommended, due to the high risk of omental entrapment.[6] No

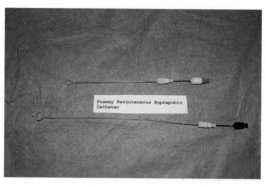

Fig. 4. Stamey percutaneous suprapubic catheter (Cook, Spencer, IN, USA).

studies have been done in veterinary medicine to evaluate the utility of any particular peritoneal dialysis catheter. In human medicine, the Tenckoff catheter is the most widely used chronic peritoneal dialysis catheter. This silicone catheter has a straight extraperitoneal portion and either a straight or curled intraperitoneal portion with multiple holes in the distal end. The Tenckhhoff catheter can have 1 or 2 cuffs (**Fig. 5**).

The Fluted T catheter (Ash Advantage peritoneal dialysis catheter; Medigroup, Aurora, IL, USA) was introduced in the 1990s, and research studies in dogs reported good results when compared with the Tenckhhoff (coiled tube) catheters.[18] This catheter is made of silicone with 2 Dacron cuffs; it is a T-shaped catheter made of long grooves or flutes (**Fig. 6**). These flutes are designed to offer minimal resistance to the efflux and influx of fluids while preventing omental adhesion.[19] The T-portion of the catheter is designed to be placed against the parietal peritoneum in a cranial-caudal direction. The fluted aspect of this catheter is 30 cm in length, but can be cut to accommodate smaller patients. This catheter has not been used widely in human medicine. Although its use has been reported in veterinary medicine, there are no studies evaluating its utility.

Other catheters that have been used in veterinary medicine include the 15F Blake surgical drain (Johnson and Johnson, Arlington, TX, USA), the Swan Neck straight or curled Missouri catheter (Kendall Healthcare, Mansfield, MA, USA), the 10-cm-length PD catheter, coaxial design (Global Veterinary Products, New Buffalo, MI, USA), Quinton Pediatric Peritoneal Dialysis catheter (Kendall Healthcare, Mansfield, MA, USA), and the Dawson-Mueller drainage catheter (Cook, Spencer, IN, USA) (**Figs. 7–10**).[20–23] These catheters are all placed surgically.

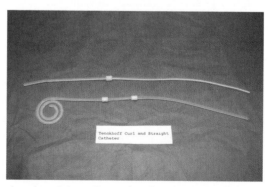

Fig. 5. Tenckhoff curl and straight catheter (Medcomp, Harleyville, PA, USA).

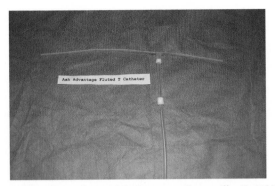

Fig. 6. Ash Advantage fluted T catheter (Medicgroup, Naperville, IL, USA).

The method of placement of peritoneal dialysis catheters is dependent on the catheter itself, the stability of the patient, and the expected length of peritoneal dialysis. In emergent situations where peritoneal dialysis is expected to be less than 72 hours, percutaneous placement of a short-term catheter is warranted. To place a percutaneous peritoneal dialysis catheter the animal is placed in dorsal recumbency, and the abdomen is shaved and sterilely prepared. It is critical that every opportunity is taken to preserve aseptic technique to prevent catheter-related infections. A stab incision is made 3 to 5 cm lateral to the umbilicus, in the direction of the pelvis.[24] The trocar is tunneled subcutaneously for several centimeters before insertion into the abdomen. The catheter is then threaded over the trocar until fully in the abdomen.[6] A purse-string suture can be placed to secure the catheter in place at its insertion site for temporary peritoneal dialysis catheters. Suture material has been reported to increase the risk of tunnel infections in human patients; therefore, peritoneal dialysis catheters with Dacron cuffs are indicated for long-term use.[6] A report in the human literature describes fluoroscopic guidance in placement of percutaneous peritoneal dialysis catheters; this technique has not been reported in veterinary medicine.[25]

When the peritoneal dialysis catheter is to be left in place for a longer period of time, a more permanent catheter should be placed. Long-term peritoneal dialysis catheters can be placed either laparoscopically (with a peritoneoscope) or surgically. Both laparoscopic and surgical catheter placement allow visualization of catheter placement, and the ability to take biopsies and to perform a partial omentectomy. The

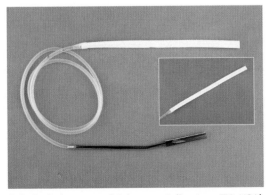

Fig. 7. Blake surgical drain (Johnson and Johnson, Arlington, TX, USA).

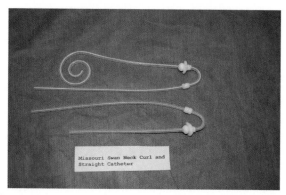

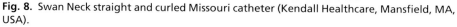

Fig. 8. Swan Neck straight and curled Missouri catheter (Kendall Healthcare, Mansfield, MA, USA).

disadvantages of these techniques include longer placement time, greater cost, and larger incision. Many of the catheters that were designed for percutaneous placement for humans are best placed surgically in dogs and cats. A recent study in healthy dogs describes a new method for implanting disk-type peritoneal dialysis catheters through small incisions, with good outcome; however, these catheters are no longer commercially available.[26] Once surgically placed, peritoneal dialysis catheters ideally should not be used for at least 10 to 14 days. This delay allows wound healing and scar formation around the cuffs, minimizing leakage of dialysate around the catheter site. This recommendation is easier to follow in human patients, in whom the peritoneal dialysis is generally used for more chronic kidney disease, rather than the acute kidney injury that is usually treated in veterinary patients. In veterinary patients that require immediate usage, the catheter should be leak tested to ensure a tight seal has been achieved. For the first 24 to 48 hours after placement large volumes of dialysate should not be used, in order to minimize intraperitoneal pressure.[5]

SYSTEM SETUP

Once the peritoneal dialysis catheter is placed, it should be attached to a closed collection system and carefully bandaged into position with dry sterile dressings. The use of topical antibiotic ointment is not recommended because it can macerate the exit-site tissue and inhibit fibroblast proliferation.[12] The peritoneal dialysis catheter

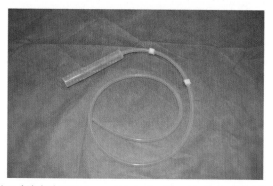

Fig. 9. Coaxial design (Global Veterinary Products, New Buffalo, MI, USA).

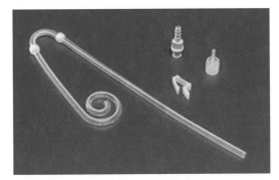

Fig. 10. Quinton Pediatric Peritoneal Dialysis catheter (Kendall Healthcare, Mansfield, MA, USA).

is connected to the dialysate bag by a length of plastic tubing called a transfer set. Older references discuss a straight transfer (straight spike), in which the same bag that contains dialysate becomes the effluent bag after the dialysate is instilled into the abdomen.[5] However, this method of performing peritoneal dialysis was associated with higher incidence of bacterial peritonitis and is not currently recommended.[27] The Y transfer set consists of a Y-shaped piece of tubing connected to both a fresh dialysate bag and a drainage container (**Fig. 11**). During the exchange, the dialysate is allowed to flow into the effluent bag. Before instilling fresh dialysate into the peritoneum, a small volume of fresh dialysate solution is drained from the dialysate bag directly into the effluent bag, bypassing the patient. This step is thought to flush bacteria that were introduced into the system at the time of connection. After the flush is done, the instillation of dialysate into the peritoneum can be performed. Newer double-bag systems have been introduced in which the Y-set is already connected to the fresh dialysate bag. This placement allows for one less connection (and opportunity for contamination) to be made at each cycle. A recent Cochrane review comparing the 3 different transfer types and the risk of peritonitis found a clear advantage over the straight spike system with both the Y-set and double-bag transfer systems. There was no significant advantage shown for the double-bag system over the Y-set system, although studies available for review were more limited.[28]

A strict sterile technique should be followed at all times when handling the peritoneal dialysis catheter and collection system. All connections should be wrapped in povidone-iodine connection shields or chlorhexidine-soaked dressings covered with sterile gauze.[12] All injection ports should be scrubbed with either chlorhexidine or povidone-iodine for 2 minutes before injections, and medication vials should be swabbed for 2 minutes before use. To reduce the risk of contamination, multiple-dose vials should not be used for dialysate additives. Hands should be washed thoroughly and sterile gloves should be worn while handling dialysate lines or bags. Catheter movement at the exit site should be minimized; the catheter site should be washed with chlorhexidine or iodine scrub and dried with sterile gauze once daily, and wrapped in dry sterile bandages. The catheter site and dry bandages should be changed more frequently should strike-through occur. The dialysis prescription should be adjusted to minimize the occurrence of exit-site leaks. The dialysate effluent should be examined for cloudiness at every exchange. Should any concern arise, the effluent should be submitted for culture. The effluent should be looked at once daily for any indication of peritonitis. These guidelines cannot be emphasized enough regarding prevention of infection during peritoneal dialysis.[19]

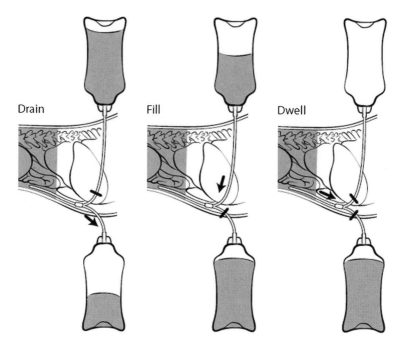

Fig. 11. An illustration of the Y-shaped drain set.

DIALYSATE

The specific composition of dialysate is an important factor to consider when performing peritoneal dialysis. Different dialysate solutions differ based on their buffer, electrolytes, and/or the osmotic agents used (**Table 1**). The ideal dialysate should promote solute clearance with little absorption of osmotic agents, provide deficient electrolytes and nutrients, correct acid-base problems, inhibit the growth of microorganisms, and be inert to the peritoneum.[29] Biocompatibility of dialysate solutions is an intensely studied field. It has been shown that the low pH, lactate buffer, high glucose content, high osmolality, and the presence of glucose degradation products (GDPs) generated during production and sterilization of dialysate can be harmful to the peritoneum.[30] Peritoneal biopsies in patients who have received long-term peritoneal dialysis showed ultrastructural changes that may be secondary to low biocompatibility of peritoneal dialysis solutions.[31] The significance of these findings is unknown, but trends are toward more biocompatible dialysate solutions.

Options for buffers in dialysate historically have included lactate, bicarbonate, and acetate. One of the initial buffers used in peritoneal dialysis solutions was acetate. Bicarbonate is generated when acetate and coenzyme A (CoA) are activated by acetate thiokinase to form acetyl CoA. The use of acetate as a buffer in dialysate solutions has fallen out of favor. Due to its low pH, acetate can produce pain during dialysate inflow. Studies have also shown that it produces vasodilation and alteration of the peritoneum, leading to loss of ultrafiltration and development of sclerosing peritonitis.[32,33] Lactate is the most common buffer used as dialysate today. The buffering effects of lactate are produced through their metabolism in the liver via the Krebs cycle or via gluconeogenesis, with the end product being bicarbonate. However, lactate has been shown in studies to be toxic to mesothelial cells when combined with a low pH, as in typical dialysate solutions.[34] Bicarbonate was not

Table 1
Composition of a commercially available peritoneal dialysate solution

	Manufacturer	pH	Osmotic Agent	Na (mM)	Ca (mM)	Mg (mM)	Lactate (mM)	Bicarb (mM)	Pouches
Dianeal PD1	Baxter	5.5	Glucose	132	1.75	0.75	35	0	1
Dianeal PD2	Baxter	5.2	Glucose	132	1.75	0.25	40	0	1
Dianeal PD4	Baxter	5.5	Glucose	132	1.25	0.25	40	0	1
Stay-Safe 2/4/3	FMC	5.5	Glucose	134	1.75	0.5	35	0	1
Stay-Safe 17/19/18	FMC	5.5	Glucose	143	1.25	0.5	35	0	1
Gambrosol Trio 10	Gambro	6.3	Glucose	132	1.75	0.25	40	0	3
Gambrosol Trio 40	Gambro	6.3	Glucose	132	1.35	0.25	40	0	3
Nutrineal	Baxter	6.5	Amino acids	132	1.25	0.25	40	0	1
Extraneal	Baxter	5.5	Icodextrin	132	1.75	0.25	40	0	1
Physioneal	Baxter	7.4	Glucose	132	1.75	0.25	10	25	2
Balance	FMC	7.4	Glucose	134	1.25	0.5	34	2	2
					1.75				
bicaVera	FMC	7.4	Glucose	134	1.75	0.5	0	34	2
bicaNova	FMC	7.4	Glucose	134	1.25	0.5	0	39	2

From Heimburger O, Blake PG. Apparatus for peritoneal dialysis. In: Daugirdas JT, Blake PG, Ing TS, editors. Handbook of dialysis. 4th edition. Philadelphia: Lippincott, Williams & Wilkins; 2007. p. 340; with permission.

initially used as a buffer for dialysate solutions because during the sterilization process calcium and magnesium would precipitate into salts. Bicarbonate solution has a higher pH than the lactate- or acetate-buffered solutions, and glucose would caramelize at the higher pH, so this solution was initially abandoned. However, because bicarbonate is a more biocompatible solution, this buffer has been studied more readily in recent years. To avoid the problems of precipitation and caramelization, bicarbonate-based solutions are formulated in 2-chambered bags. The chambers are mixed immediately before instillation of the dialysate into the peritoneum. There has been significant research describing improved biocompatibility of bicarbonate-based dialysate solutions, but no evidence has arisen that bicarbonate-based solutions improve long-term outcome.[35–37]

Commercially available dialysate solutions contain sodium, magnesium, calcium, and chloride in varying concentrations. Potassium is generally not included in dialysate solutions, but can be added if patients become hypokalemic during treatment.

Osmotic agents can be grouped into low molecular weight agents and high molecular weight agents. Low molecular weight agents that have been tried include glucose, glycerol, sorbitol, amino acids, xylitol, and fructose.[3] The standard dialysate solution contains glucose as the osmotic agent. Glucose-based dialysate comes in 3 different concentrations: 1.5%, 2.5%, and 4.25%. Dialysis performed for the removal of uremic toxins is generally done using a 1.5% solution. Use of a hypertonic glucose solution is reserved for overhydrated patients in whom the highly osmolar dialysate causes water to leave the body and enter the dialysate by osmosis. Peritoneal dialysis can be performed using commercial dextrose-based dialysate products, or dialysate may be formulated by adding dextrose to lactated Ringer solution.[12] Adding 30 mL of 50% glucose to 1 L of lactated Ringer solution will result in a 1.5% solution.

Glucose has been shown to be safe, effective, inexpensive, and readily available. However, glucose can also be readily absorbed, leading to metabolic derangements such as hyperglycemia, hyperlipidemia, hyperinsulinemia, and obesity.[38,39] Several other problems regarding the long-term safety of glucose-based products have been demonstrated. Glucose can directly and indirectly cause damage to the peritoneum. High concentrations of glucose are toxic to the mesothelium.[30] Glucose is also involved in peritoneal neoangiogenesis. These new blood vessels result in the disappearance of the osmotic gradient and a failure of ultrafiltration.[30] The acidity necessary to prevent caramelization in glucose-containing fluids can be also be harmful to the peritoneum.

GDPs are produced during heat sterilization and production of glucose-containing solutions. GDPs are toxic to fibroblasts and enhance the production of vascular endothelial growth factor by peritoneal cells.[30] These GDPs may also lead to formation of advanced glycosylation end products (AGEs).[35] AGEs are proinflammatory, and have been correlated with impaired peritoneal permeability and ultrafiltration failure.[35]

Concerns over the use of glucose-based dialysate products have led to the investigation of other osmotic agents for peritoneal dialysis in humans. Amino acid–containing peritoneal dialysis solutions have been used to improve nutrition status of peritoneal dialysis patients. Recent studies have shown improvement in nutrition status of patients when given a 1.1% solution of amino acid–containing dialysate, and work is ongoing in human medicine to establish the efficacy of supplementation.[36] A 1.1% amino acid–based solution functions osmotically similar to a 1.5% dextrose solution. Amino acid–based solutions can only be used once daily because they may cause elevations in BUN and worsen acidosis.[27]

High molecular weight osmotic agents include polymers of glucose (polyglucose), such as icodextrin. Icodextrin is a starch-derived water-soluble glucose polymer with a molecular weight of 16,800. Commercially it is available in a 7.5% solution in a lactate buffer (Extraneal; Baxter Healthcare Corp, McGraw Park, IL, USA). Icodextrin is an iso-osmolar solution (285 mOsm/kg) that produces ultrafiltration via its oncotic effect. Glucose polymers induce ultrafiltration across large pores via colloid oncotic effects, as compared with hyperosmotic dextrose solutions, which induce ultrafiltration across both small and ultrasmall pores. Absorption of icodextrin occurs via peritoneal lymphatics, so it maintains its oncotic effect much longer than dextrose-based solutions. Adverse events reported with icodextrin use include sterile peritonitis in humans.[3] Icodextrin also causes some laboratory instruments to overestimate blood glucose level, due to the presence of maltose in the bloodstream.[30] Icodextrin is used for long dwell times in humans undergoing chronic ambulatory peritoneal dialysis and continuous cyclic peritoneal dialysis, in patients with ultrafiltration failure, and in patients with diabetes mellitus.[3] The use of icodextrin in veterinary medicine has not been investigated.

Several other substances are often added to peritoneal dialysis solutions as needed. Insulin may be added to dialysate solutions in diabetics to help control hyperglycemia. Antibiotics may be added to the dialysate solution to treat peritonitis, although routine use of antibiotics is discouraged. Heparin is frequently added to the dialysate solution to prevent formation of fibrin in the peritoneal dialysis catheter. Addition of heparin to the peritoneum does not lead to systemic anticoagulation.[40]

EXCHANGE PROCEDURE

When initiating peritoneal dialysis for acute kidney injury, the goal is not to immediately normalize the azotemia. The initial objectives should be to normalize the patient's hemo-dynamic state, and acid-base and electrolyte imbalances, as well as reducing the azotemia to a BUN of less than 60 to 100 mg/dL and a creatinine of 4.0 to 6.0 mg/dL over 24 to 48 hours.[5] For this time, one-quarter to one-half of the calculated dialysate volume (30–40 mL/kg) should be instilled during each cycle. This amount allows the clinician to assess the patient for abdominal distension, respiratory impairment, and dialysate leakage. If the patient tolerates these volumes over the first 24 hours, the amount of dialysate can be increased to 30 to 40 mL/kg per cycle.[24] For patients with normal hydration status, a dialysate containing 1.5% dextrose can be used initially. For patients with volume overload or with high serum osmolality, either a 2.5% or 4.5% dialysate solution can be used for the initial cycles. When using hyperosmotic dial-ysate solutions, it is imperative to monitor the patient closely to prevent hemodynamic instability from rapid fluid shifts.

The dialysate should be warmed to 38°C to 39°C to improve permeability of the peritoneum and for patient comfort prior to instillation into the peritoneal cavity.[5] Warming should ideally be performed by heating pads or special ovens for the dialysate bags and lines. Microwaving the dialysate bags has been performed but is strongly not recommended by manufacturers because of uneven heating and potential "hot spots" that may be produced during the heating process.[27] In addition, overheating can lead to chemical alterations in the dialysate solution. Warming the dialysate by immersing the bag in warm water is also not recommended because of the risk of contamination.[27]

Most animals with acute kidney injury will have hyperkalemia, and most dialysate solutions do not have potassium added. In the initial cycles of peritoneal dialysis this is ideal; however, hypokalemia can occur with time. To prevent this, 2 to 4 mEq/L of potassium can be added to the dialysate solution after several cycles have occurred. Heparin at 100 to 500 U/L can also be added to the dialysate during the initial sessions to prevent fibrin occlusion of the catheter.[5]

To begin a peritoneal dialysis session, the fresh dialysate bag is placed above the patient while the effluent bag is placed below the patient. A small amount of dialysate is flushed from the dialysate bag directly into the effluent bag. With the first instillation, 10 mL/kg of dialysate solution is then instilled by gravity into the peritoneum over 10 minutes and is allowed to dwell for 30 to 40 minutes. The peritoneal cavity is allowed to drain by gravity into the sterile effluent bag over 20 to 30 minutes. The system is closed off to the patient and the procedure is then repeated with flushing of the line. One recent study reported achieving success using a closed intermittent negative pressure system instead of a gravity-dependent drainage period.[22] During each drainage period the effluent volume should be recorded, and the bag should be checked for color and turbidity of the fluid. If there is any blood, turbidity, or change in character of the fluid, it should be cultured immediately. After each cycle is completed a new cycle is started, making this a continuous and effective process.

Meticulous records should be kept to record details of exchange volumes and fluid balance of peritoneal dialysis patients. If the fluid balance becomes positive, or if return of dialysate effluent is less than 90%, the dialysate solution should be switched to 4.5% dextrose-containing solutions, to encourage ultrafiltration and subsequent volume removal. If the fluid balance becomes negative, hyperosmotic dialysate solution should be switched to a 1.5% solution, and steps should be taken to avoid hypovolemia.[5] Renal values, electrolytes, blood pressure, and central venous pressures should be monitored every few hours during the initial peritoneal dialysis period.

After the initial 24 to 48 hours of exchanges, the patient can be switched to a more chronic peritoneal dialysis protocol. Cycle lengths of 3 to 6 hours may be instituted, and may be increased to 3 to 4 exchanges daily as kidney function is restored. The frequency of exchanges and length of dwell time should be adjusted based on the patient's degree of azotemia, normalization of acid-base status, electrolyte disturbances, volume status, and control of uremic symptoms.[5] The amount of solute transferred across the peritoneal membrane is related to the concentration gradient for each solute and the size of the molecule. If increased removal of a larger-sized molecule such as creatinine is warranted, longer dwell times are instituted.[12] Gradual reduction of the number of exchanges and lengthening of the dwell time leading to intermittent peritoneal dialysis over 3 to 4 days with frequent reassessment is recommended before discontinuation of dialysis.[12] For example, once the patient's BUN is less than 100 mg/dL and the creatinine is less than 5.0 mg/dL, the exchanges should go from hourly to every 2 hours with a 1.5-hour dwell time. Dwell times and exchanges than can be extended on a daily basis as needed. If in the acute situation an animal receiving well-managed, aggressive peritoneal dialysis has not improved after several days, intermittent hemodialysis, renal transplantation, or euthanasia should be considered.

Continuous ambulatory peritoneal dialysis (CAPD) is the delivery technique most appropriate for animals with end-stage chronic kidney disease that require peritoneal dialysis. Long dwell times of 4 to 6 hours are instituted, permitting the animal to be ambulatory for most of the day.[5] This technique is the one most commonly used in humans with end-stage kidney disease, although it has never gained clinical acceptance in veterinary medicine for chronic kidney disease.

MONITORING

Blood volume and electrolyte changes can occur rapidly in the first few days of peritoneal dialysis. Catheter outflow obstructions can cause retention of dialysate in the abdomen and a less efficient dialysis session. For these reasons careful monitoring of patients undergoing peritoneal dialysis is critically important. Body weight and hydrations status should be monitored frequently. Body weight should be assessed in the same clinical condition (ie, without dialysate in the abdomen) during each assessment period. Central venous pressures should be checked every 4 to 6 hours and systemic arterial blood pressures should be checked every 6 to 8 hours. Urine output should be recorded every 4 hours. The patient's heart rate and respiratory rate should be recorded every 2 hours, noting whether dialysate in the abdomen causes any respiratory difficulty. Renal values, electrolytes, and acid-base status should be checked every 4 to 6 hours initially, and then at least twice daily. Magnesium should be checked at least once every 3 days if it is not evaluated in more routine bloodwork.[6] Detailed flow sheets are used at the authors' institution to assess trends in volume and electrolyte status (**Figs. 12** and **13**).

EVALUATING ADEQUACY OF PERITONEAL DIALYSIS: UREA KINETICS

The goal of urea kinetics is to provide a measure of dialysis quality and quantity. Urea kinetic modeling allows quantification of solute clearance that is delivered to the patient. Although originally conceived for the monitoring of hemodialysis, urea kinetic modeling is used as a measure of dialysis adequacy for peritoneal dialysis as well. The amount of dialysis delivered can be expressed as Kt/V, a unit-less value that measures fractional urea clearance.[41] In peritoneal dialysis, Kt/V is obtained by analyzing a 24-hour collection of the dialysate effluent, urine, and average blood urea level. When calculating urea kinetics for a patient, both the peritoneal clearance and residual renal clearance must be taken into account. Peritoneal Kt is calculated by measuring the urea content of the 24-hour dialysate effluent, and dividing the result by average plasma urea content for the same period. Residual renal Kt is calculated by measuring the urea content of the 24-hour urine collection, and dividing the result by the average urea content for the same 24-hour period. The peritoneal Kt and residual renal Kt can then be combined to obtain the total Kt. The volume of distribution of urea is represented by the letter V, and is calculated based on the patient's body size and published tables.[41] To determine Kt/V, the total Kt is then divided by V. In peritoneal dialysis, the number obtained is then multiplied by 7; by convention Kt/V is expressed in weekly periods.

The ideal Kt/V for human peritoneal dialysis patients is not entirely known and is a subject of much discussion. Recent prospective controlled studies have shown that higher clearance targets once previously recommended did not improve outcome, therefore targets have been decreased.[42–44] With human peritoneal dialysis patients, it is now recommended that the Kt/V should target 1.7 per week.[45] Those who are familiar with hemodialysis adequacy may find peritoneal dialysis Kt/V to sound small (compared with a goal hemodialysis Kt/V of 1.2 in each of 3 weekly sessions). However, because peritoneal dialysis is a continuous modality, it is much more efficient than hemodialysis and the different Kt/V values cannot be compared.[41] Evaluation of the Kt/V in veterinary peritoneal dialysis has not been reported in the literature, which may be due to the difficulty in collecting effluent and urine over 24 hours, or assessing a 24-hour average of the plasma urea.

Creatinine clearance is another method of assessing dialysis adequacy in peritoneal dialysis. The peritoneal creatinine clearance is calculated in a similar manner to the peritoneal Kt, as discussed above. The residual renal creatinine clearance is measured by taking an average of the urinary urea clearance and the urinary creatinine clearance; this is done by convention, as the residual renal creatinine clearance has been shown to markedly overestimate the true glomerular filtration rate.[41] This value is then corrected for total

Date	dialysate	#	Please note Am or PM. Also note date on each sheet inflow time	dwell time	outflow time	dialysate volume in	dialysate volume out	current exchange net balance of dialysate only (volume out - volume in = balance)	running total of balance of dialysate only	IV fluids in	Urine out	Total fluids in	Total fluid out	Current exchangeFluid difference (total fluid in - total fluids out = fluid diff)	Running total of Fluid difference	exchange	Comments
		1						0	0			0	0	0	0	1	
		2						0	0			0	0	0	0	2	
		3						0	0			0	0	0	0	3	
		4						0	0			0	0	0	0	4	
		5						0	0			0	0	0	0	5	
		6						0	0			0	0	0	0	6	
		7						0	0			0	0	0	0	7	
		8						0	0			0	0	0	0	8	
		9						0	0			0	0	0	0	9	
		10						0	0			0	0	0	0	10	
		11						0	0			0	0	0	0	11	
		12						0	0			0	0	0	0	12	
		13						0	0			0	0	0	0	13	
		14						0	0			0	0	0	0	14	
		15						0	0			0	0	0	0	15	
		16						0	0			0	0	0	0	16	
		17						0	0			0	0	0	0	17	
		18						0	0			0	0	0	0	18	
		19						0	0			0	0	0	0	19	
		20						0	0			0	0	0	0	20	
		21						0	0			0	0	0	0	21	
		22						0	0			0	0	0	0	22	
		23						0	0			0	0	0	0	23	
		24						0	0			0	0	0	0	24	
		25						0	0			0	0	0	0	25	
		26						0	0			0	0	0	0	26	
		27						0	0			0	0	0	0	27	
		28						0	0			0	0	0	0	28	

Fig. 12. Peritoneal dialysis flow sheet.

Date Parameters	Day 1	Day 2	Day 3	Day 4	Day 5	Day 6	Day 7
Wt (KG) same scale Q 8 hrs							
Creat/BUN q 12 hrs							
Na/K/CL q 12 hrs							
PCV/TS/BG Q 12 hrs							
Fluid character							
Fluid Cytology Q 24 hrs							
CVP q 8 hrs							
BP q 12 hrs							
Blood Gas q 24 hrs							
Kidney Profile EOD							
CBC EOD							
Urine output q 4 hrs							

Fig. 13. Flow chart used to monitor dialysis patient's laboratory values.

body surface area as calculated by the duBois formula.[41] The use of creatinine clearance in assessing adequacy of peritoneal dialysis in veterinary patients has not been reported in veterinary literature, likely because of the same reasons as listed here for Kt/V.

Urea reduction ratio (URR) is another measure of dialysis adequacy that is more commonly used in hemodialysis. URR is a simple calculation of the percent reduction in urea after a dialysis treatment. The formula for URR is as follows:

URR = (Pre-dialysis BUN − Post-dialysis BUN)/Pre-dialysis BUN × 100

URRs are not commonly used in CAPD in humans. Because these patients are at a steady state, meaning their urea clearance rates are similar to their urea generation rates, the URR will always approach zero. In veterinary patients with acute kidney injury and a significantly higher urea clearance rate than the urea generation rate, this measure may be useful to assess adequacy in peritoneal dialysis. Two recent studies have measured urea reduction ratios in the assessment of peritoneal dialysis adequacy.[21,23] More studies are warranted to evaluate the utility of URR for assessment of peritoneal dialysis adequacy in veterinary patients.

COMPLICATIONS

Complications of peritoneal dialysis are a frequent, but manageable, occurrence. The most common complications of peritoneal dialysis include catheter occlusion problems such as dialysate retention and subcutaneous leakage of dialysate, electrolyte disturbances, hypoalbuminemia, and bacterial peritonitis.

Dialysate retention, as defined by recovery of less than 90% of dialysate, occurred in 20% to 77% of animals reported in several retrospective studies.[20,21,23,46] Common causes of dialysate retention are catheter occlusion due to omental entrapment or fibrin accumulation in the peritoneal dialysis catheter. Performing a partial omentectomy would likely reduce the frequency of this complication. In one study, 100% (8/8) of cats with percutaneously placed peritoneal dialysis catheters developed retention of dialysate, whereas only 54.5% of cats with surgically placed peritoneal dialysis catheters developed retention of dialysate.[21] Two cats with percutaneously placed peritoneal dialysis catheters eventually required surgical placement of peritoneal dialysis catheters because of catheter outflow obstruction problems. One of these cats had a surgically placed catheter, but partial omentectomy was not performed and the cat continued to have complications involving retained dialysate. Later, a partial omentectomy was performed and fewer complications were reported postoperatively.[21] One recent retrospective study noted a low rate of dialysate retention, which was attributed to a closed intermittent negative pressure system.[22] The use of negative pressure systems for dialysate drain periods requires further investigation. Catheter design may also play a role in prevention of catheter occlusion, but not enough data are available to make any conclusions for veterinary medicine. Heparin (250–1000 U/L) can be added to the dialysate solution to try and prevent catheter obstruction from fibrin accumulation, especially in the first few days of dialysis or when the effluent is noted to be cloudy. If fibrin deposition is suspected in the catheter, treatment with a high-pressure flush of saline, urokinase (15,000 U), streptokinase, or tissue plasminogen activator has been recommended.[14]

Sequestration of dialysate subcutaneously was noted in 20% to 50% of animals in different studies.[20,21,23,46] In one study the incidence of sequestration of dialysate was similar between cats with surgical (58.3%) and percutaneously (62.5%) placed catheters. The immediate use of dialysis catheters after placement may contribute to the high rate of dialysate leakage. In humans undergoing peritoneal dialysis, it is recommended to wait for 2 to 4 weeks before the use of newly placed peritoneal dialysis catheters.[14]

The prevalence of hypoalbuminemia in animals undergoing peritoneal dialysis has been reported to be 41% to 90%.[20,21,23,46] Low dietary protein intake, gastrointestinal or renal protein loss, dialysate loss, uremic catabolism, and concurrent disease may all contribute to the hypoalbuminemia seen in animals undergoing peritoneal dialysis.[12] Protein loss may increase dramatically when peritonitis is present.[1] Usually animals that are eating well can maintain their protein levels. However, many patients undergoing peritoneal dialysis are anorexic, or nauseated secondary to their severe uremia or other concurrent disease. Enteral or parenteral nutritional supplementation is critical in these patients to help maintain protein levels. A 1.1% amino acid dialysate solution may also be used for additional nutritional supplementation. Electrolyte abnormalities are commonly reported in peritoneal dialysis. Hyponatremia, hypochloremia, hypomagnesemia, hypokalemia, hyperkalemia, and hyperglycemia have all been reported in veterinary studies to varying extents.[20–22,46]

Peritonitis is diagnosed when 2 of the following 3 criteria are recognized: (1) cloudy dialysate effluent, (2) greater than 100 inflammatory cells/μL of effluent or positive culture results, and (3) clinical signs of peritonitis.[6] Peritonitis has previously been reported as a common side effect in veterinary medicine. The most common source of peritonitis is contamination of the bag spike or tubing by the handler, but intestinal, hematogenous, and exit-site sources of infection do occur.[1] Several more recent retrospective studies have reported a significantly lower rate (4%, 0%, and 0%) of peritonitis.[20–22] The lower rate of peritonitis may be due to the use of the Y-Set transfer system as opposed to the straight-spike transfer system, or increased vigilance and adherence to aseptic technique. In one study *Escherichia coli* was the major contaminant, but other studies have reported a variety of bacteria, including *Klebsiella*, *Pseudomonas*, *Enterococcus*, *Mycoplasma*, *Acinetobacter*, and *Providencia*.[21,23,46]

Pleural effusion and dyspnea are uncommon side effects of peritoneal dialysis in humans and animals. Pleural effusion can be caused by overhydration or pleuroperitoneal leakages. Careful and frequent monitoring of the patient's hydration status, central venous pressures, urine output, and weight can decrease the incidence of overhydration. If overhydration is suspected, the dialysate should be changed to a more hyperosmotic solution to promote ultrafiltration. The concentration of blood glucose can be tested in the pleural fluid, as elevated glucose levels would indicate a pleuroperitoneal leak. Pleuroperitoneal leaks are a contraindication for peritoneal dialysis, so the procedure should be immediately discontinued if a pleuroperitoneal leak is diagnosed. Respiratory distress due to increased intra-abdominal pressure can occur, and careful attention to the patient's respiratory rate in relation to dialysate inflows should be noted. Dialysate volumes should be decreased if increased intra-abdominal pressure is contributing to ventilatory dysfunction.

Dialysis disequilibrium is a rare complication of peritoneal dialysis, characterized by dementia, seizures, coma, and/or death.[1] It is thought to occur secondary to rapid drops in blood osmolality that often occur during the first cycles of dialysis. Rapid solute removal causes influx of water into the brain and neurologic dysfunction.[12] Animals that have severe azotemia, hypernatremia, hyperglycemia, or acidosis may be at increased risk.[1] Dialysis disequilibrium was suspected in 2 dogs.[20,46] Clinical signs exhibited included head tremors or head-bobbing in each respective animal. One of the dogs developed clinical signs after the third cycle, and temporary discontinuation of peritoneal dialysis helped resolve clinical signs.[46] The other dog developed clinical signs after 2 days of peritoneal dialysis and had a documented drop in measured osmolality of 42 mOsm from the start of dialysis to the onset of clinical signs.[20] If there is suspicion for disequilibrium, the dialysate prescription should be adjusted to include fewer exchanges or longer dwell times to remove urea and small solutes at a slower rate. Osmolality should be monitored closely, especially during the first few days of dialysis, to make sure that changes are not occurring too rapidly.

In human medicine, peritoneal membrane changes and loss of ultrafiltration are significant complications associated with peritoneal dialysis. Such conditions have not been reported in veterinary patients. It is possible that in the short duration of peritoneal dialysis in veterinary patients, peritoneal membrane changes do not have time to occur, or that it is not noted in veterinary patients because monitoring dialysis adequacy is not routinely done. If dialysis adequacy is more routinely examined, it is possible that these complications will begin to be noted.

PERITONEAL DIALYSIS IN VETERINARY MEDICINE

There have been several case reports[47–51] and retrospective studies on peritoneal dialysis in dogs and cats. The earliest large retrospective study performed by Crisp and colleagues[46] looked at peritoneal dialysis in 25 dogs and 2 cats. Animals enrolled in this study had either chronic kidney disease or acute kidney injury. Of 21 animals with acute kidney injury, 11 had ethylene glycol toxicity, 4 had gentamicin toxicity, 3 had leptospirosis, 1 dog had a ureteral laceration, 1 dog had thiacetarsemide toxicosis, 1 dog had *E coli* pyelonephritis, and 1 dog had acute kidney injury of unknown cause. Of the dogs diagnosed with chronic kidney disease, 3 had chronic interstitial nephritis, 1 had chronic interstitial nephritis and pyelonephritis, and 1 had glomerular amyloidosis. Peritoneal dialysis was effective in decreasing the magnitude of azotemia, but the overall survival rate was very low. No data were evaluated to predict outcome of peritoneal dialysis in this study.

Beckel and colleagues[20] looked at peritoneal dialysis in a small group of dogs that had acute kidney injury secondary to leptospirosis. This study reported a high survival rate of 80%, which is similar to that reported in studies of dogs with leptospirosis treated with conservative management (82%) and with hemodialysis (86%).[52] The outcome is also similar to an older retrospective study from Europe in which dogs with acute kidney injury secondary to leptospirosis and treated with peritoneal dialysis had a survival rate of 73%.[53]

Two recent studies have looked at peritoneal dialysis exclusively in feline populations. A study by Dorval and Boysen[22] looked at 6 cats with acute kidney injury. The cause of acute kidney injury was determined in 4 cats, which included pyelonephritis in 1, suspected pyelonephritis in 1, Easter lily toxicity in 1, and traumatic acute kidney injury following bilateral pyelectomies in 1. Five cats (83%) were discharged from the hospital, and all 4 of the cats with 1-year follow-up had no residual renal disease noted. A study by Cooper and Labato[21] (pending publication) looked at 22 cats with acute kidney injury that received peritoneal dialysis. Causes of renal disease included acute-on-chronic kidney disease in 7 cats, ureterolithiasis in 5, spay complications in 4 (bilateral ureteral ligation in 3 cats and hypotension under anesthesia in 1), and 4 with Easter lily toxicity. Ten cats (45.5%) were discharged from the hospital. There was no significant difference noted among indications for peritoneal dialysis in predicting survival, but it should be noted that 0% of cats with toxicities were discharged and 100% of cats with spay complications were discharged. Overall it seemed that animals with surgically treatable disease that needed peritoneal dialysis for stabilization and support had better prognoses than cats with nontreatable disease.

Another recent study by Nam and colleagues[23] looked at 20 dogs treated with peritoneal dialysis for acute kidney injury and chronic kidney disease. The survival rate was higher for the dogs with acute kidney injury (67%) than for chronic kidney disease (37.5%).

More veterinary studies are needed to evaluate which catheters, indications for dialysis, and prescriptions are most ideal for veterinary patients to achieve the fewest complications and the best outcomes.

SUMMARY

Although hemodialysis and continuous renal replacement therapy are emerging as safe and effective therapies for acute kidney injury, they are not readily available in many places. Peritoneal dialysis is labor intensive, but is technically simpler than hemodialysis and may be performed in any clinic with adequate technical assistance and supervision. Peritoneal dialysis is an effective treatment option for veterinary patients with acute kidney injury refractory to fluid therapy. It can be used an adjunctive therapy to medical management, or can be used as a temporary means to stabilize a patient prior to a surgical procedure. Peritoneal dialysis can also be used to manage a variety of other conditions in humans, and these may be applicable in veterinary medicine as well. Peritoneal dialysis has a high rate of complications, but most are manageable with intense nursing care and careful attention to aseptic technique. Understanding the physiology of dialysis and fluid transport through the peritoneal membrane allows the clinician to make informed decisions regarding dialysate dose and treatment regimen. Peritoneal dialysis is an important modality in the treatment of acute kidney injury and toxicities in veterinary patients.

REFERENCES

1. Labato MA. Peritoneal dialysis in emergency and critical care medicine. Clin Tech Small Anim Pract 2000;15(3):126–35.

2. Blake PG, Daugirdas JT. Physiology of peritoneal dialysis. In: Daugirdas JT, Blake PG, Ing TS, editors. Handbook of dialysis. 4th edition. Philadelphia: Lippincott Williams & Wilkins; 2007. p. 323–38.

3. Teitelbaum I, Burkart J. Peritoneal dialysis. Am J Kidney Dis 2003;42(5):1082–96.

4. Flessner MF. Peritoneal transport physiology: insights from basic research. J Am Soc Nephrol 1991;2(2):122–35.

5. Cowgill LD. Application of peritoneal dialysis and hemodialysis in the management of renal failure. In: Osborne CA, editor. Canine and feline nephrology and urology. Baltimore (MD): Lee and Fiberger; 1995. p. 573–84.

6. Dzyban LA, Labato MA, Ross LA, et al. Peritoneal dialysis: a tool in veterinary critical care. J Vet Emerg Crit Care 2000;10(2):91–102.

7. Gotloib L, Fudin R. Use of peritoneal dialysis and mesothelium in non primary renal conditions. Adv Perit Dial 2009;25:2–5.

8. Winchester JF, Boldur A, Oleru C, et al. Use of dialysis and hemoperfusion in treatment of poisoning. In: Daugirdas JT, Blake PG, Ing TS, editors. Handbook of dialysis. 4th edition. Philadelphia: Lippincott Williams & Wilkins; 2007. p. 300–19.

9. Garcia-Lacaze M, Kirby R, Rudloff E. Peritoneal dialysis: not just for renal failure. Compend Cont Educ Pract Vet 2002;24(10):758–72.

10. Chen CY, Chen YC, Fang JT, et al. Continuous arteriovenous hemodiafiltration in the acute treatment of hyperammonemia due to ornithine transcarbamylase deficiency. Ren Fail 2000;22:823–36.

11. Gotloib L, Fundin R, Yakubovich M, et al. Peritoneal dialysis in refractory end-stage congestive heart failure: a challenge facing a no-win situation. Nephrol Dial Transplant 2005;20(Suppl 7):vii32–6.

12. Pendse S, Singh A, Zawada E. Initiation of dialysis. In: Daugirdas JT, Blake PG, Ing TS, editors. Handbook of dialysis. 4th edition. Philadelphia: Lippincott Williams & Wilkins; 2007. p. 14–21.

13. Ross LA, Labato MA. Peritoneal dialysis. In: DiBartola SP, editor. Fluid, electrolyte, and acid-base disorders in small animal practice. 3rd edition. St Louis (MO): Elsevier; 2006. p. 635–49.

14. Ash SR, Daugirdas JT. Peritoneal access devices. In: Daugirdas JT, Blake PG, Ing TS, editors. Handbook of dialysis. 4th edition. Philadelphia: Lippincott Williams & Wilkins; 2007. p. 356–75.

15. Thodis E, Passadakis P, Lyrantzopooulos N, et al. Peritoneal catheters and related infections. Int Urol Nephrol 2005;37:379–93.

16. Eklund B, Honkanen E, Kyllonen L, et al. Peritoneal dialysis access: prospective randomized comparison of single-cuff and double-cuff straight Tenckhoff catheters. Nephrol Dial Transplant 1997;12(12):2664–6.

17. Gokal R, Alexander S, Ash S, et al. Peritoneal catheters and exit-site practices toward optimum peritoneal access: 1998 update. Perit Dial Int 1998;18(1):11–33.

18. Ash SR, Janle EM. T-fluted peritoneal dialysis catheter. Adv Perit Dial 1993;9(1):223–6.

19. Dzyban LA, Labato MA, Ross LA, et al. CVT update: peritoneal dialysis. In: Bonagura JD, editor. Kirk's current veterinary therapy XIII. Philadelphia: Saunders; 2000. p. 859–60.

20. Beckel NF, O'Toole TE, Rozanski EA, et al. Peritoneal dialysis in the management of acute renal failure in 5 dogs with leptospirosis. J Vet Emerg Crit Care 2005; 15(3):201–5.

21. Cooper RL, Labato MA. Peritoneal dialysis in cats with acute kidney injury [abstract 325]. In: Proceedings of the American College of Veterinary Internal Medicine Forum. San Antonio (TX): The American College of Veterinary Medicine; June 4–7, 2008.

22. Dorval P, Boysen SR. Management of acute renal failure in cats using peritoneal dialysis: a retrospective study of six cases (2003–2007). J Feline Med Surg 2009; 11:107–15.
23. Nam SJ, Choi R, Oh WS, et al. Peritoneal dialysis in dogs: 20 cases (2006-2008). Journal of Veterinary Clinics 2009;26(1):23–8.
24. Parker HR. Peritoneal dialysis and hemofiltration. In: Bovee KC, editor. Canine nephrology. Media (PA): Harwal; 1984. p. 723–53.
25. Reddy C, Dybbro PE, Guest S. Fluoroscopically guided percutaneous peritoneal dialysis catheter placement: single center experience and review of the literature. Ren Fail 2010;32:294–9.
26. Harada K, Uechi M, Yamano S, et al. New procedure for implanting peritoneal dialysis catheters in small animals [abstract 324]. Proceedings of the American College of Veterinary Internal Medicine Forum. Anaheim (CA): The American College of Veterinary Medicine; June 9–12, 2010.
27. Heimbürger O, Blake PG. Apparatus for peritoneal dialysis. In: Daugirdas JT, Blake PG, Ing TS, editors. Handbook of dialysis. 4th edition. Philadelphia: Lippincott Williams & Wilkins; 2007. p. 339–55.
28. Daly C, Campbell MK, Cody JD, et al. Double bag or Y-set versus standard transfer systems for continuous ambulatory peritoneal dialysis in end-stage renal disease. Cochrane Database Syst Rev 2009;1:CD003078.
29. Vanholder RC, Lameire NH. Osmotic agents in peritoneal dialysis. Kidney Int Suppl 1996;56:S86.
30. Vardham A, Zweers MM, Gokal R, et al. A solutions portfolio approach to peritoneal dialysis. Kidney Int 2003;64:S114–23.
31. Williams JD, Craig KJ, Topley N, et al. Peritoneal dialysis: changes to the structure of the peritoneal membrane and potential for biocompatible solutions. Kidney Int Suppl 2003;84:S158–61.
32. Faller B, Marichal JF. Loss of ultrafiltration in CAPD: a role for acetate. Perit Dial Bull 1984;4:10–3.
33. Slingeneyer A, Mion C, Mourad G, et al. Progressive sclerosing peritonitis. A late and severe complication of maintenance peritoneal dialysis. Trans Am Soc Artif Intern Organs 1983;29:633–40.
34. Topley N, Coles GA, Williams JD. Biocompatibility studies on peritoneal cells. Perit Dial Int 1994;14(Suppl 3):S21–8.
35. Witowski J, Jorres A, Korybalska K, et al. Glucose degradation products in peritoneal dialysis fluids: do they harm? Kidney Int Suppl 2003;84:S148–51.
36. Tjiong HL, Swart R, van den Berg JW, et al. Amino acid-based peritoneal dialysis solutions for malnutrition: new perspectives. Perit Dial Int 2009;29(4): 384–93.
37. Topley N. In vitro biocompatibility of bicarbonate based peritoneal dialysis solutions. Perit Dial Int 1997;17(1):42–7.
38. Fusshoeller A, Plail M, Grabensee B, et al. Biocompatibility pattern of a bicarbonate/lactate-buffered peritoneal dialysis fluid in APD: a prospective, randomized study. Nephrol Dial Transplant 2004;19(8):2101–6.
39. Sitter T, Sauter M. Impact of glucose in peritoneal dialysis: saint or sinner? Perit Dial Int 2005;25:415.
40. Goel S, Misra M, Saran R, et al. The rationale for, and role of, heparin in peritoneal dialysis. Adv Perit Dial 1998;14:11–4.
41. Blake PG. Adequacy of peritoneal dialysis and chronic peritoneal dialysis prescription. In: Daugirdas JT, Blake PG, Ing TS, editors. Handbook of dialysis. 4th edition. Philadelphia: Lippincott Williams & Wilkins; 2007. p. 387–409.

42. Paniagua R, Amato D, Vonesh E, et al. Effects of increased peritoneal clearances on mortality rates in peritoneal dialysis: ADEMEX, a prospective, randomized, controlled trial. J Am Soc Nephrol 2002;13:1307–20.

43. Goldberg R, Yalavarthy R, Teitelbaum I. Adequacy of peritoneal dialysis: beyond small solute clearance. Contrib Nephrol 2009;163:147–54.

44. Golper TA, Churchill D, Blake P, et al. NKF-K/DOQI clinical practice guidelines for peritoneal dialysis adequacy: update 2000. Am J Kidney Dis 2001;37(1):S9–64.

45. Heimbürger O. How should we measure peritoneal dialysis adequacy in the clinic. Contrib Nephrol 2009;163:140–6.

46. Crisp MS, Chew DJ, DiBartola SP, et al. Peritoneal dialysis in dogs and cats: 27 cases (1976–1987). J Am Vet Med Assoc 1989;195(9):1262–6.

47. Dorfelt R. Peritoneal dialysis in a dog. Kleinterpraxis 2007;52(3):151–61.

48. Fox LE, Grauer GF, Dubielzig RR, et al. Reversal of ethylene glycol-induced nephrotoxicosis in a dog. J Am Vet Med Assoc 1987;191:1433.

49. Jackson RF. The use of peritoneal dialysis in the treatment of uremia in dogs. Vet Rec 1964;76:1481.

50. Kirk RW. Peritoneal lavage in uremia in dogs. J Am Vet Med Assoc 1957;131:101.

51. Thornhill JA, Ash SR, Dhein CR, et al. Peritoneal dialysis with the Purdue column disc catheter. Minn Vet 1980;20:27.

52. Adin CA, Cowgill LD. Treatment and outcome of dogs with leptospirosis: 36 cases (1990-1998). J Am Vet Med Assoc 2000;216(3):371–5.

53. Avellini G, Fruganti G, Morettini B, et al. Peritoneal dialysis in the treatment of canine leptospirosis. Atti Soc Italiana Sci Vet 1973;27:341–77.

Intermittent Hemodialysis for Small Animals

Carly Anne Bloom, DVM[a], Mary Anna Labato, DVM[b],*

KEYWORDS

- Hemodialysis • Intermittent • Dialyzer • Acute kidney injury
- Chronic kidney disease

Intermittent hemodialysis (IHD) is a renal replacement modality that is defined by short, efficient hemodialysis sessions with the goal of removing endogenous or exogenous toxins from the bloodstream. Common indications for IHD include drug or toxin ingestion, acute or acute-on-chronic kidney injury, and chronic kidney disease (CKD). Sessions can be performed once, as is common with toxin ingestion, or can be repeated daily or every other day for several days or longer, as is often done for acute kidney injury (AKI). Sessions can be planned 2 or 3 times per week for the duration of the patient's life, as may be selected for CKD. Sessions are traditionally 1 to 6 hours in length, but can be longer depending on stability of the patient and efficiency of the session. IHD is designed as a more efficient modality than continuous renal replacement therapy (CRRT), meaning that IHD sessions remove small dialyzable molecules (including blood urea nitrogen [BUN], creatinine, phosphorus, electrolytes, and certain drugs and toxins) from the bloodstream more rapidly than CRRT. Between treatments (the interdialysis period), these dialyzable molecules may again increase in the bloodstream. IHD is commonly performed in university or private practice specialty referral centers, and cases are most often overseen by Diplomates of the Colleges of Veterinary Internal Medicine or Emergency and Critical Care.

PRINCIPLES OF HEMODIALYSIS

The main forces used during IHD are diffusion, convection, and adsorption. The magnitude of exchange of fluids and solutes is determined by the characteristics of the solute as well as the pore size and structural characteristics of the dialyzer

[a] Small Animal Internal Medicine, University of Queensland School of Veterinary Science, Small Animal Hospital, Therapies Road, St Lucia, QLD 4072, Australia
[b] Small Animal Medicine, Department of Clinical Sciences, Cummings School of Veterinary Medicine, Tufts University, 200 Westboro Road, North Grafton, MA 01536, USA
* Corresponding author.
E-mail address: mary.labato@tufts.edu

Vet Clin Small Anim 41 (2011) 115–133
doi:10.1016/j.cvsm.2010.11.001
0195-5616/11/$ – see front matter © 2011 Elsevier Inc. All rights reserved.

membrane. In IHD, diffusion is the most prevalent force for exchange of solutes and fluids; convection and adsorption generally play a minor role.

During diffusion, solutes move from areas of high to low concentration. In moving, solutes leave the blood or dialysate fluid compartment in which they had been dissolved, cross the dialysis membrane, and enter the opposite fluid compartment. Blood solutes such as BUN, creatinine, and electrolytes diffuse across the semipermeable dialyzer membrane into dialysate, which is discarded. Solutes in high concentration in dialysate, such as bicarbonate and selected electrolytes, may diffuse across the dialyzer membrane according to their concentration gradient into blood. The rate of solute transfer via diffusion is determined by the concentration gradient of the solutes, kinetic energy in solution (mainly determined by molecular weight), and membrane permeability. Diffusion is best at removing molecules with low molecular weight from the blood, including BUN and creatinine, sodium, potassium, phosphorus, and magnesium (**Box 1**).

During convection, water is removed from the blood along with dissolved solutes. Blood traveling in semipermeable membranes of the dialyzer is exposed to positive transmembrane pressure, which pushes fluid (ultrafiltrate) and dissolved solutes out of blood, across the dialyzer membrane, and into the dialysate, which is discarded. The rate of fluid and solvent transfer via convection is determined by transmembrane hydrostatic pressure between the blood and dialysate, and the surface area of the dialysis membrane. Convection, a prevalent force in CRRT but not IHD, is best at removing molecules with low and middle molecular weight from the blood. Middle

---

Box 1
Molecular weights of selected uremic toxins

Low molecular weight (<500 Da)

- Creatinine
- Hydrogen
- Magnesium
- Oxalic acid
- *p*-Cresol
- Phosphate
- Potassium
- Sodium
- Urea (60)

Middle and high molecular weight (>500 Da)

- β_2-Microglobulin
- Parathyroid hormone
- Carbamylated proteins
- Granulocyte inhibitory proteins
- Other peptides and proteins

Data from Yeun JY, Depner TA. Principles of hemodialysis. In: Owen WF, Pereira BJG, Sayegh M, editors. Dialysis and transplantation: a companion to Brenner & Rector's the kidney. Philadelphia: WB Saunders; 2000. p. 1–31.

molecules include many inflammatory mediators, as well as uremic toxins (see **Box 1**).

INDICATIONS FOR IHD
Acute and Acute-on-chronic Kidney Injury

AKI occurs as a result of acute damage to the hemodynamic, filtration, or excretory functions of the kidney (**Table 1**). The subsequent acute decrease in glomerular filtration rate leads to accumulation of uremic toxins and metabolic wastes in the blood stream, resulting in dysregulation of fluid, electrolyte, and acid-base balance.

A diagnostic algorithm that includes the following criteria may be used to establish the clinical definition of AKI.

Main criteria for diagnosis of AKI
- Acute onset of clinical signs (<7 days)
- Increased creatinine or increased BUN levels despite fluid correction of prerenal azotemia.

Supportive criteria for diagnosis of AKI
- Known normal creatinine within past 1 month
- Known recent ischemia or nephrotoxicant ingestion
- Morphologic confirmation of acute renal lesions
- Return of creatinine to normal values.

In dogs, the most common causes of AKI include ischemia and toxin ingestion.[1] Ischemic events may be caused by pancreatitis, hypovolemia, sepsis, disseminated intravascular coagulopathy, hospital procedures (general anesthesia), or other causes.[2,3] The most common ingested nephrotoxicant in dogs is ethylene glycol, though AKI has been reported from many other toxins, including grapes and raisins, aminoglycoside antibiotics, chemotherapy agents such as cisplatin and ifosfamide, and nonsteroidal antiinflammatory medications (NSAIDs).[1,4,5] Leptospirosis is a common cause of AKI in dogs, and peritoneal or hemodialysis seems to improve outcome in dogs with severe infections.[6,7]

In cats, the most common causes of AKI include toxic and ischemic insults. The most common ingested nephrotoxicant in cats is the lily plant of the genera *Lilium* and *Hemerocallis*, although AKI has been reported from ethylene glycol, as well as a variety of medications such as aminoglycoside antibiotics, NSAIDs, and chemotherapy agents.[8,9] Partial or complete ureteral obstruction can lead to acute or chronic kidney injury, most commonly as a result of calcium-based urolithiasis, the incidence of which is rising.[10,11] Recently, dried solidified blood calculi have been shown to cause ureteral obstruction in cats.[12] Some clinicians define urethral obstruction in cats as an indication for hemodialysis.[13]

In both dogs and cats, bacterial pyelonephritis, ureteral obstruction, and urinary tract rupture can cause AKI. Bacterial pyelonephritis is commonly caused by ascending lower urinary tract infection, but may be caused by hematogenous spread. Ureteral obstruction is most common in cats and small dogs caused by calcium-based ureteroliths, or less commonly ureteral trauma, neoplasia, or inflammation.[10] Urinary tract rupture may be caused by trauma, pressure necrosis from urolithiasis, or surgery.[14] A combination of melamine and cyanuric acid caused AKI in both dogs and cats during an outbreak of contaminated pet food from China in March of 2007.[15,16]

Initial management of acute or acute-on-chronic injury includes intravenous fluid administration, correction of hypovolemia, correction of mineral, electrolyte, and acid-base imbalances, supportive care of the clinical signs of uremia, and nutritional

Table 1
Renal indications for hemodialysis in the veterinary literature

Reference	Indication for Hemodialysis
Cowgill and Elliott,[17] 2000	Acute renal failure
	When the clinical consequences of the azotemia, fluid, electrolyte, and acid-base disturbances cannot be managed with medical therapy
	When severe oliguria or anuria in which an effective diuresis cannot be maintained with replacement fluids, osmotic or chemical diuretics, and renal vasodilators
	Chronic renal failure
	When severe, chronic uremia (BUN level >90, creatinine level >7) exceeds the efficacy of medical management, and owners wish for short periods of dialytic support to ameliorate the azotemia and other complications of CKI
	Finite periods of hemodialysis may be indicated for the preoperative management of animals awaiting renal transplantation
Langston,[28] 2002	Acute renal failure
	Uncontrolled biochemical or clinical manifestations of uremia
	Life-threatening electrolyte disturbances: hyperkalemia, hyponatremia, hypernatremia
	Life-threatening fluid overload: pulmonary edema, congestive heart failure, systemic hypertension
	Severe or refractory azotemia (BUN level >100 mg/dL; creatinine level >10 mg/dL) that is unresponsive to aggressive medical management for 12 to 24 hours
	Chronic renal failure
	Refractory uremia (BUN level >100 mg/dL; creatinine level >8 mg/dL)
	Intractable clinical signs related to uremia
	Preoperative stabilization for renal transplantation
Elliott,[23] 2000	Refractory azotemia (BUN level >90 mg/dL, creatinine level >6 mg/dL)
	Intractable uremic signs
	Hyperkalemia
	Fluid overload
	Severe metabolic acidosis
	Preoperative conditioning for renal transplantation
	Postoperative delayed graft function
	Acute renal graft rejection
	Acute exacerbations of chronic renal failure
Groman,[19] 2010	Fluid overload
	Immune-mediated diseases
	Removal of inflammatory mediators
	Apheresis
	Artificial liver

support. Treatment also includes removal of the inciting cause of renal injury, if possible. Many causes of AKI are potentially reversible; animals may die of complications of uremia before sufficient renal recovery occurs.

IHD may be an appropriate consideration when medical management fails to achieve the goals outlined earlier. Therefore, IHD is indicated in cases of significant or rising azotemia, electrolyte abnormalities, or acidosis unresponsive to medical management. IHD is also indicated in cases of oliguria and anuria in the face of appropriate medical management.

Before IHD is considered, consider the following questions in your patient:

- Have I adequately rehydrated my patient?
- Have I corrected hypovolemia and hypotension using fluid therapy or pressor medications?
- Have I challenged my anuric or oliguric patient with diuretic therapy?

If the answers are yes to these questions and medical management still fails to improve the patient's clinical and clinicopathologic picture, or if the life-threatening severity of disease precludes attention to each question, consideration of IHD is warranted. These questions should be addressed in a matter of hours, not days, because early intervention improves the chance of a successful outcome.[13,17]

CKD

IHD is commonly used in the management of humans with CKD.[18] IHD is an uncommon but available therapy for management of CKD in veterinary patients. Indications for IHD in patients with CKD include reduction of chronic progressive azotemia, hyperkalemia, and fluid overload, as well as stabilization before renal transplantation.

Future indications for IHD therapy

In the future, IHD may become part of the treatment offered for liver failure via liver dialysis, in which a specialized dialyzer membrane acts as an artificial liver. IHD may become part of a routine treatment of patients with systemic inflammatory response syndrome, sepsis, or other severe inflammatory conditions via filtration and removal of inflammatory mediators, or fluid overload and congestive heart failure via ultrafiltration and removal of excess intravascular fluid volume as well as apheresis.[19]

HEMODIALYSIS EQUIPMENT
Venous Access

Hemodialysis removes blood volume from the patient, cleanses it using the extracorporeal dialysis membrane, and returns it to the patient. Therefore, dependable venous access is a cornerstone of IHD success. In veterinary medicine, recirculating blood access and return is generally obtained using a double-lumen intravenous jugular catheter (see the article on vascular access by Chalhoub and colleagues elsewhere in this issue for further exploration of this topic).

When first selecting a dialysis catheter, consider both the lumen width and the catheter length. Select the largest lumen width appropriate for your patient, which enables higher blood flow, increased dialysis efficiency (if desired), and theoretically fewer complications such as blood stasis and clotting. Select the length of your catheter by measuring from the expected insertion point to the junction of the cranial vena cava and right atrium of the patient. Vascular access may be impaired if catheters are too short and are unable to draw blood from the vena cava or right atrium, or if they are too long and result in increased resistance to flow.

Dialysis catheters can be temporary or permanent. Temporary catheters are appropriate for treatment of acute intoxications, acute and acute-on-chronic injury, and in patients too unstable to receive a permanent catheter. Temporary catheters are placed using a modified Seldinger technique.[20,21] All personnel involved in catheter placement should wear a cap, mask, and sterile gloves. The doctor or technician placing the catheter should also wear a sterile gown. First, the patient is lightly sedated; we often use butorphanol 0.2 mg/kg intravenously. Comatose patients should not be sedated. Next, clip and drape the area in a sterile manner, and perform a sterile preparation of the area using a chlorhexidine scrub and alcohol. The temporary dialysis catheter is then placed as follows.

The vessel is punctured with a trocar or 16 G over-the-needle catheter, using a cutdown technique if appropriate. The guidewire is advanced through the lumen of the trocar, and the trocar is withdrawn. The dilator sheath is placed over the guidewire into the vessel, and the guidewire is withdrawn. The catheter is placed through the dilator sheath into the vessel, the sheath is withdrawn, and the catheter is sutured into place. Alternatively, the dilator sheath can be removed before placement of the catheter over the guidewire. A lateral radiograph of the thorax is always taken to make sure the catheter is placed appropriately and the tip is at the level of the right atrium. The catheter is wrapped in a sterile manner, and is used only for hemodialysis. The catheter is locked with heparin (1000 units/mL) when not in use, to prevent clotting.

Permanent dialysis catheters that are surgically placed are recommended for those patients who receive chronic IHD. Permanent catheters are also chosen based on lumen width and catheter length, as explained earlier. Both types of catheters are heparin locked when not in use, are used exclusively for hemodialysis, and are always handled in a sterile manner. Differences between temporary and permanent catheters include the following[17,22]:

- Material
  Temporary catheters can be polyurethane or silicone
  Permanent catheters should be silicone, which is softer and less reactive than polyurethane
- Placement
  Temporary catheters are placed percutaneously in a clean room using the modified Seldinger technique
  Permanent catheters are placed surgically, and the catheter is tunneled subcutaneously from insertion site to the skin exit site to reduce motion, decrease infection risk, and keep the catheter in place
- Cuffing
  Temporary catheters do not contain cuffs
  Permanent catheters may contain cuffs to help keep the catheter in place for long periods; the cuff is placed in the subcutaneous tunnel.

THE DIALYZER OR ARTIFICIAL KIDNEY

The hemodialyzer is a compact, disposable extracorporeal unit that acts as an artificial kidney. The dialyzer unit is a sealed compartment with connections on either end to allow for flow of blood and dialysate through the unit (**Fig. 1**). Within the most common type of dialyzer are thousands of hollow straws (called hollow fiber design). Blood flows within the straws, whereas dialysate flows around the straws, in a concurrent or countercurrent direction. The surface of the straw acts as both a physical barrier separating the blood and dialysate compartments, and as a semipermeable

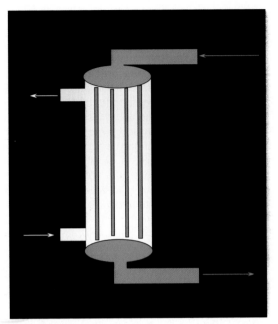

Fig. 1. A dialyzer. (*Courtesy of* Dr Cathy Langston, New York.)

membrane allowing transfer of fluid and solutes according to the principles of diffusion and convection (**Fig. 2**).

When first selecting a dialyzer unit, consider the membrane type, and the size of the dialyzer unit. Membranes come in a wide variety of types, and both the membrane material and the pore size are important. At our dialysis center, we generally use dialyzer membranes made of polysulfone, a synthetic material. Synthetic dialyzer membranes are less reactive, and are less likely to induce complement activation than the older, cellulose-based dialyzer membranes. Dialyzers are classified broadly by pore size as low flux (small pore size that allows passage of small solutes), or high flux (larger pore size that allows passage of water and small and middle molecules).

The larger the dialyzer unit, the greater the membrane surface area for exchange of water and solutes, and, potentially, the more efficient the dialysis session. However, with larger dialyzer units comes greater extracorporeal blood volume, meaning that

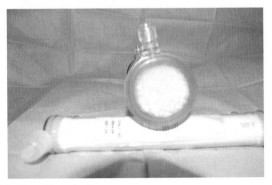

Fig. 2. Close-up of hollow fiber design.

more blood is outside the patient's body during the dialysis session. Therefore, the size of the dialyzer unit must be carefully chosen to maximize efficiency and minimize excessive extracorporeal blood volume. In addition, each dialyzer unit comes with a set of blood tubing. The dialyzer unit plus the associated blood tubing is called the blood circuit, and each blood circuit has a predetermined, consistent, and labeled blood volume that fills the circuit. Therefore, when choosing a dialyzer unit, consider the volume of the blood circuit, which equals the total extracorporeal blood volume. The total extracorporeal blood volume should be less than 10% of the patient's blood volume to minimize patient hypotension and hypovolemia.[17,23] The smallest blood circuits that are commonly used in veterinary medicine are neonatal circuits, which necessitate an extracorporeal blood volume of at least 50 mL. For small patients less than 7.0 kg, this circuit contains more than 10% of the patients' blood volume, and it is advantageous to prime the circuit with type-matched whole blood, colloidal fluids, or other volume-expanding fluids to minimize hypotension and hypovolemia.[17]

THE IHD MACHINE

The IHD machine is the foundation of the dialysis session (**Fig. 3**). The machine allows the doctor or technician to control the following parameters:

- Blood flow rate
- Dialysate flow rate
- Direction of blood flow with respect to dialysate flow (concurrent vs countercurrent)
- Dialysate composition
- Treatment length

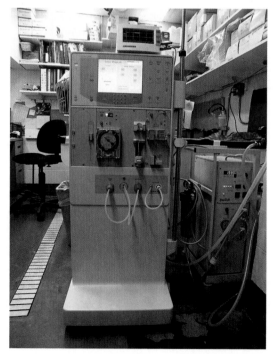

Fig. 3. IHD machine.

- Sodium profiling, a method to regulate plasma osmolality and stabilize fluid shifts
- Anticoagulant administration rate, including bolus and continuous rate infusion (CRI) capabilities
- Temperature of returning blood
- Fluid removal from the bloodstream.

Careful attention to these parameters allows you to control the efficiency of the dialysis session and maximize the safety and stability of the patient. The IHD machine manufactures dialysate during each session, according to your prescription. The basic ingredients include a concentrated solute solution, a concentrated bicarbonate solution, and purified water. The concentrated solute solution may contain sodium, potassium, and calcium, as well as dextrose, chloride, and magnesium in amounts that approximate plasma concentrations. Solute solutions are available without potassium for use with hyperkalemic patients. Solute solutions are also available with different calcium concentrations and even without calcium, for use with hypercalcemic patients or patients anticoagulated with citrate, as discussed later. Most modern IHD machines allow you to sodium profile during the session. The most commonly used method of sodium profiling keeps dialysate sodium slightly higher than patient plasma sodium at the start of the session, with a gradual decrease in dialysate sodium during the session. The high dialysate/plasma sodium ratio allows sodium to diffuse from dialysate into patient plasma early in the dialysis session, when diffusion of urea out of patient plasma into dialysate is most rapid.[22] Using the equation for plasma osmolality

$$2 (Na^+ + K^+) + BUN/2.8 + BG/18$$

we see that increasing plasma sodium during times of rapid decrease in plasma urea can help stabilize patient plasma osmolality, which lowers the risk of a serious IHD side effect called dialysis disequilibrium syndrome (DDS), as discussed later. As the session progresses, dialysate sodium is lowered to avoid patient plasma hypernatremia.[22]

The bicarbonate solution is initially separate from the concentrated solute solution to avoid precipitation with calcium and magnesium, and is mixed by the IHD machine in diluted states to avoid precipitation.[17] Acetate, an alternative to bicarbonate, is more stable in solution but is not recommended, because it can cause vasodilation, hypotension, and reduced cardiac contractility in veterinary patients.[17]

The blood path is defined by the path of the extracorporeal circuit (**Fig. 4**). Blood is pulled from one of the 2 ports of the dialysis catheter, and travels through the

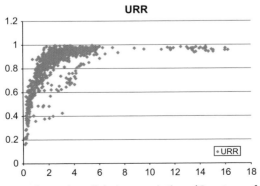

Fig. 4. Graph of URR to determine dialysis prescription. (*Courtesy of* Dr Cathy Langston, New York.)

extracorporeal circuit being pulled (prepump) and then pushed (postpump) by the clockwise circling of the blood pump. Blood then enters the straws of the dialyzer and runs the length of the dialyzer, separated from the dialysate by the semipermeable dialyzer membrane. Filtered blood is then returned to the patient via the second port of the dialysis catheter. IHD can be performed with a single-lumen catheter if needed; the IHD machine alternates pull and return of blood, and the session is less efficient.[22] Along the extracorporeal circuit are instruments to detect air and leaks, a filter to catch thrombi, pressure pods for measuring occlusion or disconnection in the circuit, and sampling ports from which blood may be drawn and medications given.

Other monitoring equipment helpful or essential to an IHD session include a continuous electrocardiogram, activated clotting time (ACT) machine, blood warmer cuff to warm the returning blood line, pulse oximeter, blood pressure monitoring, and supplemental oxygen. In-line blood-volume profiling equipment monitors hematocrit and oxygen saturation, and is a helpful adjunct to pulse oximetry and indirect blood pressure monitoring in the vigilance against hypotension and hypoxemia, 2 complications of IHD. It is essential to have equipment and staff capable of initiating cardiopulmonary cerebral resuscitation in the event of an arrest.

Patients should be positioned and lightly restrained on a cushioned, comfortable table, with a heating pad positioned under the patient. We generally keep a harness on our patients, and restrain them lightly to the table. Cats sit in the well-cushioned bottom half of a cat carrier. Absorbent pads help keep the patient clean and dry.

ANTICOAGULATION

Extracorporeal blood must be anticoagulated when processing through the dialysis tubing and dialyzer unit. The dialyzer membrane initializes the contact activation pathway of the coagulation cascade[24,25]; therefore, IHD is a prothrombotic procedure, and anticoagulation is almost always used during each session. The 2 most common methods of anticoagulation are unfractionated heparin and citrate. Unfractionated heparin inhibits coagulation by binding antithrombin; together, this complex binds and inactivates multiple coagulation factors, including IIa (thrombin), IXa, Xa, XIa, and XIIa.[26] Unfractionated heparin is infused directly into the blood of the extracorporeal circuit before the filter, and is often given as a bolus followed by a CRI. The initial bolus is given at 25 to 50 units/kg, and the heparin CRI is adjusted based on ACT readings.[22] The goal is to keep the ACT 1.6 to 2 times more than normal, or approximately 160 to 200 seconds.[22] Heparin CRI is discontinued 30 minutes before the end of the IHD session, and the patient is considered heparinized for at least 6 to 8 hours after the session. If intervals between dialysis sessions are short the patient is considered heparinized in the interdialytic period. Citrate inhibits coagulation by binding calcium, which is an important cofactor in the amplification and propagation phases of the cell-based model of coagulation.[25] Citrate anticoagulation differs from heparin because citrate anticoagulation is considered regional; the extracorporeal circuit is anticoagulated, but the patient ideally is not. Citrate is infused directly into the blood of the extracorporeal circuit before the filter, and anticoagulates the extracorporeal circuit. The citrate infusion is adjusted based on the postfilter ionized calcium in the extracorporeal blood.[22] Before the filtered and citrated blood returns to the patient, calcium is infused into the patient's blood, binding and inactivating the citrate.

STAFFING

IHD sessions last from 1 to 6 hours; sessions may be extended for increased efficiency in certain cases. At our dialysis center, IHD takes place in a quiet, dedicated room directly across the hall from the intensive care unit (ICU). At least 2 dedicated hemodialysis personnel work on each IHD case: at least one is in the dialysis room monitoring the patient at all times, whereas the other is in the dialysis room or immediately accessible. If not in the same room, personnel are in contact via walkie-talkie. ICU staff, although separate from dialysis staff, are alerted that there is a dialysis session and are available to assist if needed.

Our dialysis staff consists of a dedicated day and evening dialysis technician, whose primary allegiance is the hemodialysis unit, in which they are highly trained in both IHD and CRRT. One dialysis technician helps run nearly every dialysis session. Between session and patients, they run the IHD machine daily, oversee water purification and testing, stock and organize the dialysis room, and participate in continuing education with the dialysis team. One technician is on call at all times; therefore, dedication and dependability of technicians are essential to running a dialysis unit. Between dialysis duties, our technicians work with in- and outpatients, and both are employed full time by the university.

The second part of our hemodialysis team is the clinicians: all internal medicine residents, plus interested interns and emergency and critical care residents, are trained in IHD and CRRT. They participate in a rotating on-call schedule to assist referring veterinarians, clients, and house doctors in deciding whether to pursue hemodialysis on a given case, and plan and run each session. Dialysis plans, prescriptions, and sessions are overseen by 2 dedicated faculty members who specialize in renal medicine. A small team of interested veterinary students are trained to assist during hemodialysis sessions. Building a dialysis unit takes the dedication, training, continuing education, and commitment of many.

FORMULATING AN IHD PRESCRIPTION

The dialysis prescription refers to the parameters that are set for each session to deliver a particular dose of dialysis to a patient. The prescription is different for each patient and for each session; however, some general principles apply. Choosing a dialysis prescription includes consideration of the following parameters such as uremia, the hemodialyzer, blood flow rate, length of session and frequency of sessions (**Box 2**).[23]

Box 2
Decision parameters for creating a dialysis prescription
Severity of uremia
Expected frequency of IHD sessions
Choice of hemodialyzer
Volume of extracorporeal circuit
Dialysate composition
Dialysate flow rate
Blood flow rate
Length of dialysis session
Anticoagulant dosage
Choice of priming solution
Ultrafiltration rate
Ultrafiltration volume

BLOOD FLOW RATE AND LENGTH AND FREQUENCY OF DIALYSIS SESSIONS

For acute and acute-on-chronic kidney injury, initial BUN level is often markedly increased. Although IHD is capable of lowering BUN level quickly, a rapid decrease in BUN and/or sodium levels leads to marked decreases in plasma osmolality. Consequent rapid fluid shifts can result in DDS. Therefore, initial sessions are designed to be less efficient.[27] Methods to decrease diffusion efficiency include shorter sessions, slower blood flow rates, and concurrent (rather than countercurrent) flow of blood and dialysate.

One way to calculate desired efficiency of the initial session based on severity of uremia is via the urea reduction ratio (URR) to determine the volume of blood that needs to be processed through the dialyzer to achieve a certain percent reduction in BUN level.[22] URR and the corresponding blood flow rate (L/kg body weight) needed to achieve that particular URR have been determined for dogs and cats using empirical data from the Companion Animal Hemodialysis Unit at the Veterinary Medical Teaching Hospital at the University of California-Davis. In IHD, blood flow rate is the primary determinant of small molecule clearance, including BUN and potassium clearance.[22] Therefore, one way to begin a dialysis prescription is to determine a desired URR (**Box 3**), determine the volume of blood per kilogram body weight the machine must process to achieve that desired URR (see **Fig. 4**), and determine the desired length of the session, which is often 1.5 to 2 hours for the first session, 3 hours for the second session, and 4 hours (cats) to 5 hours (dogs) for the third or fourth sessions.[28] Using the patient's body weight, desired blood volume to be processed, and desired length of the session, you can set your blood flow rate in mL/kg/min accordingly. Blood flow rate is often set low at

---

Box 3
A simplified method built on the URR criteria

- First session

  Blood flow rate 5 mL/kg/min

  > Note: Cowgill and Elliott[17] recommend blood flow rates as low as 1 to 2 mL/kg/min for animals with predialysis BUN level greater than 180 mg/dL

  Length of session approximately 1 to 2 hours

  > Note: Cowgill and Elliott[17] recommend prolonged, slow treatment sessions of up to 8 hours for small patients with severe uremia (BUN level >250 mg/dL), using blood flow rates less than 2 mL/kg/min

- Second session

  Blood flow rate 10 mL/kg/min

  Length of session approximately 3 hours

- Additional sessions

  Blood flow rate 15 to 20 mL/kg/min

  Length of session

  Cats approximately 4 hours

  Dogs approximately 5 hours

Data from Cowgill LD, Elliott DA. Hemodialysis. In: DiBartola SP. Fluid therapy in small animal practice. 3rd edition. Philadelphia: WB Saunders; 2000. p. 528–47; and Langston C. Hemodialysis in dogs and cats. Compendium 2002;24:540–9.

the start of the session and is slowly increased to the prescribed blood flow rate in the first 30 minutes of the session, to avoid hypotension or nausea.[23]

For IHD of patients with CKD, sessions are performed 2 or preferably 3 times per week, with twice-weekly sessions appropriate only for those patients with sufficient residual renal function to avoid significant rebound solute accumulation between dialysis sessions.[29] Blood flow rate targets can be set at 15 to 25 mL/kg/min if the patient's starting BUN level and vascular access can tolerate this high rate. Targets for length of session are 4 hours in cats and 5 hours in dogs, again, if well tolerated by the patient.[28,29] For acute and chronic IHD, longer sessions may be both feasible and desirable, depending on treatment goals.

Between dialysis sessions, solutes do reaccumulate. Therefore, bloodwork must always be taken at the start and end of the dialysis session and between dialysis sessions, so that appropriate dialysis prescriptions and interdialysis treatments are optimized for each individual patient.

PRIMING SOLUTION

Priming solution is often saline, but colloids can be used for patients whose extracorporeal blood volume approaches or exceeds the 10% blood volume guideline, or for patients who are anemic or hypovolemic at the start of the session. Useful colloids include typed whole blood and Hetastarch diluted 50% with saline.[22]

DIALYSATE FLOW RATE

Dialysate flow rate is, by convention, 500 mL/min. This rate can be altered if needed. A faster dialysis flow rate provides a modest increase in clearance, whereas a slower dialysis flow rate provides a modest decrease in clearance.[17,22]

ULTRAFILTRATION

Much of the discussion of hemodialysis focuses on removal of solutes, such as urea, creatinine, and potassium, from the uremic patient's bloodstream. However, during IHD, fluid can also be removed from the bloodstream. This process is called ultrafiltration, and is of great benefit to overhydrated patients. The amount of fluid to remove during an IHD session can be calculated as follows[22]: % overhydration × kilograms body weight × 10 = milliliters of fluid to remove during the dialysis session.

Once you know the milliliters of excess patient fluid you wish to remove and the length of the session, you can calculate the number of milliliters of plasma fluid your machine should remove, which is programmed in milliliters per hour. The rate of patient fluid removal should not exceed 20 mL/kg/h.[22] Ultrafiltration can be modeled to remove more plasma fluid toward the end of the dialysis session, when dialysis efficiency has decreased and the patient is at less risk for solute and corresponding fluid shifts.[27]

MEASURING EFFICACY

URR, which was estimated before the start of the dialysis session, can be measured after the session using the following equation:

$$URR = (BUN_{pre} - BUN_{post})/BUN_{post}$$

If the URR is higher than anticipated, the session has been more efficient than expected, and you may wish to change your dialysis prescription for the next session.

If the URR is lower than anticipated, there may be clotting or clogging of the dialysis membrane, causing reduced efficiency. It is also possible that there is catheter recirculation, meaning that a significant portion of the returned blood is rapidly removed again for filtration, rather than joining the body blood pool. This situation can happen with dual-lumen catheters with staggered ends in which blood is being drawn from the distal lumen and returned through the proximal lumen; such reduced efficiency can be ameliorated if the direction of blood flow is reversed.[22] Target URRs should be no greater than 0.1 URR per hour.

Kt/V can also be used to calculate session efficiency and is discussed in detail in another article by Cowgill elsewhere in this issue. It is a commonly used measure of urea removal and is a kinetically modeled index reflecting the fractional clearance of urea from its distribution volume during a single dialysis session. This index refers to the delivered dose of dialysis that is equal to delivered clearance. In this index, K is the urea clearance of the dialyzer (mL/min), t is the time of the dialysis session (min), and V is the volume of urea distribution (L) that approximates total body water. Essentially, $Kt/V = \ln(BUN_{pre}/BUN_{post})$. The higher the Kt/V value, the greater the dose of dialysis and efficacy of the dialysis treatment. Kt/V values between 1.2 and 1.4 are considered adequate hemodialysis doses in human patients, but conventional dialysis prescriptions in animals often result in Kt/V values between 2.5 and 3, reflecting highly effective dialysis treatment.[17,30] (See the article by Cowgill elsewhere in this issue for further exploration of this topic.)

COMPLICATIONS

Complications of IHD have been widely reported, and include hypotension and hypovolemia; problems with vascular access; and neurologic, respiratory, hematologic, and gastrointestinal complications.[17,23]

Hypotension and hypovolemia occur during IHD sessions as a result of ultrafiltration and large extracorporeal blood volumes and can persist during or between sessions as a result of blood loss (from bleeding secondary to uremic ulceration, overheparinization, or coagulopathy, or blood loss secondary to filter or line clotting in which not all extracorporeal blood volume can be returned to the patient). Treatments include decreased ultrafiltration, crystalloid or colloid therapy, pressor therapy, or cessation of the IHD session in severe cases. Approximately 50% of feline IHD cases have problems with hypotension and hypovolemia.[9,31]

Problems with vascular access are common and include thrombosis, failure to provide adequate blood flow, and less commonly bleeding and infection.[17,29] Thrombosis is countered by filling each catheter lumen with heparin between dialysis sessions; however, incorrect dosage of heparin locks can predispose the patient to bleeding.[17] Failure to provide adequate flow can be countered with careful attention to catheter size choice, as explained earlier. The goal is to choose the largest bore catheter you can safely place in your patient, and to choose the proper length catheter positioned in the right atrium or vena cava.

Neurologic complications can be caused by uremic encephalopathy, intracranial bleeding or thrombosis, or DDS. DDS is caused by rapid shifts in sodium, urea, or bicarbonate, leading to cerebral edema. Clinical signs include agitation, disorientation, vomiting, seizure, coma, and death during or after a dialysis session. We find that dogs often vocalize or become agitated, whereas cats often do not display obvious premonitory signs and may die suddenly. Prevention includes mannitol infusion during the dialysis session, sodium modeling, and limited-efficiency sessions; treatment includes mannitol and diazepam. In a review of IHD in cats, Langston and colleagues[31] report DDS in 38% of cats. Clinical signs included disorientation, agitation, vocalization, dilated pupils, acute blindness, or coma. Seventy-eight percent of affected cats responded to treatment with mannitol, whereas 13% did not respond to mannitol, and 8% died despite DDS treatment. Suspected DDS has also been reported in dogs undergoing IHD.[5]

Respiratory signs can occur in IHD patients as a result of underlying disease, complications or IHD, or both. Respiratory complications include uremic pneumonitis and pulmonary hemorrhage, pleural effusion and pulmonary edema, hypoxemia, hypoventilation, and pulmonary thromboembolism (PTE).[23] We suspect that we see pulmonary hemorrhage secondary to leptospirosis infection, as well as because of uremic or iatrogenic coagulopathy. Adin and Cowgill[7] report that 50% of leptospiremic dogs in one study were thrombocytopenic, likely because of vasculitis. Fluid gain, or failure to correct overhydration, during IHD sessions can lead to pleural effusion and pulmonary edema; cardiac disease can cause or contribute to this complication. Hypoxemia and hypoventilation can be caused by ventilatory failure in the critically ill or neurologically impaired patient; whereas hypoxemia can be caused by diffusion failure as a result of pulmonary hemorrhage, pneumonitis, infectious pneumonia, or edema, or ventilation-perfusion mismatch caused by PTE.[32]

Hematologic complications including anemia, thrombocytopenia, and leucopenia are also common in patients with IHD. Again, these complications can be caused by primary disease; anemia is a common sequela of CKD. Anemia and thrombocytopenia result from coagulopathy and vasculitis common with systemic inflammatory response syndrome, and leucopenia can result from infectious or inflammatory processes. Anemia is also common as a result of frequent blood sampling, loss through the extracorporeal circuit, and bleeding, as described earlier. Thrombocytopenia can occur secondary to contact activation with the dialysis membrane, and promotion of the coagulation cascade as a result of disease-specific or iatrogenic coagulopathy, whereas leucopenia can occur transiently as a result of white blood cell interaction with the dialysis membrane.[23] Clinical anemia and thrombocytopenia may be corrected by addressing the underlying cause, and providing compatible colloid, whole-blood, packed red blood cells, or plasma transfusions.

Gastrointestinal complications such as nausea, vomiting, and inappetance are common in uremic animals, and can also be a complication of dialysis-induced hypotension, DDS, dialysate contaminants, and incompatible blood transfusion reactions.[23] Complications can be addressed using histamine-2 receptor blockers or proton-pump inhibitors, antiemetics, and appetite stimulants as appropriate. Many dialysis centers place esophageal feeding tubes at the time of dialysis catheter placement, to help ensure proper nutrition, hydration, and oral medication during interdialysis periods.[27,33] Parenteral nutrition must be considered when enteral nutrition is not possible.

OUTCOME

Outcome of medical management for AKI in dogs, cats, and humans routinely averages around 50% to 60%.[1,2,8] Indications to forego continued medical management in favor of hemodialysis include worsening azotemia, worsening hyperkalemia, and anuria or oliguria despite appropriate medical management, as discussed earlier. The cause of AKI can influence the success of both medical and dialytic therapy.

Adin and Cowgill[7] report on the outcome of 14 dogs treated with IHD for AKI secondary to leptospirosis. Twelve of the 14 dogs were oliguric or anuric despite appropriate medical therapy. Survival rate was excellent at 86%, with only one of 14 dogs necessitating chronic hemodialysis. Prognosis for AKI caused by grape or raisin toxicity in dogs treated medically is 53%, and Eubig and colleagues[4] and Stanley and Langston[5] report successful reversal of currant-induced AKI in a dog with progressive azotemia and oliguria despite appropriate medical management. In cats, AKI caused by lily inges- tion can be fatal, with recent articles showing 0% survival for anuric lily-intoxicated cats, but that survival after oliguria may be possible with early and aggressive dialysis therapy.[28,34] Worwag and Langston[8] discuss successful IHD in 25% (2 of 8) of feline AKI cases but do not specify the criteria for dialysis in these 8 cats; it may be the dialyzed cats were significantly more uremic or more critically ill than the successfully medically managed cats, because overall survival for all cats treated for AKI in this study was 61%. Kyles and colleagues[10] report on the use of IHD to stabilize 13% of cats undergoing surgery for ureteral calculi; although these investigators do not relate IHD to outcome, the outcome of cats that had surgery to correct ureteral obstruction caused by calculi was better than the outcome of cats treated medically for this problem, with 91% of surgically treated cats and 72% of nonsurgically treated cats surviving for 1 month. In a review article on IHD in cats, Langston and colleagues[31] found that the average survival rate for cats treated with IHD for AKI is 60%, similar to the survival rates in human patients with AKI treated with IHD. Pyelonephritis carried the best prognosis (100% survival), whereas ethylene glycol ingestion had 60% survival but necessitated a more prolonged course of dialysis (mean of 12 ± 7 sessions compared with 3 sessions for cats with pyelo- nephritis), and resulted in higher BUN and creatinine levels at the termination of dialysis. AKI had better outcomes than acute on CKD (13% or 1 of 8 cats recovered and survived) or CKD (no cats survived).

SUMMARY

IHD is a useful and feasible modality to improve outcome in dogs and cats with kidney injury that do not respond adequately to medical management. The decision to pursue hemodialysis in patients with acute or acute-on-chronic kidney injury should be made as quickly as possible to improve the likelihood of a successful outcome . IHD requires thorough understanding of renal physiology, as well as the principles and machinery involved in dialysis. It also requires a trained and dedicated staff 24 hours a day, 7 days a week, to field questions, identify appropriate cases, develop tailored dialysis prescriptions, perform the technical duties involved during and between dialysis sessions, attend to the patient and client in a holistic and compassionate manner, and be prepared to act in emergency situations that may arise in the care of these often critically ill patients. We encourage readers to become familiar with dialysis facilities near them, and to reach out to these facilities to learn more about dialysis, and indica- tions and preparations to refer. If you are considering referring a patient for hemodial- ysis, please contact your local dialysis facility to discuss the case (Appendix); avoid venipuncture of the jugular veins so they remain intact for dialysis catheter placement; and be prepared to address the clients' expectations and financial and emotional investment involved in performing dialysis in our veterinary patients.

APPENDIX: LIST OF IHD FACILITIES

Animal Medical Center, 510 East 62nd Street, New York, NY 10065, USA
   Tel: +1 212 329 8618
   Dr Cathy Langston: cathy.langston@amcny.org
   www.amcny.org/dialysis

AVETS, 4224 Northern Pike, Monroeville, PA 15146, USA
   Tel: +1 412 373 4200

Dr Merilee Costello
www.avets.us

Companion Animal Hemodialysis Unit, Veterinary Medical Teaching Hospital, University of California-Davis, Davis, CA 95616, USA
Tel: +1 530 752 1393
Dr Larry Cowgill: ldcowgill@ucdavis.edu
http://www.vetmed.ucdavis.edu/vmth/small_animal/hemo

Louisiana State University, Veterinary Medical Teaching Hospital, Baton Rouge, LA 70803, USA
Tel: +1 225 578 9600
Dr Mark Acierno
www.dialysis@vetmed.lsu.edu

Tufts University, Cummings School of Veterinary Medicine, Foster Hospital for Small Animals, 200 Westboro Road, North Grafton, MA 01545, USA
Tel: +1 508 839 5395x84538
Dr Mary Labato
Dr Linda Ross
www.tufts.edu/vet

Aubi Companion Animal Hospital, Strada Genova 299/A, 10024 Moncalieri, Italy
Tel: +39 011 6813033
Dr Claudio Brovida
www.anubi.it

Centro Nefrologico Veterinario, Clinica Veterinaria Citta di Catania, Via Vittorio Veneto 313, 95126 Catania, Italy
Tel: +39 095 503924
Dr Angelo Basile
www.nefrovet.com

Clinica Veterinaria Roma Sud, Via Pilade Mazza 24, Rome 00173, Italy
Tel: +39 06 72672403
Dr Daniela Mignacca
www.clinicaveterinariaromasud.it

Vetsuisse Faculty University of Berne, Laenggass-Strasse 128, PO Box 8466, Berne, Switzerland
Tel: +41 (0)31 631 2943
Dr Thierry Francey
www.vetdialyse.unibe.ch

Tierarztliche Klinik fur Kleintiere, Kabels Stieg 41, D-22850 Norderstedt, Germany
Tel: +49 (0)40 5298940
www.tierklinik-norderstedt.de

Hospital Veterinario Montenegro, Rua Pereira Reis, 191, 4200-447 Porto, Portugal
Tel: +351 225 089 639/+351 225 089 989
www.hospvetmontenegro.com

Renal Vet Rio de Janeiro, Rua Tereza Guimaraes, 42, Botafogo, Rio de Janeiro - RJ, CEP 22280-050, Brazil
Tel: +55 21 22752391/39027158
www.veterinariaonline.com

Renal Vet Sao Paulo, Rua Heitor Penteado, 99, Sumare, Sao Paulo - SP, CEP 00000000, Brazil

Tel: +55 11 38752666

www.veterinariaonline.com

Manhattan Animal Hospital, 1 Fl NO 77, Sec 4, Civic Boulevard, Taipei, Taiwan
Tel: +886 229 815203
Dr David Tan

REFERENCES

1. Vaden SL, Levine J, Breitschwerdt EB. A retrospective case-control of acute renal failure in 99 dogs. J Vet Intern Med 1997;11(2):58–64.
2. Behrend EN, Grauer GF, Mani I, et al. Hospital-acquired acute renal failure in dogs: 29 cases (1983–1993). J Am Vet Med Assoc 1996;208(4):537–41.
3. Stokes JE, Bartges JW. Causes of acute renal failure. Compend Contin Educ Pract Vet 2006;28:387–96.
4. Eubig PA, Brady MS, Gwaltney-Brant SM, et al. Acute renal failure in dogs after the ingestion of grapes or raisins: a retrospective evaluation of 43 dogs (1992–2002). J Vet Intern Med 2005;19(5):663–74.
5. Stanley SW, Langston CE. Hemodialysis in a dog with acute renal failure from currant toxicity. Can Vet J 2008;49:63–6.
6. Beckel NF, O'Toole TE, Rozanski EA, et al. Peritoneal dialysis in the management of acute renal failure in 5 dogs with leptospirosis. J Vet Emerg Crit Care 2005; 15(3):201–5.
7. Adin CA, Cowgill LD. Treatment and outcome of dogs with leptospirosis: 36 cases (1990–1998). J Am Vet Med Assoc 2000;216(3):371–5.
8. Worwag S, Langston CE. Acute intrinsic renal failure in cats: 32 cases (1997–2004). J Am Vet Med Assoc 2008;232(5):728–32.
9. Langston CE. Acute renal failure caused by lily ingestion in six cats. J Am Vet Med Assoc 2002;220(1):49–52.
10. Kyles AE, Hardie EM, Wooden BG, et al. Management and outcome of cats with ureteral calculi: 153 cases (1984–2002). J Am Vet Med Assoc 2005;226(6):937–44.
11. Cannon AB, Westropp JL, Ruby AL, et al. Evaluation of trends in urolith composition in cats: 5,230 cases (1985–2004). J Am Vet Med Assoc 2007;231:570–6.
12. Westropp JL, Ruby AL, Bailiff NL, et al. Dried solidified blood calculi in the urinary tract of cats. J Vet Intern Med 2006;20:828–34.
13. Diehl SH, Seshadri R. Use of continuous renal replacement therapy for treatment of dogs and cats with acute or acute-on-chronic renal failure: 33 cases (2002–2006). J Vet Emerg Crit Care 2008;18(4):370–82.
14. Bjorling DE. Traumatic injuries of the urogenital system. Vet Clin North Am Small Anim Pract 1984;14(1):61–76.
15. Cianciolo RE, Bischoff K, Ebel JG, et al. Clinicopathologic, histologic, and toxicologic findings in 70 cats inadvertently exposed to pet food contaminated with melamine and cyanuric acid. J Am Vet Med Assoc 2008;233(5):729–37.
16. Rumbeiha WK, Agnew D, Maxie G, et al. Analysis of a survey database of pet food-induced poisoning in North America. J Med Toxicol 2010;6:172–84.
17. Cowgill LD, Elliott DA. Hemodialysis. In: DiBartola SP, editor. Fluid therapy in small animal practice. 2nd edition. Philadelphia: WB Saunders; 2000. p. 528–47.
18. Yeun JY, Depner TA. Principles of hemodialysis. In: Owen WF, Pereira BJG, Sayegh M, editors. Dialysis and transplantation: a companion to Brenner & Rector's the kidney. Philadelphia: WB Saunders; 2000. p. 1–31.
19. Groman R. Apheresis in veterinary medicine: therapy in search of a disease. In: Proceedings of the Advanced Renal Therapies Symposium. 2010. p. 26–32.

20. McLaughlin K, Jones B, Mactier R, et al. Long-term vascular access for hemodialysis using silicon dual lumen catheters with guidewire replacement of catheters for technique salvage. Am J Kidney Dis 1997;29(4):553–9.
21. Taylor RW, Palagiri AV. Central venous catheterization. Crit Care Med 2007; 35(5):1390–6.
22. Langston CA, Poeppel K, Mitelberg E. AMC dialysis handbook. New York: Animal Medical Center; 2010. p. 3.
23. Elliott DA. Hemodialysis. Clin Tech Small Anim Pract 2000;15:136–48.
24. Fischer KG. Essentials of anticoagulation in hemodialysis. Hemodial Int 2007;11: 178–89.
25. Smith SA. The cell-based model of coagulation. J Vet Emerg Crit Care 2009; 19(1):3–10.
26. Dunn M, Brooks MJ. Antiplatelet and anticoagulant therapy. In: Bonagura JD, Twedt DC, editors. Kirk's current veterinary therapy XIV. St Louis (MO): Saunders Elsevier; 2009. p. 24–8.
27. Fischer JR, Pantaleo V, Francey T, et al. Veterinary hemodialysis: advances in management and technology. Vet Clin North Am Small Anim Pract 2004;34(4): 935–67.
28. Langston C. Hemodialysis in dogs and cats. Compendium 2002;24:540–9.
29. Cowgill LD. Management of the chronic hemodialysis patient. In: Proceedings of the Advanced Renal Therapies Symposium. 2008. p. 1–18.
30. Daugirdas JT, Van Stone JC. Physiologic principles and urea kinetic modeling. In: Daugirdas JT, Blake PG, Ing TS, editors. Handbook of dialysis. 3rd edition. Philadelphia: Lippincott Williams & Wilkins; 2001. p. 15–45.
31. Langston CE, Cowgill LD, Spano JA. Applications and outcomes of hemodialysis in cats: a review of 29 cases. J Vet Intern Med 1997;11(6):348–55.
32. West JB. Respiratory physiology: the essentials. Philadelphia: Lippincott Williams & Wilkins; 2008. p. 13–73.
33. Ross S. Dialysis complications. In: Proceedings of the Advanced Renal Therapies Symposium. 2010. p. 53–4.
34. Berg RIM, Francey T, Segev G. Resolution of acute kidney injury in a cat after lily (*Lilium lancifolium*) intoxication. J Vet Intern Med 2007;21:857–9.

Continuous Renal Replacement Therapy in Dogs and Cats

Mark J. Acierno, MBA, DVM

KEYWORDS

- Continuous renal replacement therapy • CRRT
- Acute kidney injury • Dialysis

In the early 1900s, a young pharmacologist at the Johns Hopkins University School of Medicine performed a series of experiments that would lay the foundation for all extracorporeal blood purification technologies developed during the next 100 years. Abel and colleagues[1] directed arterial blood from animal patients, mixed it with an anticoagulant, passed it through a device that divided the blood into strawlike semipermeable membranes that were suspended in fluid, and then directed the blood back to the patient (**Fig. 1**). Abel demonstrated that the subject's blood could be altered by changing the composition of the fluid. This process, referred to as vividif-fusion, relied on the properties of diffusion and became the basis for intermittent hemodialysis (IHD).

Continuous renal replacement therapy (CRRT) is a more recently developed blood purification modality. As the name implies, CRRT is a continuous process, and once treatment begins, therapy continues until renal function returns or the patient is transitioned to intermittent dialysis. CRRT is similar to IHD because patient blood is divided into thousands of strawlike semipermeable membranes contained within a dialyzer; however, whereas IHD is primarily a diffusive therapy, CRRT uses diffusion, convection, and, to a lesser extent, adhesion.

CRRT has several significant advantages compared with IHD. The slow and gradual nature of the technique provides better control of electrolytes and acid-base balance.[2] The continuous operation more closely approximates the functioning of a normal kidney.[3] Use of convection in CRRT provides a significant advantage in the removal of larger molecules than can be achieved with diffusion. These larger molecules are closer in size to those that are normally filtered by the kidney. The goal of IHD is to make dramatic changes in a patient's uremic, acid-base, and fluid status over short periods using diffusion; therefore, significant quantities of pure dialysate must be produced onsite. This technique requires a sizeable investment in the purchase and

The author has nothing to disclose.

Department of Veterinary Clinical Science, School of Veterinary Medicine, Louisiana State University, Skip Bertman Drive, Baton Rouge, LA 70803, USA

E-mail address: acierno@pocketdvm.com

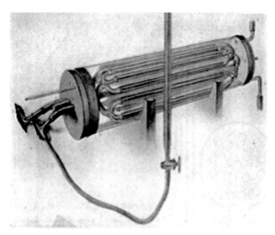

Fig. 1. Dr John Abel directed arterial blood from animal patients, mixed it with an anticoagulant, directed it through the device that divided the blood into strawlike semipermeable membranes that were suspended in fluid, and then directed the blood back to the patient. He demonstrated that the subject's blood could be altered by changing the composition of the fluid. (*From* Abel J, Rowntree L, Turner B. On the removal of diffusible substances from the circulating blood of living animals by dialysis. J Pharmacol Exp Ther 1914;5:285; with permission.)

maintenance of specialized water treatment facilities.[4] In contrast, the efficient use of diffusion and convection in CRRT allows for the use of prepackaged sterile fluids and makes CRRT units virtually free of maintenance between treatments.

INDICATIONS

The most common indication for CRRT is the treatment of acute kidney injury (AKI) in cases in which renal function is expected to return in the near future or for patients who are to be transitioned to IHD. The author has used CRRT for patients with leptospirosis, tumor lysis syndrome, heatstroke, pre- and postsurgical support of ureteral obstructions, as well as aminoglycoside and melamine toxicities. CRRT can also be used to remove certain drugs and toxins. The ability of any extracorporeal therapy to remove a substance depends on the size of the molecule, its volume of distribution, as well as its degree of protein binding.[5] A small molecule with a minimal volume of distribution and low protein binding would be most amenable to removal. The extent to which many drugs, toxins, and substances of abuse can be removed by CRRT or IHD has been published.[6] CRRT has also been used to treat people with diuretic-resistant congestive heart failure; however, this treatment has not yet been evaluated in companion animals.[7]

BLOOD PURIFICATION

The basis of all extracorporeal blood purification is the dividing of a patient's blood into thousands of strawlike semipermeable membranes contained in the dialyzer. While traveling through the dialyzer's semipermeable membranes, blood is purified by diffusion, convection, and, to a lesser extent, adhesion. Diffusion is the tendency of molecules in solution to move from an area of higher concentration to that of lower concentration.[7] As Abel demonstrated almost a century ago, by bathing the dialyzer's semipermeable membranes in solution, the movement of substances can be facilitated in or out of the patient's blood by altering the solution's composition. This principle remains the basis of IHD.

Convection also takes place in the strawlike semipermeable membranes of the dialyzer; however, convection involves exposing the blood to a positive transmembrane pressure. This can be accomplished by creating a relative negative pressure around the membranes, a positive pressure within the membranes, or a combination of the 2 processes. Fluid, called ultrafiltrate, is pushed out of the blood and across the semipermeable membrane. Toxins, electrolytes, and other small molecules are then carried with the ultrafiltrate, which is then discarded.[7,8] Fluids and electrolytes must be replaced with great accuracy because dehydration, overhydration, or severe electrolyte imbalances can quickly develop. The benefits of convection are 2-fold. First, convection makes more economical use of fluids than diffusion. Second, larger molecules are more effectively cleared by convection than by diffusion.[9]

Adsorption also plays a role in blood purification and occurs when molecules adhere to the membrane and are removed from circulation. Human patients with systemic inflammatory response syndrome who undergo CRRT experience a significant decrease in circulating inflammatory mediators.[10] Some of these mediators leave the blood by diffusion or convection, whereas others become adhered to the semipermeable membrane. Although this technique has attracted interest as a possible treatment of systemic inflammatory syndrome, it is not clear if the reduction in mediators correlates to decreased morbidity or mortality.

MODES OF OPERATION

CRRT combines diffusion and convection to produce 4 distinct treatment modalities: slow continuous ultrafiltration (SCUF), continuous venovenous hemofiltration (CVVH), continuous venovenous hemodialysis (CVVHD), and continuous venovenous hemodiafiltration (CVVHDF). SCUF is the least complicated of the treatment modalities (**Fig. 2**). It is a purely convective modality in which blood enters the dialyzer, is divided into thousands of strawlike semipermeable membranes, and is exposed to a positive transmembrane pressure. Ultrafiltrate is forced out of the blood into the intermembrane space and is then discarded as effluent, and the hemoconcentrated blood is returned to the patient.[11] SCUF is used in human medicine for patients with nondiuretic responsive congestive heart failure.[7]

Similar to SCUF, CVVH is also a purely convective modality in which blood enters the dialyzer, is divided into thousands of strawlike semipermeable membranes, and then exposed to a positive transmembrane pressure; however, in CVVH, a sterile balanced electrolyte solution is used to replace the ultrafiltrate (**Fig. 3**).[11] The electrolyte solution can be added before or after the dialyzer, but in either case it is called the replacement fluid. When the replacement fluid is added before the dialyzer (predialyzer configuration), the patient blood is diluted and then convection within the dialyzer restores the blood to its normal physiologic volume. When the replacement fluid is added after the dialyzer (postdialyzer configuration), the blood is first hemoconcentrated within the dialyzer and then a sterile balanced electrolyte solution is added before the blood is returned to the patient. The benefit of operating in postdialyzer configuration is that it is efficient; however, as the blood becomes increasingly concentrated within the dialyzer, there is a risk of sludging and clotting.[12] Although the predialyzer configuration has a lower risk of clotting, it is much less efficient.[13] Because a filtration fraction [(ultrafiltrate rate mL/min $\times$ 100)/(blood flow rate mL/min $\times$ [1-hematocrit value])] of 25% to 30% can be achieved before the risk of clotting significantly increases. Other

SCUF

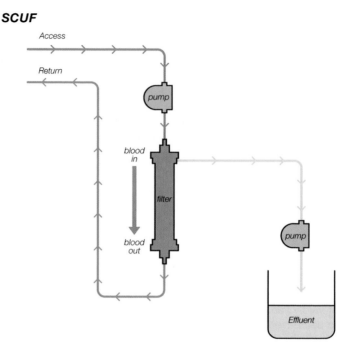

Fig. 2. SCUF, a purely convective modality, generates ultrafiltrate that is not replaced. (*From* Acierno MJ, Maeckelbergh V. Continuous renal replacement therapy. Compend Contin Educ Vet 2008;30(5):269, copyright 2008, Veterinary Learning Systems, Yardley, Pennsylvania; with permission.)

investigators report good success using the predialyzer configuration (Cathy Langston, personal communication, 2010).

CVVHD is a diffusive therapy that closely resembles IHD (**Fig. 4**).[14] Blood enters the dialyzer and is divided into thousands of strawlike semipermeable membranes that are bathed in a solution (dialysate) that flows countercurrent to the blood flow. Toxins that are in high concentration in the blood diffuse across the membrane and enter the dialysate, whereas substances in a high concentration in the dialysate (eg, bicarbonate) diffuse into the blood. The exhausted dialysate is then disposed of as effluent. Although CVVHD is similar to IHD, the slow dialysate flow rates of CVVHD allow the use of prepackaged sterile dialysate.[15]

CVVHDF combines the diffusive characteristics of CVHD with the convective properties of CVVH (**Fig. 5**).[14] Blood enters the dialyzer and is divided into thousands of strawlike semipermeable membranes, which are bathed in the dialysate, while the blood is exposed to a positive transmembrane pressure. Diffusion guides the movement of smaller uremic toxins and electrolytes, whereas the positive transmembrane pressure facilitates the movement of fluid and larger molecules. A sterile balanced electrolyte solution is used to replace the ultrafiltrate. Because the amount of convection and diffusion can be adjusted independently, this modality offers the greatest treatment flexibility.

At present, it is not clear which CRRT modality is most effective in the treatment of AKI. Although convective modalities (CVVH, CVVHDF) have an advantage in the clearance of larger molecules,[16] diffusive therapies (CVVHD) are just as effective in the clearance of smaller molecules such as urea and creatinine.[17] The exact role that larger

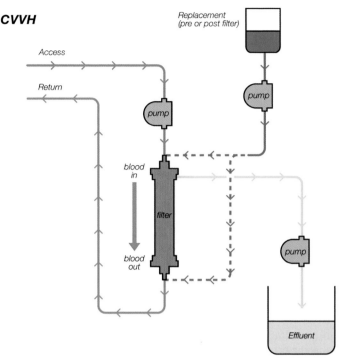

Fig. 3. CVVH is a purely convective modality in which ultrafiltrate is replaced with a sterile balanced electrolyte solution. (*From* Acierno MJ, Maeckelbergh V. Continuous renal replacement therapy. Compend Contin Educ Vet 2008;30(5):269, copyright 2008, Veterinary Learning Systems, Yardley, Pennsylvania; with permission.)

molecules play in the pathogenesis of AKI or signs associated with uremia is not known. In addition, diffusive therapies are associated with lower incidence of CRRT circuit clotting.[13] Nevertheless, in most instances, convective therapies (CVVH or CVVHDF) are used, with good results.

EQUIPMENT

Gambro Renal Systems (Lakewood, CO, USA) manufactures virtually all CRRT systems used in veterinary medicine. Although most veterinary facilities use the older Prisma unit, the new more advanced Prismaflex has replaced it. These units are highly integrated and computerized. A central computer coordinates the movement of 4 peristaltic pumps: a blood pump, a dialysis solution pump, a replacement solution pump, and an effluent pump. The actual speed of these pumps is electronically verified and adjusted. All fluids (dialysate, replacement, effluent) are continuously weighed and compared with calculated expected weights. Any difference between the actual and expected weight results in a system alarm. Dozens of system parameters are continuously calculated, monitored, and displayed. These systems incorporate a heparin infusion system, although the Prismaflex also has integrated supports for citrate anticoagulation.

BLOOD ACCESS

In all but the smallest patients, a dual-lumen temporary dialysis catheter is placed in the jugular vein using the Seldinger technique.[18,19] These specialized catheters are

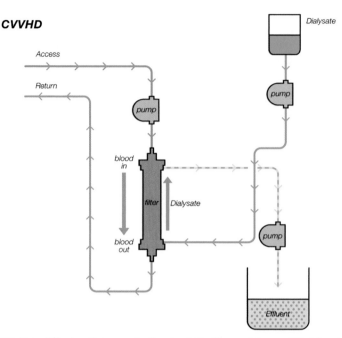

Fig. 4. CVVHD is a diffusive therapy similar to IHD. (*From* Acierno MJ, Maeckelbergh V. Continuous renal replacement therapy. Compend Contin Educ Vet 2008;30(5):270, copyright 2008, Veterinary Learning Systems, Yardley, Pennsylvania; with permission.)

designed to maximize blood flow and minimize blood recirculation. Typically, an 11.5F dual-lumen temporary dialysis catheter is placed in very large dogs, whereas an 8F catheter is placed in smaller dogs. In the smallest patients, a single-lumen 5F dialysis catheter is placed in each jugular vein. A more extensive discussion of the proper selection and care of vascular access catheters by Chalhoub and colleagues can be found elsewhere in this issue.

ANTICOAGULATION

Although CRRT tubing and dialyzers are made from highly biocompatible material, clotting is inevitable in the absence of adequate anticoagulation. Formation of clots in the CRRT circuit results in a significant loss of patient blood, requires the replacement of an expensive CRRT circuit, and results in time that the patient is not receiving treatment. Anticoagulation of the CRRT circuit is usually accomplished with heparin or citrate.

A constant rate infusion (CRI) of heparin has historically been the most widely used method of anticoagulation in patients undergoing CRRT,[19] and most CRRT systems have integrated heparin syringe pumps. Heparin increases the activity of antithrombin, a circulating protease inhibitor. Because the patient's blood is systemically anticoagulated, there is a risk of uncontrolled bleeding; however, monitoring activated clotting time (ACT) and actively managing heparin infusion rates can minimize this risk (**Box 1**). Because of the low per-sample cost and minimal blood volume requirements, ACT devices manufactured by Medtronic (Minneapolis, MN, USA) are the most commonly used for monitoring ACT in veterinary CRRT.

Calcium is an essential cofactor required throughout the clotting cascade. Before the patient's blood enters the CRRT circuit, citrate is infused, which chelates the

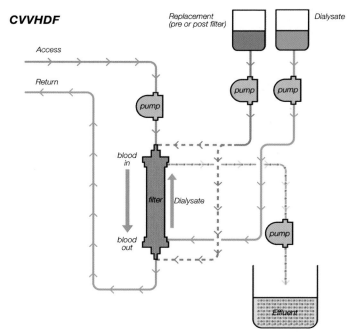

Fig. 5. CVVHDF combines the diffusive aspects of CVVHD with the convective properties of CVVH. (*From* Acierno MJ, Maeckelbergh V. Continuous renal replacement therapy. Compend Contin Educ Vet 2008;30(5):270, copyright 2008, Veterinary Learning Systems, Yardley, Pennsylvania; with permission.)

calcium and renders the blood unable to clot. Many of the resulting calcium-citrate complexes are lost through the dialyzer as effluent, while the remaining citrate returns to the patient and is metabolized by the liver into bicarbonate. The patient's physiologic calcium levels are maintained by infusing calcium directly to the patient. Citrate anticoagulation has advantages in that anticoagulation is limited to the CRRT unit and circuit lifespan may be extended[20]; however, alkalosis from citrate metabolism as well as hypocalcemia and hypercalcemia are common life-threatening complications in both human and veterinary patients.[21,22] Therefore, the patient's serum calcium concentration and acid-base status must be frequently monitored.[21] Because of lower cost and ease of use and based on personal experience, heparin anticoagulation is used at the author's facility.

TREATMENT ADEQUACY

Although the toxins responsible for the uremia are not known, serum urea is easily measured and commonly used as a surrogate for all small molecules removed in CRRT.[23] The formula Kt/V is a commonly used measure of CRRT treatment adequacy. It represents the urea clearance over time, normalized for the patient's volume of distribution. In this calculation, K represents urea clearance in milliliters per minute. Total solute removal per period (Kt) is the product of clearance (K in milliliters per minute) and time (t in minutes) that the patient receives treatment per day. Kt is then normalized by dividing urea clearance over time by the patient's volume of distribution (V in milliliters). Urea is approximately equally distributed in all body fluid compartments, and its removal by CRRT is so gradual that significant differences

---

Box 1
Louisiana State University heparin work sheet

Start of therapy

  Check ACT

  In the absence of coagulopathy (ACT>150), give 25-unit/kg heparin bolus

  Record total units given _____

  Recheck ACT. If less than 180, repeat bolus (maximum 3 total boluses)

  Record number of boluses given _____

  ACT at start of therapy _____

During CRRT

  Start heparin infusion, 20 units/kg/h

  If ACT<180, increase heparin by 1 unit/kg/h

  If ACT>220, decrease heparin by 1 unit/kg/h

  If ACT<170, bolus 10 unit/kg heparin and increase CRI

  If ACT<160, bolus 15 unit/kg heparin and increase CRI

  Monitor ACT every 30 minutes after any change

  Monitor ACT every 2 hours once stable

---

do not develop between compartments; therefore, V is equal to total body water in milliliters (60% of body weight in kilograms $\times$ 1000). Studies in humans suggest that a Kt/V of 1.4 or more may be associated with decreased morbidity and mortality.[23,24] Although studies in companion animals are lacking, the author has found that a Kt/V of 1.4 produces satisfactory reductions in the concentration of urea and provides adequate control of acid-base and electrolyte balance in oliguric and anuric patients. Values for K can be estimated before treatment starts (K_{calc}) and then actual K calculated (K_{del}) once treatment begins.

As an example, a male neutered pit bull weighing 27 kg presents for treatment of AKI secondary to tumor lysis syndrome. A decision is made to treat the patient with CVVH in a postdialyzer replacement fluid configuration. To optimize treatment, it is ensured that the calculated Kt/V is at least 1.4. As a starting point, blood flow rate (Qb) is estimated to be set at 100 mL/min (a little more than 3 times the weight in kg), and ultrafiltration rate is 20%; therefore, ultrafiltrate production rate is 20 mL/min. Although CRRT is theoretically an uninterrupted modality, patients need to be walked and the system needs attending. From experience, it was estimated that the patient should receive 1320 minutes (22 hours) of therapy per day. From **Box 2**, the formula for $K_{calc\ CVVH}$ = ultrafiltrate (20 mL/min). Therefore Kt/V$_{calc\ CVVH}$ = 1.65 (20 mL/min $\times$ 1320 min)/16,000 mL. Although this is an acceptable Kt/V, it should be ensured that the filtration fraction is not greater than 25% to 30%. If the packed cell volume of the patient is 30, the filtration fraction is 28% [(20 mL/min $\times$ 100)/(100 mL/min $\times$ [1−0.30])]. By decreasing the ultrafiltration rate to 17% (Q_{uf} = 17 mL/min), $K_{calc\ CVVH}$ would be a respectable 1.4, whereas filtration fraction decreases to a more comfortable 24%.

Once treatment has begun, actual Kt/V$_{del}$ can be calculated to determine if treatment parameters require adjustment. To calculate K_{del} for the aforementioned patient, urea and ultrafiltrate values are needed. According to the laboratory tests, patient

---

Box 2
Kt/V formula

K_{calc} = Calculated (estimated) urea clearance

K_{del} = Actual delivered urea clearance

CVVH: postdialyzer replacement fluid

   K_{calc} = Ultrafiltrate rate (mL/min)

   K_{del} = Ultrafiltrate urea concentration (mg/dL) $\times$ Ultrafiltration rate (mL/min)/Predialyzer urea concentration (mg/dL)

CVVH: predialyzer replacement fluid

   K_{calc} = Ultrafiltration rate (mL/min)/(1+[Fluid replacement (mL/min)/Blood flow rate (mL/min)])

   K_{del} = Ultrafiltrate urea concentration (mg/dL) $\times$ Ultrafiltration rate (mL/min)/Predialyzer urea concentration (mg/dL)

CVVHD

   K_{calc} = Dialysate rate (mL/min)

   K_{del} = Postdialyzer dialysate urea concentration (mg/dL) $\times$ Dialysate rate (mL/min)/Prefilter blood urea level (mg/dL)

CVVHDF: postdialyzer replacement fluid

   K_{calc} = Ultrafiltration rate (mL/min) + Dialysate rate (mL/min)

   K_{del} = Ultrafiltrate urea concentration (mg/dL) $\times$ (Ultrafiltration rate [mL/min] + Dialysate rate [mL/min])/Predialyzer blood urea level (mg/dL)

---

serum urea nitrogen was 88 mg/dL and ultrafiltrate 80 mg/dL. Using the formula in **Box 2**, K_{del} = 15.45 mL/min (ie, [80 mg/dL $\times$ 17 mL/min]/88 mg/dL), and therefore, Kt/V_{DEL} = 1.27. Because this value is less than the ideal, the blood flow rate can be increased to 110 mL/min. Ultrafiltration rate will continue to be 17%; therefore, ultra-filtrate production will be 18.7 mL/min, and Kt/V = 1.54 ([18.7mL/min $\times$ 1320 min]/16,000 mL). Filtration fraction will continue to be an acceptable 24% [(18.7 mL/min $\times$ 100)/(110 mL/min $\times$ [1−0.30])].

COMPLICATIONS

The most significant complications involve coagulation. Despite appropriate heparin management, clotting of the CRRT circuit is inevitable. To minimize treatment disruptions and the unavoidable loss of patient blood caused by an unexpected circuit clot, system parameters, such as filter and transmembrane pressure, are monitored carefully and the entire circuit is replaced if values unexpectedly change. Although the author has had success with circuits lasting more than 70 hours, the entire CRRT blood pathway is routinely replaced every 48 hours. Clots forming in or around the dialysis catheter can present a challenge to maintaining adequate blood flow. Proper care and troubleshooting of these catheters has been covered elsewhere. Some patients develop bleeding or oozing at the catheter site. This complication is most pronounced in cases in which previous jugular vein trauma precluded placement of the catheter by the Seldinger technique; however, this has not proved to be clinically significant except in small patients. Hypotension is another potential complication. Although the cause of the blood pressure drop at the start of therapy is likely to be multifactorial, the amount of blood needed to fill the CRRT circuit is at least partly the reason.[25]

SPECIAL CONSIDERATIONS FOR SMALL PATIENTS

Continuous renal replacement circuits typically require 50 mL to 84 mL of blood to fill the tubing and dialyzer. This volume can represent a significant portion of a smaller patient's total blood volume and can lead to an unsafe drop in blood pressure at the start of treatment. One way to overcome this problem is to prime the CRRT circuit with whole blood or fresh frozen plasma and packed cells before the start of therapy. As blood is taken from the patient, they simultaneously receive a transfusion so that they have no change in blood volume. A problem arises because the strawlike semi-permeable membranes of most CRRT dialyzers are composed of acrylonitrile and sodium methallyl sulfonate copolymer (AN69). When exposed to acidic blood, these membranes activate bradykinins, which can potentiate life-threatening hemodynamic instability.[26,27] Because stored blood products typically have a low pH, such blood primes can prove fatal. This problem can be circumvented by attaching both the CRRT patient-access and patient-return lines to the bag containing stored blood products and allowing the CRRT machine to correct the pH and remove the activated bradykinins. Thus, the bag of blood receives treatment as if it were a patient (**Fig. 6**). After approximately 30 minutes, the treatment is paused, the bag is disconnected, and the patient is connected. Using this strategy, patients weighing as little as 2.5 kg have been treated. It is important to properly anticoagulate the blood being treated because the replacement fluids/dialysate typically contain calcium. A similar hemodynamic instability has been reported in human patients who are treated with

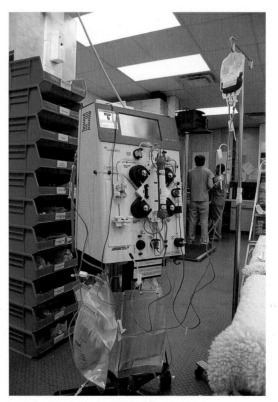

Fig. 6. Whole blood being dialyzed to correct pH.

angiotensin-converting enzyme inhibitors and receive CRRT[28]; therefore, care should be taken when treating such patients.

PATIENT CARE

Providing properly trained, technically competent patient care is the most challenging aspect of providing CRRT. Once the patient has begun therapy, there is an obligation to continue treatment 24 hours a day until the patient recovers, is transitioned to IHD, or is euthanized. Advanced knowledge of renal physiology and the mechanics of the CRRT unit are essential for treatment decisions. The pool of adequately trained doctors and support staff is likely to be limited even in the largest practice. When patients require more than a few days of treatment, the staffing issues can become challenging. In the author's hospital, a doctor and a specially trained veterinary student constantly attend to the patient. These professionals are busy ensuring not only that the functioning of the CRRT unit is being monitored and analyzed but also that the hydration status of the patient is carefully scrutinized. Overhydration is an independent predictor of death in people with AKI. This overhydration is likely to be true in companion animals as well; therefore, attempt is made to account for every milliliter of fluid that enters or leaves patients undergoing CRRT on a continuous basis. There are likely to be a limited number of centers throughout the country that can provide the necessary level of care.

SUMMARY

CRRT is a relatively new extracorporeal blood purification modality for the treatment of AKI, fluid overload, and toxin exposure. Although CRRT has both therapeutic and operational advantages compared with IHD, its intensive nature and the need for specialized 24-hour care will likely limit the availability of this modality to a small number of referral institutions.

REFERENCES

1. Abel J, Rowntree L, Turner B. On the removal of diffusible substances from the circulating blood of living animals by dialysis. J Pharmacol Exp Ther 1914;5: 275–316.
2. Bellomo R, Farmer M, Parkin G, et al. Severe acute renal failure: a comparison of acute continuous hemodiafiltration and conventional dialytic therapy. Nephron 1995;71:59–64.
3. Clark WR, Mueller BA, Alaka KJ, et al. A comparison of metabolic control by continuous and intermittent therapies in acute renal failure. J Am Soc Nephrol 1994;4:1413–20.
4. Langston C. Hemodialysis in dogs and cats. Compendium 2002;24:540–9.
5. Johnson C, Simmons W. Dialysis of drugs. Ann Arbor (MI): Nephrology Pharmacy Associates; 2006.
6. Johnson C. 2007 Dialysis of drugs. Verona (WI): Nephrology Pharmacy Associates; 2007.
7. Clark WR, Ronco C. Continuous renal replacement techniques. Contrib Nephrol 2004;144:264–77.
8. Golpher T. Solute transport in CRRT. In: Bellomo R, Baldwin I, Ronco C, et al, editors. Atlas of hemofiltration. London: WB Saunders; 2002. p. 15–8.
9. Ronco C, Bellomo R, Ricci Z. Continuous renal replacement therapy in critically ill patients. Nephrol Dial Transplant 2001;16(Suppl 5):67–72.

10. De Vriese AS, Colardyn FA, Philippe JJ, et al. Cytokine removal during continuous hemofiltration in septic patients. J Am Soc Nephrol 1999;10:846–53.

11. Bellomo R, Ronco C. An introduction to continuous renal replacement therapy. In: Bellomo R, Baldwin I, Ronco C, et al, editors. Atlas of hemofiltration. London: WB Saunders; 2002. p. 1–9.

12. Henderson LW. Pre vs. post dilution hemofiltration. Clin Nephrol 1979;11:120–4.

13. Parakininkas D, Greenbaum LA. Comparison of solute clearance in three modes of continuous renal replacement therapy. Pediatr Crit Care Med 2004;5:269–74.

14. Bellomo R, Ronco C. Nomenclature for continuous renal replacement therapy. In: Bellomo R, Baldwin I, Ronco C, et al, editors. Atlas of hemofiltration. London: WB Saunders; 2002. p. 11–4.

15. Davenport A. Replacement and dialysate fluids for patients with acute renal failure treated by continuous veno-venous haemofiltration and/or haemodiafiltration. Contrib Nephrol 2004;144:317–28.

16. Cerda J, Ronco C. Modalities of continuous renal replacement therapy: technical and clinical considerations. Semin Dial 2009;22:114–22.

17. Ricci Z, Ronco C, Bachetoni A, et al. Solute removal during continuous renal replacement therapy in critically ill patients: convection versus diffusion. Crit Care 2006;10:R67.

18. Seldinger SI. Catheter replacement of the needle in percutaneous arteriography; a new technique. Acta Radiol 1953;39:368–76.

19. Davenport A. Anticoagulation for continuous renal replacement therapy. Contrib Nephrol 2004;144:228–38.

20. Kutsogiannis DJ, Gibney RT, Stollery D, et al. Regional citrate versus systemic heparin anticoagulation for continuous renal replacement in critically ill patients. Kidney Int 2005;67:2361–7.

21. Tolwani AJ, Wille KM. Anticoagulation for continuous renal replacement therapy. Semin Dial 2009;22:141–5.

22. Diehl S, Seshadri R. Use of continuous renal replacement therapy for treatment of dogs and cats with acute or acute-on-chronic renal failure. J Vet Emerg Crit Care 2008;18:370–82.

23. Ricci Z, Salvatori G, Bonello M, et al. In vivo validation of the adequacy calculator for continuous renal replacement therapies. Crit Care 2005;9:R266–73.

24. Ronco C, Bellomo R, Homel P, et al. Effects of different doses in continuous veno-venous haemofiltration on outcomes of acute renal failure: a prospective randomised trial. Lancet 2000;356:26–30.

25. Sulowicz W, Radziszewski A. Pathogenesis and treatment of dialysis hypotension. Kidney Int Suppl 2006;S36–9.

26. Hackbarth RM, Eding D, Gianoli Smith C, et al. Zero balance ultrafiltration (Z-BUF) in blood-primed CRRT circuits achieves electrolyte and acid-base homeostasis prior to patient connection. Pediatr Nephrol 2005;20:1328–33.

27. Brophy PD, Mottes TA, Kudelka TL, et al. AN-69 membrane reactions are pH-dependent and preventable. Am J Kidney Dis 2001;38:173–8.

28. Verresen L, Fink E, Lemke HD, et al. Bradykinin is a mediator of anaphylactoid reactions during hemodialysis with AN69 membranes. Kidney Int 1994;45:1497–503.

Vascular Access for Extracorporeal Renal Replacement Therapy in Veterinary Patients

Serge Chalhoub, DVM, Cathy E. Langston, DVM*,
Karen Poeppel, LVT

KEYWORDS

• Hemodialysis • CRRT • Catheter

Vascular access is the first and most basic requirement of successful extracorporeal renal replacement therapy (ERRT). An adequately functioning dialysis catheter allows for smooth and efficient patient management, whereas a poorly functioning catheter frustrates the technician, doctor, and patient. In veterinary medicine, central venous catheters are the predominant form of vascular access. Much thought and care should go into appropriate catheter selection, placement, and maintenance. In humans and animals, these catheters can be placed fairly quickly; however, they remain a major cause of morbidity for dialysis patients. Therefore, it is important to understand their limitations and to respect guidelines on proper placement techniques and care.

CATHETER COMPOSITION AND CHARACTERISTICS

Various materials can be used to make a catheter that is minimally thrombogenic, flexible, and nonirritating to the vessel wall. Synthetic polymers, such as polyurethane, polyethylene, polytetrafluoroethylene (PTFE), silicone, and carbothane, are suitable choices. Most of these materials are stiff (at least initially), which makes their percutaneous placement possible. Polyethylene is stiff and kinks when bent. These catheters can be used for temporary catheters but are not appropriate for long-term use.[1] Polyurethane has some rigidity at room temperature, which assists in placement, but it becomes softer and more flexible at body temperature. Alcohol-containing antibiotic ointments weaken the material.[1]

To allow simultaneous removal and return of blood, a dialysis catheter has 2 lumens. Although catheters are placed in a central vein, the lumen that provides blood egress

---

Renal Medicine Service, The Animal Medical Center, 510 East 62nd Street, New York, NY 10065, USA
* Corresponding author.
E-mail address: Cathy.langston@amcny.org

Vet Clin Small Anim 41 (2011) 147–161
doi:10.1016/j.cvsm.2010.09.007
0195-5616/11/$ – see front matter © 2011 Elsevier Inc. All rights reserved.

from the body is generally referred to as the *arterial* port or access port, and the lumen that provides blood return to the body is termed the *venous* port or return port. The arterial lumen is usually shorter than the venous return lumen to avoid uptake of blood returning from the dialyzer (access recirculation), which would decrease the efficiency of treatment (**Fig. 1**). In some situations, 2 single-lumen catheters are placed in separate vessels or in the same vessel to provide blood egress and return.

In lumens with a single opening (at the tip or a side port), partial occlusion from thrombosis or a fibrin sheath can decrease catheter function to the point of it being unable to provide adequate dialysis. The risk of complete occlusion is lessened by having multiple ports (**Fig. 2**). If the ports are positioned circumferentially around the catheter, even if the vessel wall is drawn against the ports on one side of the catheter, blood flow can continue on the opposite side. If the side ports are small, blood preferentially flows through the tip, making the side ports superfluous. If the side ports are large, they weaken the catheter, and increase the amount of heparin that diffuses out of the catheter between dialysis treatments.[2]

A double-D configuration provides the highest lumen volume with the lowest surface area in contact with the blood to diminish shear stress while maintaining a modest outer circumference[1]; however, other configurations are commonly used, including round or C-shaped lumens (**Fig. 3**).[3]

TEMPORARY CATHETERS

Temporary catheters should more precisely be called nontunneled, noncuffed catheters (**Fig. 4**). Depending on the type, a temporary catheter may function for up to 4 weeks. In most cases, a temporary catheter is the appropriate choice unless there is suspicion of preexisting chronic kidney disease and the owners are interested in chronic dialysis. Temporary catheters are designed with a tapering tip to facilitate percutaneous placement and are placed via Seldinger technique (**Box 1**). Because these catheters may need to remain in place for weeks, strict attention to aseptic technique during placement is essential. Catheter placement must be done in a clean procedure room with restricted traffic, and all personnel involved in the procedure should wear caps and masks. A large barrier drape and sterile gloves are mandatory. Because of the springiness of the guidewire, a surgical gown is recommended to decrease the risk of contaminating the guidewire during placement. Sedation and/or local anesthetic may be necessary depending on the patient's clinical status and demeanor.

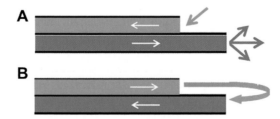

Fig. 1. In the correct configuration, blood enters the catheter through the proximal lumen and is returned via the distal lumen (*Panel A*). If the direction of flow is reversed (*Panel B*), blood returning via the proximal lumen is likely to be recirculated by reuptake at the distal lumen.

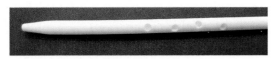

Fig. 2. Multiple ports of a temporary dialysis catheter.

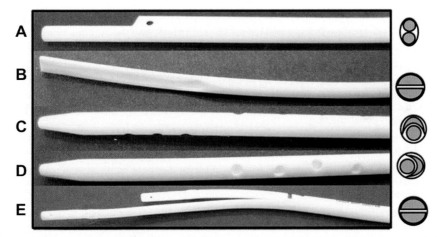

Fig. 3. (A–E) Multiple catheter tips with cross section of lumen configuration on right. Catheter (D) is a rotated view of catheter (C), showing placement of multiple openings. (Reprinted from Bartges J, Polzin D, editors. Nephrology and urology of small animals. Wiley-Blackwell; 2011; with permission.)

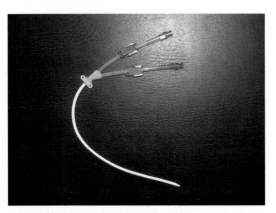

Fig. 4. A temporary, noncuffed and nontunneled catheter.

Box 1
Seldinger technique for nontunneled catheter placement

- Clip a wide area, including dorsal cervical area.

- Position pet for catheter placement. For lateral recumbency, pull the front legs back and place a bolster (ie, stack of paper towels) under the neck to expose the jugular vein. If needed, dorsal recumbency with the legs pulled back allows access to both jugular veins without repositioning but generally requires heavier sedation or anesthesia.

- Perform a surgical scrub of the area.

- Place Steri-Drape (3M, St Paul, MN, USA) over site (it helps to dry the site with sterile gauze first). Extend the coverage with 4 quadrant drapes.

- Fill both lumens of the catheter with heparinized saline (500 units in 250 mL saline, usually in a bowl; sterilely drawn from a bag is tedious but acceptable). Wet the outside of the catheter.

- Prepare the guidewire by retracting the J-wire part back into the introducer segment.

- Use a #11 blade to nick the skin over the venipuncture site. Place the introducer needle into the jugular vein. Some prefer placing a small catheter (ie, Jelco [Smiths Medical, St Paul, MN, USA] comes with most catheter kits) into the vessel. Some kits come with a Raulerson bulb. If using it, place the small plastic bulb on the needle and squeeze it to evacuate the air before inserting it under the skin.

- Once the needle is in the vessel, let go of the bulb and the vacuum draws blood into the bulb without spilling it on the fingers. This was designed to decrease risk of contagious diseases.

- If unable to hit the vessel with the needle, a cutdown may need to be done. It may be advisable to put surgical silk or umbilical tape under the vessel to help mobilize, stabilize, and provide hemostasis.

- With either method, once there is flashback of blood, advance the guidewire through the needle or introducer catheter into the vessel. Frequently, the front legs need to be pulled forward to allow the wire to cross over the clavicle. Watch the electrocardiogram; if artifacts are seen, the wire may be "tickling" the myocardium.

- Remove the needle, but be careful not to let the guidewire back out. Apply pressure to avoid excessive bleeding.

- Pass the smaller dilator down the guidewire. Be careful not to contaminate the guidewire or allow it to back out. Advance the dilator with a push and twist motion. Hold it as close to parallel to the vessel as possible (ie, lay the dilator flat against the body). The dilator should go at least halfway.

- Remove the dilator, applying pressure to decrease blood loss, and pass the larger dilator (if present) in the same way.

- Remove the dilator and pass the catheter down the guidewire. Be careful to keep hold of the guidewire and do not let it advance into the patient as the catheter is advanced.

- Once the catheter is in place, remove the guidewire.

- Check each lumen of the catheter for free flow of blood. Flush with heparinized saline when catheter placement is optimal.

- If a cutdown was needed, close the subcutaneous tissue, then the skin. The method of securing the catheter to the skin varies with model. If a large amount of catheter is outside the body, drape it in a gentle curve over the dorsal cervical region and suture there as well as near the skin exit site.

- Wrap the catheter sufficiently to travel to radiology and back without dislodging.

PERMANENT CATHETERS

Permanent hemodialysis catheters have an external cuff which is usually made of Dacron (**Fig. 5**). The catheter is placed with a portion in a subcutaneous pocket, which separates the site where the catheter exits the skin from the site where the catheter enters the vessel by several centimeters (**Figs. 6** and **7**). The Dacron cuff is positioned in this subcutaneous pocket and allows fibroblasts to adhere, thus securing the catheter in place and decreasing bacterial migration to the vessel. These catheters are intended to be used for up to 2 years and are generally placed using a surgical technique (**Box 2**). The ends of the catheter are usually blunt, so an introducer sheath is necessary for percutaneous placement. Ideally, the catheter would be placed in an operating room under fluoroscopic guidance. Permanent catheters may have the ends of the lumens separated, so that the intravenous portion acts like 2 separate catheters placed in the same vein. By having separated tips, side ports can be placed circumferentially on each lumen, and the increased flexibility of the tips and their movement with each cardiac cycle may help decrease fibrin sheath formation.[2]

OTHER VASCULAR ACCESS

An arteriovenous (AV) fistula or graft is the preferred access in people receiving chronic hemodialysis. An artery is surgically anastomosed to a vein with a section of autologous vein or synthetic graft (typically PTFE). Within approximately one month, endothelial cells line the graft, and the endothelial cells of the autologous vein segment take on characteristics of arterial endothelium instead of venous. The graft/fistula is then accessed by percutaneous puncture of the arterial and venous segments with large-gauge needles at each dialysis treatment. Between treatments, no anticoagulant is needed because blood is continually flowing through the graft/fistula. Because it is completely enclosed under the skin, the infection rate is extremely low in comparison to catheters. A model of AV fistula has been developed for canine hemodialysis, and a brachial-cephalic access could be considered for dogs receiving chronic dialysis.[4]

CATHETER FLOW CHARACTERISTICS

Because flow is proportional to catheter diameter and inversely proportional to catheter length, it is desirable to select the largest diameter catheter that can be placed. Minor changes in catheter diameter cause very large changes in flow, based on the Poiseuille equation:

$$Q_b = \frac{(K \cdot P \cdot D^4)}{(L \cdot V)}$$

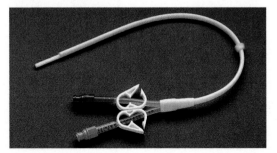

Fig. 5. Permanent, tunneled, cuffed catheter.

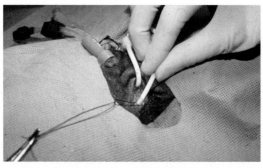

Fig. 6. A permanent catheter has been tunneled under the skin and is being inserted into the jugular vein through a separate skin incision.

where Q_b is blood flow; K, a proportionality constant; P, the change in pressure; D, the luminal diameter; L, the catheter length, and V, the blood viscosity. A 19% increase in catheter diameter doubles the blood flow; a 50% increase causes a fivefold increase in blood flow.[2] Approximate blood flow rates for various catheters are presented in **Table 1**. For intermittent treatment, the catheter should ideally provide more than 15 mL/kg/min blood flow. Flow rates of 3 to 5 mL/kg/min are adequate for continuous renal replacement therapy.

With any method of placement, flow through both lumens of the catheter should be brisk when aspirated with a large syringe. Fluoroscopic guidance is helpful in ensuring that the tip of the catheter is appropriately placed at the junction of the cranial vena cava and right atrium. If fluoroscopy is not used during placement, a postprocedure radiograph to confirm accurate placement should be performed (**Fig. 8**).

CATHETER CARE AND MAINTENANCE

The ERRT catheter should be used only for ERRT procedures and handled only by ERRT personnel. At each ERRT treatment, the exit site should be inspected and cleaned with antiseptic solution (**Box 3**). When the ERRT catheter is accessed at the beginning and end of each treatment or at any other time, the catheter ports should receive an aseptic scrub for 3 to 5 minutes. The ERRT technician should wear

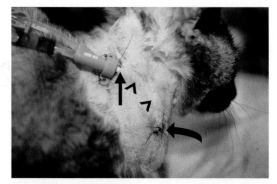

Fig. 7. Permanent (tunneled, cuffed) catheter in place. Skin exit site indicated by straight arrow. The catheter is tunneled under the skin (*arrowheads*), and the point of insertion into the jugular vein is indicated by the curved arrow.

examination gloves and a mask when opening or closing the catheter. When not in use, the catheter is bandaged in place and completely covered.

Between ERRT treatments, each lumen of the catheter is filled with an anticoagulant solution. Unfractionated heparin is currently used most commonly. A concentration of 500 to 1000 U/mL is generally used for cats, and 1000 to 5000 U/mL, for dogs. A portion (15%–20%) of the instilled heparin diffuses out of the tip of the catheter.[5] An alternative locking solution is sodium citrate. A 4% trisodium citrate solution has similar rates of catheter thrombosis, dysfunction, and infection compared with 5000 U/mL heparin locking solution, with fewer episodes of major systemic bleeding.[6,7] Higher citrate concentrations (>30%) are also antimicrobial.[8,9] Some veterinary units routinely incorporate an antibiotic (eg, cefazolin, 10 mg/mL) into the heparin used as the locking solution. Any locking solution should be removed before the next use of the catheter; however, catheter malfunction sometimes makes this impossible. This is especially problematic when using citrate, because injection of a highly concentrated (46.7%) citrate solution may cause symptomatic hypocalcemia and sudden death. Aspirin is routinely used in veterinary patients as an antiplatelet agent (0.5–2 mg/kg by mouth every 24 hours in dogs, every 48 hours in cats) to decrease catheter-associated thrombosis.

CATHETER PERFORMANCE

Catheter function can decrease over time if thrombosis or stenosis occurs gradually, or performance can decline abruptly. A simple way of monitoring function at each dialysis treatment is to record the blood speed when the pressure in the arterial chamber (prepump) is −200 mm Hg. A gradual decline in the blood speed at a standardized pressure predicts catheter malfunction. The arterial pressure should be maintained above −200 to −250 mm Hg, because at more negative values, the pump speed indicated on the machine is probably higher than the actual blood flow.[2]

Access recirculation decreases the efficiency of treatment by "diluting" the blood being withdrawn with blood that has just returned from the dialyzer. With the extracorporeal circuit blood lines attached in the normal configuration, recirculation is usually less than 5%, but reversing the connections such that blood is withdrawn from the distal port (venous) increases recirculation to 13% to 24%.[10] Sometimes, this reversed configuration is necessary, because a decrease in access pressure may allow an increase in the blood flow rate. If the blood flow rate that can be achieved in this configuration is much greater than the normal configuration, the increase in flow more than offsets the decrease in efficiency.[10] During initial intermittent hemodialysis treatments, when efficiency is purposefully limited to decrease complications, the blood lines may be reversed to create recirculation.

Access recirculation can be measured by various techniques, all of which seek to alter the venous line blood in some fashion and then detect the presence of altered blood in the arterial line blood. Some alterations include dilution with saline (detected by ultrasound or light transmission), change in temperature (cooling) or conductivity (added hypertonic saline), and hemoconcentration (via ultrafiltration).[11] The indicator dilution method is the most accurate method of determining access recirculation (Transonic Systems, Inc, Ithaca, NY, USA). Ultrasound detectors are placed on the access and return lines. Injection of a bolus of saline in the venous line just past the access line detector dilutes the blood, and this dilution is detected by an ultrasonic sensor placed on the venous blood line. If there is recirculation, the blood entering the arterial line is also diluted to a smaller degree, which is measured by the arterial line ultrasonic sensor. The percentage of blood recirculation is then calculated by the machine.

Box 2
Surgical placement of a tunneled cuffed "permanent" catheter

- Permanent catheter placement should ideally occur in an operating room with fluoroscopic guidance and full barrier precautions (large drape, gown, gloves, cap, mask, and so forth).

- With the patient under general anesthesia in left lateral recumbency, clip a wide area over the right jugular vein from the angle of the mandible to beyond the thoracic inlet and from the dorsal midline to past the ventral midline.

- Pull the pet's front legs back and secure them to provide optimal exposure of the jugular vein. A rolled towel under the neck helps with positioning. Sterilely prepare the area. Place 250 mL of sterile saline in the bowl and add 500 units of heparin (0.5 mL).

- After the drapes have been positioned, make a skin incision over the jugular vein as close to the thoracic inlet as possible. Dissect down to the jugular vein and isolate it with moistened umbilical tape in dogs and silk in cats. Use the umbilical tape to free some of the fascia off the vein for a distance of about 2.5 cm. Ligate any tributaries that may be entering the jugular vein in this segment.

- Preplace (but do not tie) silk ligatures at the most proximal and distal ends of the exposed vessel. Carefully clear all the fascia off the vessel using fine forceps without teeth. Any fascia left on the vessel decreases its expandability and makes it more difficult to pass the catheter. Excessive handling of the vessel can promote vasospasms that make passing the catheter much more difficult.

- Once the vessel is adequately exposed and cleaned, have an assistant place 0.25 to 0.5 mL of lidocaine on the vessel to decrease vasospasm.

- Have an assistant open the catheter pack, being careful not to let the injection caps fall out. Fill both lumens with heparinized saline and close the clamps.

- To determine where to make the exit site, set the tip of the catheter at the level of the right atrium (roughly at the point of the elbow) and determine where the cuff is to lie. The catheter needs to fall in a gentle arch toward the dorsal aspect of the neck, with the ports facing more toward the back of the animal.

- After determining the exit site, set the catheter aside and make a stab incision in the skin. If necessary, use hemostats to get through the subcutaneous layer.

- Use the tunneling device to make a subcutaneous tunnel for the catheter. Initially, direct the device toward the head to the angle of the mandible, then direct it back to make it exit through the skin incision at the jugular vein. Attach the catheter to the device and pull the catheter through the tunnel.

- To place the catheter in the vessel, gently grasp the vein with the thumb forceps. Holding a #11 blade almost parallel to the vessel, insert the tip of the blade into the vessel and gently pull the blade up to make a very small incision into the vessel. Have the assistant control hemostasis with the umbilical tape or silk ligatures.

- Place the tip of the catheter into the lumen of the vessel. At the point where the arterial port starts, the catheter has to be turned to allow this area to fit into the incision without snagging. The vessel can then be grasped with a moistened gauze sponge at the distal end.

- Pass the catheter into the vessel with gently steady movements to the predetermined level. In cats, particularly, passing the catheter may be a slow process.

- Once the catheter is in position, check blood flows by aspirating each port with a 12-mL syringe. There should be no resistance to flow and no stopping or "stickiness." If the catheter does not flow well, reposition it and check again.

- Use intraoperative fluoroscopy to confirm positioning. If for some reason, excellent flows cannot be obtained simultaneously for both ports, make sure the arterial side works well.

- Ligate the proximal jugular vein with the preplaced suture. Ligate the distal vein over the catheter to prevent backflow. Tie this suture snuggly, but do not compress the lumen of the catheter.

- Close the incision in 2 layers. Close the exit site stab incision with one suture. Suture each port to the skin separately. If the catheter is not to be used immediately, fill each lumen with the exact filling volume of 500 to 5000 units/mL heparin. Bandage the catheter in place.

Hemoglobin monitors (ie, Critline III TQA, Hemametrics, Kaysville, UT, USA) can detect access recirculation by injection of saline first in the venous line, followed by the arterial line, but they are not accurate measures of recirculation compared with the ultrasonic dilution technique.[12] Some dialysis machines have incorporated technology to automate measurement, using changes in dialysate in lieu of injection of a substance directly into the blood line, and include use of temperature or conductivity changes. These measurements can be made repeatedly throughout the dialysis treatment.

COMPLICATIONS

Despite using the least thrombogenic materials possible, hemodialysis catheters have a high rate of thrombosis. Thrombosis may be intraluminal or extraluminal (**Fig. 9**).

Table 1
Common ERRT catheter specifications and approximate blood flow rates[a]

Manufacturer	Type	Lumens	French Size	Length (cm)	Max Qb (mL/min)
Quinton PermCath (Covidien, Mansfield, MA, USA)	Cuffed	2	15	45	370
Quinton PermCath	Cuffed	2	15	40	400
Quinton PermCath	Cuffed	2	15	36	410
MedComp Pediatric (Medical Components Inc, Harleysville, PA, USA)	Cuffed	2	8	18	120
MedComp Temporary	Noncuffed	2	11.5	24	360[b]
Mila International Inc, Erlanger, KY, USA	Noncuffed	2	7	20	
[c]Arrow International Inc, Reading, PA, USA	Noncuffed	2	7	20	100
[c]Arrow, 20 ga lumen	Noncuffed	3	5.5	13	40
[c]Arrow, 22 ga lumen	Noncuffed	3	5.5	13	20
[c]Arrow, 20 ga lumen	Noncuffed	3	5.5	8	50
[c]Arrow, 22 ga lumen	Noncuffed	3	5.5	8	30
[c]Intracath (BD, Franklin Lakes, NJ, USA) through the needle	Noncuffed	1	19 ga	30.5	20

[a] Maximum blood flows determined in vitro using canine packed red blood cell solution (29% packed cell volume). Arterial chamber pressure maintained at −250 mm Hg or higher. Maximum blood flow rates in vivo may be lower.
[b] Maximum blood flow determined in vivo.
[c] Not designed for dialysis.

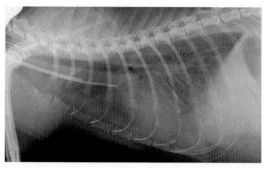

Fig. 8. Appropriate positioning of hemodialysis catheter, with the distal tip of the catheter positioned at the junction of the cranial vena cava and the right atrium.

Both ports of the catheter should be flushed with saline or heparinized saline after every use (approximately 10–12 mL for a large catheter, 3 to 6 mL for smaller catheters) to prevent intraluminal thrombosis. Each port is then filled with the locking solution (heparin, citrate, or other). Systemic anticoagulation has not been shown to decrease intraluminal thrombosis.[13]

Treatment of thrombosis should be initiated as soon as detected. Delays in treatment may decrease the adequacy of dialysis and may allow the thrombus to enlarge. Signs of intraluminal thrombosis include inadequate blood flow during dialysis or an inability to aspirate the catheter. Forceful flushing of the catheter with saline should be attempted first. Dislodgement of the thrombus does not seem to cause clinically relevant pulmonary thromboembolic disease.[14]

If a saline flush does not restore catheter flow, tissue plasminogen activator (tPA) can be instilled in the occluded lumen (Alteplase, CathFlow, Genentech, Inc, San Francisco, USA). The lumen is aspirated after a 30- to 45-minute dwell time, and if the thrombus is not aspirated, the dwell time is prolonged to 1 to 2 hours, with intermittent aspiration. If the catheter can be cleared sufficiently to perform a dialysis treatment but flow remains suboptimal, tPA can be instilled in the catheter lumen for up to 48 hours and removed at the start of the next dialysis treatment.[15] In the authors' experience, tPA dwell protocols are successful in allowing sufficient blood flow to perform a dialysis treatment, but the effects are short-lived, with retreatment or catheter replacement being necessary within a week.

Other methods of improving function of an occluded or partially occluded catheter include mechanical disruption. A guidewire can be placed in the catheter to dislodge a thrombus at the tip of the catheter but is less effective at dislodging thrombi that have formed at side ports.

Extraluminal thrombi include thrombi that form around the tip of the catheter and may be attached to the vessel wall and thrombi in the right atrium. These thrombi may act as a ball valve, allowing infusion but occluding the catheter and preventing aspiration. Thrombi in the right atrium and in the cranial vena cava near the heart may be imaged with echocardiography. Risk factors of thrombosis include venous stasis (from volume depletion, hypotension, immobilization, congestive heart failure), enhanced coagulability, and vessel wall trauma.[16] In the authors' experience, more than 50% of patients with a catheter in place for more than 3 weeks have thrombus formation, based on routine surveillance. Thrombi can be detected echocardiographically in about 20% of their patients within 1 week of catheter placement, although catheter flow problems become apparent around 2 weeks after catheter placement.

Box 3
Dialysis catheter care

- Unwrap the catheter bandage by cutting it on the opposite side of the neck from the catheter—be *very* careful not to cut the catheter.
- Clean the area around the catheter exit site and between catheter and skin.
- Assess the catheter exit site for redness, swelling, odor, or discharge, and assess the subcutaneous tunnel for signs of infection or excessive bruising.
- Remove the cohesive bandage (Vetrap; 3M Animal Care Products, St Paul, MN, USA) and the tape that is on the clamps.
- Place a sterile barrier around the catheter to prevent ports from touching the fur or skin.
- Wear examination gloves and a mask from this point until the catheter is wrapped again.
- Perform a surgical-type scrub on both ports, extending from the clamps to the tops of the injection ports.
- Spray the ports with dilute Nolvasan or Betadine.
- Place another sterile barrier around the catheter.
- Have 2 squares of *sterile* gauze within reach, as well as all syringes that are needed.
- Open the arterial/proximal port by removing the injection cap.
- Wipe the port opening with sterile gauze.
- Withdraw the exact volume (which is printed on the catheter for each side) of the lumen and discard it—this is the citrate lock, so *never* flush the catheter first.
- Flush the lumen with 6 mL fresh (mixed within 24 hours) heparinized saline or normal saline.
- Repeat this procedure on the venous/distal side.
- Replace the citrate locks by injecting the exact volume of each lumen.
- Replace the injection cap; use a new injection cap even when just changing the citrate lock.
- At this point, gloves and mask can be removed.
- Tape both clamps shut to ensure that they do not pop open inadvertently.
- Place a piece of cohesive bandage around both ports to keep ports clean in case the outer bandage becomes wet or soiled.
- Place a gauze square with triple antibiotic ointment over the catheter exit site.
- Wrap the catheter with cast padding, cling wrap, then cohesive bandage; the trick is to wrap tightly enough so that the bandage stays in place but not too tightly.
- Place a strip of porous white tape around both ends of the bandage to anchor it to the skin and prevent slipping; this is especially important for active animals.
- Place a final piece of tape with the words "Do Not Cut/Do Not Use" on the outside of the wrap.

Prophylactic administration of aspirin or warfarin decreases catheter thrombosis compared with no treatment. Bleeding complications were more common with warfarin, and its routine use is not recommended.[17]

If a small mural or right atrial thrombus is detected, the recommendation for humans is 6 months of systemic anticoagulation. If the thrombus is large, the catheter should be removed and systemic anticoagulation started with unfractionated or low–molecular weight heparin for 5 to 7 days and warfarin for at least 1 month. If the thrombus is large and infected, surgical thrombectomy is recommended.[16] In veterinary patients, a

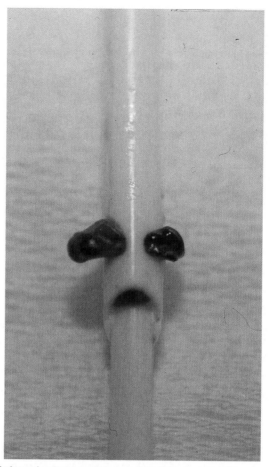

Fig. 9. Intraluminal thrombosis in a permanent catheter, extending through multiple side ports.

long-standing thrombus may become covered with endothelium or fibrous tissue. Surgical removal has not been attempted in them.

A sheath of fibrin may form around the catheter within 24 hours of placement, and this form of obstruction accounts for 38% to 50% of catheter malfunctions in people.[16] In people, tPA infusion through the dialysis catheter over 2 to 3 hours during or after a dialysis treatment may be effective in disrupting a fibrin sheath.[15] Thrombolytic infusion to dissolve extraluminal thrombi or a fibrin sheath has been used with variable results in veterinary patients. A technique of fibrin sheath stripping involves placement of a femoral catheter advanced to the cranial vena cava. A snare is used to encircle the fibrin sheath around the dialysis catheter and gently remove the sheath. This technique has not been attempted in veterinary medicine.

Replacement of the catheter over a guidewire is a simple and effective method of treating intraluminal thrombosis or fibrin sheath formation. A guidewire is placed in the dysfunctional catheter. If angiography is desired, the catheter is partially removed, leaving the tip within the vessel, and contrast agent is injected through the catheter (**Fig. 10**). If a fibrin sheath is detected, the old catheter is removed and a balloon

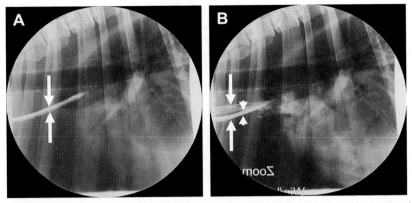

Fig. 10. Angiogram demonstrating fibrin sheath. (*Panel A*) Dialysis catheter is visible between the arrows. (*Panel B*) The catheter has been partially removed and is not visible in this view. A fibrin sheath of the same diameter as the catheter is filled with contrast (*arrowheads*), whereas the full extent of the vena cava is marked by the large arrows. A thrombus (filling defect in contrast) is present at the tip of the fibrin sheath.

catheter inserted over the guidewire. The balloon is inflated to disrupt the fibrin sheath. A new catheter is placed over the guidewire through the same exit site and subcutaneous tunnel (if present). Disrupting the fibrin sheath with catheter replacement has better results than catheter replacement alone in humans.[18] Careful attention to asepsis is necessary during the entire procedure. If angiography is not performed, catheter replacement over a guidewire can be performed in the dialysis unit if needed.

Central venous stenosis occurs in 27% to 38% of human patients but is frequently asymptomatic.[16] The incidence and significance of this condition in veterinary patients is unknown, but facial edema, which can be a sign of cranial vena caval stenosis or obstruction, is a common finding in dogs receiving hemodialysis and may cause a marked decrease in dialysis treatment efficiency (**Fig. 11**).

Infections are the most frequent catheter complication in humans[19] and are most probably the predominant cause of morbidity in veterinary patients as well. Catheter-related infections can be minimized by following strict aseptic guidelines when

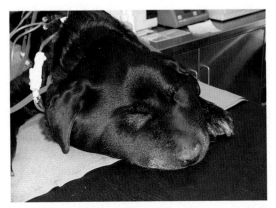

Fig. 11. Example of a Labrador retriever with a cranial vena caval obstruction associated with his dialysis catheter resulting in severe facial edema.

placing and using dialysis catheters and by inspecting the catheter entry site daily while in hospital and before every dialysis treatment. The authors routinely culture the tip of dialysis catheters on their removal for surveillance purposes. Biofilm develops fairly quickly in the lumens of central venous catheters and is known to be a major source of catheter-related bacteremia in humans. Instillation of antimicrobial solutions, such as citrate or heparin combined with an antibiotic, may reduce the risk of bacteremia.[20]

Inadvertent catheter dislodgement is an infrequent complication. During each dialysis treatment, the extracorporeal tubing is securely taped to a harness placed on dogs or attached directly to the forelimb in cats, so that exuberant motion of the patient does not unduly stress the sutures anchoring the catheter in place. On rare occasions, patients are sedated to prevent them from removing their catheters.

SUMMARY

Dual-lumen catheters are the most commonly used method of vascular access for extracorporeal renal replacement therapy. They are fairly quick to place but require meticulous care for optimal function. The most common complications are thrombosis and infection. Monitoring catheter performance should be a routine part of dialysis patient care.

ACKNOWLEDGMENTS

The authors would like to thank Eleanora Mitelberg, LVT for her assistance in article preparation and image acquisition.

REFERENCES

1. Ash SR. Fluid mechanics and clinical sussess of central venous catheters for dialysis - answers to simple but persisting problems. Semin Dial 2007;20:237.
2. Depner TA. Catheter performance. Semin Dial 2001;14:425.
3. Wentling AG. Hemodialysis catheters: materials, design and manufacturing. Contrib Nephrol 2004;142:112.
4. Adin CA, Gregory CR, Adin DB, et al. Evaluation of three peripheral arteriovenous fistulas for hemodialysis access in dogs. Vet Surg 2002;31:405.
5. Sungur M, Eryuksel E, Yavas S, et al. Exit of catheter lock solutions from double lumen acute haemodialysis catheters - an in vitro study. Nephrol Dial Transplant 2007;22:3533.
6. Grudzinski L, Quinan P, Kwok S, et al. Sodium citrate 4% locking solution for central venous dialysis catheters - an effective, more cost-efficient alternative to heparin. Nephrol Dial Transplant 2007;22:471.
7. MacRae JM, Dojcinovic I, Djurdjev O, et al. Citrate 4% versus heparin and the reduction of thrombosis Study (CHARTS). Clin J Am Soc Nephrol 2008;3:369.
8. Weijmer MC, Debets-Ossenkopp YJ, van de Vondervoort FJ, et al. Superior antimicrobial activity of trisodium citrate over heparin for catheter locking. Nephrol Dial Transplant 2002;17:2189.
9. Weijmer MC, van den Dorpel MA, Van de Ven PJG, et al. Randomized, clinical trial comparison of trisodium citrate 30% and heparin as catheter-locking solution in hemodialysis patients. J Am Soc Nephrol 2005;16:2769.
10. Carson RC, Kiaii M, MacRae JM. Urea clearance in dysfunctional catheters is improved by reversing the line position despite increased access recirculation. Am J Kidney Dis 2005;45:883.

11. Sherman RA, Kapoian T. Dialysis access recirculation. In: Nissenson AR, Fine RN, editors. Handbook of dialysis therapy. 4th edition. Philadelphia: Saunders Elsevier; 2008. p. 102.

12. Lopot F, Nejedly B, Sulkova S, et al. Comparison of different techniques of hemodialysis vascular access flow evaluation. Int J Artif Organs 2003;26:1056.

13. Beathard G. Catheter thrombosis. Semin Dial 2001;14:441.

14. Beathard G. The use and complications of catheters for hemodialysis vascular access: introduction. Semin Dial 2001;14:410.

15. Lok CE, Thomas A, Vercaigne L, et al. A patient-focused approach to thrombolytic use in the management of catheter malfunction. Semin Dial 2006;19:381.

16. Liangos O, Gul A, Madias NE, et al. Long-term management of the tunneled venous catheter. Semin Dial 2006;19:158.

17. Willms L, Vercaigne L. Does warfarin safely prevent clotting of hemodialysis catheters? Semin Dial 2008;21:71.

18. Oliver MJ, Mendelssohn DC, Quinn RR, et al. Catheter patency and function after catheter sheath disruption: a pilot study. Clin J Am Soc Nephrol 2007;2:1201.

19. Himmelfarb J, Dember LM, Dixon BS. Vascular access. In: Pereira BJ, Sayegh MH, Blake P, editors. Chronic kidney disease, dialysis, transplantation. 2nd edition. Philadelphia: Elsevier Saunders; 2005. p. 341.

20. Donlan RM. Biofilm formation: a clinically relevant microbiological process. Clin Infect Dis 2001;33:1387.

Anticoagulation in Intermittent Hemodialysis: Pathways, Protocols, and Pitfalls

Sheri Ross, DVM, PhD

KEYWORDS

• Anticoagulation • Hemodialysis • Coagulation

The safety and efficiency of intermittent hemodialysis have improved dramatically over the past several decades. Despite this advancement, prevention of thrombosis in the extracorporeal blood circuit remains a significant challenge in many cases. During intermittent hemodialysis, the patient's blood is exposed to many substances, including the dialysis catheter, blood tubing, chambers and headers, and the large surface area of the dialyzer membrane. These surfaces exhibit variable degrees of thrombogenicity.[1] In order to deliver a safe and effective dialysis treatment, an appropriate level of anticoagulation must be achieved to prevent thrombosis of the extracorporeal circuit without causing excessive bleeding in the patient.

COAGULATION

Since the 1960s, the understanding of homeostasis has been based on the coagulation cascade model.[2] In this model, clotting mechanism is divided into 2 pathways. In each pathway, the clotting factors are proenzymes that can be converted to active enzymes. Coagulation may be initiated via an intrinsic pathway, so named because all the components are present within the blood, or an extrinsic pathway, in which tissue factor (TF), a subendothelial cell membrane protein, is required in addition to the circulating components. The initiation of either pathway results in activation of factor X and the eventual generation of a fibrin clot through a common pathway.[3]

The most recent model of coagulation is known as the cell-based model of coagulation. In this model, coagulation involves 3 phases: initiation, amplification, and propagation. A recent review of this subject has been provided elsewhere.[4] This model is

The author has nothing to disclose.
Departments of Nephrology, Urology, Hemodialysis, University of California Veterinary Medical Center – San Diego, 10435 Sorrento Valley Road, Suite 101, San Diego, CA 92121, USA
E-mail address: sro@ucdavis.edu

Vet Clin Small Anim 41 (2011) 163–175
doi:10.1016/j.cvsm.2010.12.001

a result of the discovery that exposure of blood to cells that express TF on their surface is both necessary and sufficient to initiate blood coagulation in vivo.[5] In the cell-based model, coagulation requires a cell, or cellular debris expressing TF and platelets. TF is not present on the surface of vascular endothelium but is present within the membranes of cells surrounding the vasculature, where it is exposed to blood only by disruption of the endothelium or activation of the endothelial cells or monocytes. Cellular microparticles (MPs) are membrane fragments derived from many different cell types during various states including remodeling, activation, and apoptosis.[6] These MPs have been shown to express TF, which may contribute significantly to thrombosis.[7] MP levels are already increased in patients with renal disease, but an even more dramatic increase occurs in patients undergoing hemodialysis; this further increase is primarily caused by platelet-derived MPs. Possible explanations for the increase in MP levels include complement activation within the dialyzer, shear effect of cells during transit through the catheter and extracorporeal circuit, and to a lesser extent, the presence of endotoxins in the dialysate.[8]

EFFECTS OF UREMIA ON COAGULATION

Although dialysis requires anticoagulation to prevent clotting in the extracorporeal circuit, it is important to recognize that many uremic patients have a bleeding diathesis. The pathogenesis of uremic bleeding is multifactorial and includes defects in all stages of platelet hemostasis, including adhesion, secretion, and aggregation. The platelet count is usually within the normal range or just slightly low in uremic patients (**Box 1**).[9,10] Although levels of von Willebrand factor (vWf) are usually normal or slightly elevated in patients with kidney disease, a functional defect in the interaction of vWf with glycoprotein IIb/IIIa complex in uremic patients inhibits platelet–vessel wall interactions, contributing to bleeding.[11] When compared with healthy controls, uremic patients also produce excessive prostacyclin and nitric oxide, and these elevated levels contribute to the bleeding diathesis.[12] Prostacyclin is a potent inhibitor of platelet aggregation and the most important modulator of the production of platelet cyclic AMP.[13] Nitric oxide is a potent modulator of vascular tone that limits platelet adhesion to the endothelium and platelet-platelet interaction by increasing the formation of cellular cyclic GMP.[14] In addition to uremia-associated bleeding diathesis, patients with uremia may also have comorbid conditions and/or receive medications that affect hemostasis and are therefore predisposed to bleeding complications.

COAGULATION AND EXTRACORPOREAL CIRCUITS

Both the TF and contact activation pathways may trigger clotting in the extracorporeal circuit. Turbulence and shear stress can cause platelet activation via the contact pathway and can ultimately lead to release of TF, or TF may be triggered directly through the TF pathway.[15] When the blood flow is slow, platelets can bind to fibrinogen adherent to the extracorporeal circuit thus precipitating clotting. During hemodialysis, platelets and leukocytes may aggregate on the dialyzer membrane. Once they adhere to the artificial surface, both cell types become activated and may express TF on their surface. The composition of the dialyzer membrane seems to influence the extent of adherence and activation.[16]

Within the extracorporeal circuit, not only the dialyzer membrane but also the dialysis catheter, blood lines, dialyzer headers, and arterial and venous pressure chambers contribute to the risk of thrombogenesis. The arterial and venous pressure chambers are particularly thrombogenic because of the blood-air interface and the potential for stagnation of blood flow. The likelihood of circuit clotting also increases

Box 1
Some factors affecting hemostasis in uremic patients
Platelet-related factors
Defective activation of glycoprotein IIb-IIIa receptors
Abnormal intracellular calcium mobilization
Reduced intracellular ADP and serotonin levels
Decrease in dense granule content
Vessel wall–related factors
Abnormal platelet adhesion
Decreased von Willebrand factor activity
Enhanced nitric oxide and prostacyclin production
Blood-related factors
Anemia
Erythropoietin deficiency
Altered blood rheology
Other factors
Drugs: β-lactam antibiotics, nonsteroidal antiinflammatory drugs, antiplatelet agents, anticoagulants
Comorbid conditions: gastrointestinal ulceration
Invasive procedures: surgery, biopsy, feeding tube, intravenous catheter placement
Uremic toxins

with hemoconcentration caused by dehydration, excessive ultrafiltration, or the administration of packed red blood cells (**Box 2**).[15]

PARAMETERS FOR ASSESSING CLOTTING IN THE EXTRACORPOREAL CIRCUIT

Careful monitoring of the extracorporeal circuit during dialysis may provide many indicators of potential clotting problems (**Box 3**). The simplest method of evaluation is visual inspection (**Fig. 1**). Very dark blood within the circuit, streaks within the dialyzer, or the presence of fibrin on the walls of the arterial or venous chambers may indicate clotting and should be further evaluated by flushing the circuit with saline while temporarily occluding the arterial blood line. Flushing the circuit allows not only for a better assessment of the degree of clotting in the dialyzer and chambers but also the inspection of the arterial header. After every treatment, the patient's dialyzer should be closely inspected and the degree of fiber clotting recorded. This information may be used to adjust the anticoagulation regime for subsequent treatments. The degree of dialyzer clotting for 2356 individual dialysis treatments at 3 veterinary dialysis centers (University of California Davis College of Veterinary Medicine, University of California Veterinary Medical Center – San Diego, and Animal Medical Center) is presented in **Fig. 2**.

The extracorporeal circuit pressures, typically measured in the arterial and venous pressure chambers, may also indicate clotting problems. An increase in the postpump arterial pressure combined with a decrease in the venous pressure indicates the

---

Box 2
Technical or mechanical factors that may contribute to clotting in the extracorporeal circuit

Blood-related factors

Low blood flow rates

Inadequate blood flow due to catheter positioning or access recirculation

Frequent interruption of blood flow due to machine alarm conditions

High ultrafiltration rate

High hematocrit

Intradialytic transfusion of blood products

Circuit-related factors

Retained air in dialyzer or lines due to inadequate priming

Inadequate priming of heparin infusion line

Biocompatibility of dialyzer membrane

Anticoagulation-related factors

Inadequate loading dose of heparin

Insufficient time lapse after loading the dose for systemic anticoagulation

Inadequate dose/setting of the heparin constant rate infusion pump

Delayed starting of heparin pump/failure to release line clamp

Early termination of heparin constant rate infusion

---

presence of clotting in the arterial chamber or the dialyzer. An increase in the venous pressure could indicate clotting in the venous return line or a problem at the venous port on the dialysis catheter.

A more accurate way of assessing clotting within the dialyzer involves the measurement of the fiber bundle volume (FBV) or the residual volume within the blood compartment of the dialyzer. The FBV is easy to measure in vitro and has been the main criterion used to determine if a dialyzer is suitable for reuse in human dialysis units practicing reuse.[17] During the dialysis treatment, FBV may be measured to provide

---

Box 3
Signs of clotting in the extracorporeal circuit

Very dark blood

Dark streaks in the dialyzer

Foaming or clot formation in the venous trap

Clots at the arterial header

Increased arterial pressure with a decrease in venous pressure

    Clotting in arterial chamber or dialyzer

Increase in venous pressure

    Clotting in venous return

Decrease in fiber bundle volume

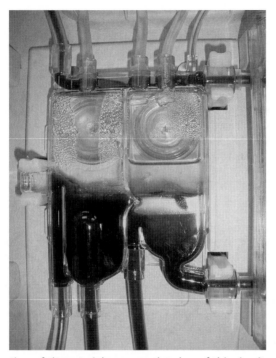

Fig. 1. Visual inspection of the arterial pressure chamber of this circuit reveals a fibrin clot that has formed at the blood-air interface. The blood level in the chamber has been lowered, and saline may be seen trapped above the clot.

a real-time assessment of dialyzer fiber clotting. Ultrasonic flow-dilution sensors are placed immediately predialyzer and immediately postdialyzer and connected to a hemodialysis monitoring system Transonic HD01 Hemodialysis Monitor (Transonic Systems Inc, Ithaca, NY, USA) and computer with appropriate software. There are 2 methods to measure FBV using this system. The first method is based on a bolus injection of saline and requires measurements from both sensors, whereas the second

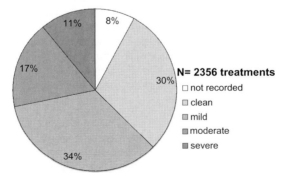

Fig. 2. Severity of clotting in hollow fiber dialyzers in 2356 intermittent hemodialysis treatments. Data were collected from 3 veterinary intermittent dialysis units in the United States (University of California Davis College of Veterinary Medicine, University of California Veterinary Medical Center – San Diego, and Animal Medical Center).

method is based on a step change in ultrafiltration and only requires the venous sensor. The obvious advantage of real-time assessment of clotting in the dialyzer is the ability to alter the dose of anticoagulant or stop the treatment before significant clotting and subsequent blood loss in the dialyzer.

HEPARIN

Unfractionated (UF) heparins include a family of highly sulfated polysaccharides composed of anionic glycosaminoglycans with molecular weights ranging from 4 to 40 kDa. UF heparin is by far the most frequently used anticoagulant for preventing thrombosis in the extracorporeal circuit in intermittent hemodialysis because of its low cost, relatively short biologic half-life, and ease of administration. UF heparin is highly negatively charged and binds nonspecifically to endothelium, platelets, macrophages, proteins, and some plastic surfaces. When given intravenously, UF heparin has a half-life of approximately 1.5 hours.[18] UF heparin has both hepatic and renal clearance and is also metabolized by the endothelium.

Heparin binds to antithrombin, causing a conformational change that results in activation.[19] Heparin-bound antithrombin inactivates multiple coagulation factors including thrombin and factor Xa and to a lesser degree factors VII, IXa, XIa, and XIIa. The binding of heparin may increase the rate of inactivation of these proteases by up to 1000-fold. Only UF heparin with more than 18 repeating saccharide units inhibits both thrombin and factor Xa, whereas shorter chains just inhibit factor Xa. Too much heparin may result in excessive bleeding, whereas inadequate administration leads to thrombosis in the extracorporeal circuit, with subsequent blood loss in the dialyzer and a decrease in the efficiency of the treatment.

In human medicine, the most important adverse effect of UF heparin administration is heparin-induced thrombocytopenia (HIT) syndrome. There are 2 documented syndromes of HIT. HIT type I is a transient reduction in platelet count, occurs in 10% to 20% of patients, and generally resolves within a few days. HIT type II involves an immune reaction and is typically a more serious condition. In the acute phase, there is a very high risk for both thrombocytopenia and thromboembolic disease. If left untreated, there is a more than 50% risk for the development of venous thrombosis within a month. In patients who develop HIT type II, use of all heparin-containing products must be discontinued and the patient must be systemically anticoagulated to prevent thrombosis. HIT type II has been reported in 3% to 12% of human patients who undergo hemodialysis.[20] Although there is a significantly lower risk for development of HIT syndrome with the exclusive use of low-molecular-weight heparins (LMWHs), once a patient develops HIT syndrome secondary to UF heparin, there is more than 90% cross-reactivity with LMWH.[21] Although this is by far the most significant obstacle to the use of UF heparin in human medicine, the HIT syndrome has not been recognized in veterinary medicine. Other adverse effects attributed to UF heparin include changes to lipid metabolism, alopecia, mild hyperkalemia, and osteoporosis.

MEASURING ANTICOAGULATION

The heparin dose and administration regime are an important part of the dialysis prescription. The unpredictable pharmacokinetics of UF heparin and its narrow therapeutic window make optimal dosing strategies difficult to define. Therefore, measuring the heparin concentration in the blood of a patient undergoing hemodialysis is ideal for inducing optimal anticoagulation. However, in clinical practice, it is not practical to measure blood levels of heparin directly; thus, the dose of heparin is managed by measuring its anticoagulant effect. The anticoagulant effect of heparin is measured as the increased time taken for clot formation under controlled conditions. To be practical in the clinical setting of a dialysis unit, the clotting time assay must be inexpensive and convenient and, most importantly, it must provide rapid results at clinically relevant concentrations of heparin to allow for the adjustment of the heparin concentration during the dialysis treatment.

Both the activated partial thromboplastin time (aPTT) and activated clotting time (ACT) have been used to measure the anticoagulant effect of UF heparin in clinical practice. However, the aPTT seems to produce inconsistent results, especially at high blood levels of heparin required for adequate anticoagulation in extracorporeal therapies.[22] When using the aPTT to monitor UF heparin anticoagulation, it is recommended that a reagent-specific therapeutic range be established using heparin concentrations in blood.

The ACT is a point-of-care test that was first described in 1966 to screen for disorders of coagulation and as a tool for monitoring UF heparin therapy.[23] In this assay, whole blood is mixed with an activator of the extrinsic clotting cascade, and the time necessary for blood to congeal is measured. In the 1980s, use of the ACT to monitor UF heparin therapy gained clinical acceptance.[24–26]

For intermittent hemodialysis, the goal of anticoagulant therapy is to limit clotting in the dialyzer and circuit without causing excessive bleeding in the patient. To establish this goal, an ACT of 170 to 220 seconds has been recommended.[27] An alternative goal is an increase in ACT in the range of 140% to 180% of baseline. Increases of this magnitude in the ACT generally prevent visible clotting in the dialyzer and blood tubing.[28]

STANDARD HEPARIN PROTOCOL

In veterinary medicine, anticoagulation in routine intermittent hemodialysis typically consists of the systemic administration of a standard dose of heparin (10–50 U/kg) as a bolus 5 minutes before starting the dialysis treatment. Using frequent ACT monitoring (every 15–30 minutes), adequate anticoagulation is then maintained with a continuous infusion of heparin (10–50 U/kg/h) into the arterial limb of the circuit to maintain an ACT of 160 to 200 seconds (reference range: 90–140 seconds). Less commonly, boluses of heparin (10–50 U/kg) given every 30 minutes may be used in lieu of a constant rate infusion to achieve the same ACT goal or to more rapidly increase ACT in patients with a low ACT. The heparin infusion or bolus administration may be discontinued up to 30 minutes before the end of the treatment or continued throughout the treatment, depending on the patient's bleeding risk and the degree of clotting in the extracorporeal circuit. Careful observation of the patient and the extracorporeal circuit and careful ACT determinations ensure adequate systemic anticoagulation throughout the dialysis treatment (**Table 1**, **Fig. 3**).

Table 1 Suggested heparinization protocol for dogs and cats for intermittent hemodialysis		
	Dogs	**Cats**
UF heparin bolus administered intravenously 5 min before initiating dialysis (U/kg)	25–50	10–25
Constant rate infusion of UF heparin during treatment	50–100 U/kg/h	20–50 U/cat/h
Target ACT during treatment (s)	160–180	150–180

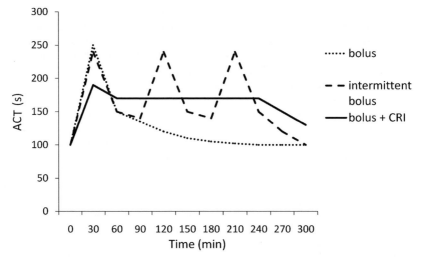

Fig. 3. Examples of anticoagulation profiles obtained from the administration of UF heparin during intermittent hemodialysis. The dotted line shows the prolongation of ACT obtained with a single loading dose of UF heparin. The dashed line shows the expected clotting time profile with intermittent bolus administration of heparin. The solid line shows the expected clotting time profile with an initial bolus followed by a CRI of UF heparin. In all these illustrations, heparin administration was discontinued 30 minutes before the end of the dialysis treatment. CRI, constant rate infusion.

STRATEGIES FOR HIGH-RISK PATIENTS

In some patients presented for hemodialysis, systemic anticoagulation may be contraindicated. Patients who have recently (<48 hours) undergone surgery, biopsy, or some other invasive procedure or patients with gastrointestinal hemorrhage, possible cranial trauma, pulmonary contusions, or any evidence of active bleeding should not receive systemic anticoagulation because of the risk of inducing or exacerbating bleeding. In these patients, alternate strategies must be used to prevent clotting in the extracorporeal circuit.

No-Heparin Hemodialysis

In human medicine, no-heparin hemodialysis is now the most common method of providing dialysis to patients at high risk of bleeding. This procedure was initially developed for use in patients with high bleeding risks.[29] The protocol for no-heparin hemodialysis requires pretreatment of the extracorporeal circuit with 2000 to 5000 units of UF heparin during the recirculation phase of preparation of the dialysis machine. Before beginning the dialysis treatment, the heparinized saline is flushed from the circuit with saline to prevent the patient from receiving a heparin bolus. Once the treatment is initiated, the blood flow rate is quickly increased to more than 300 mL/min and maintained at this rate for the duration of the treatment. Approximately every 15 to 30 minutes during the treatment, a saline bolus of 30 to 50 mL is flushed into the arterial side of the circuit. These boluses of saline help to wash fibrin strands through the dialyzer and into the venous pressure chamber, thus minimizing clotting. The volume status of the patient must be carefully monitored, and the volume of saline administered during the flushes must be removed via ultrafiltration, if necessary, to prevent hypervolemia. In addition, the arterial and venous pressures must be monitored closely. If signs of early clotting are detected, the treatment should be stopped or switched to a low-dose heparin treatment to prevent more extensive clotting. No-heparin hemodialysis treatments have been used successfully in human medicine without a significant difference in treatment adequacy as compared with patients receiving standard anticoagulation therapy.[30] This method has also been used successfully in high-risk veterinary patients.

Heparin/Protamine Regional Anticoagulation

One of the first methods used to prevent coagulation in high-risk patients involved regional anticoagulation using heparin and protamine.[31] This method involves the constant infusion of UF heparin into the arterial limb of the extracorporeal circuit, with simultaneous infusion of protamine into the blood just before it is returned to the patient. The use of regional anticoagulation requires frequent checks of the ACT from the arterial and venous lines, with adjustments of the heparin and protamine infusion rates to maintain the ACT in the extracorporeal circuit at approximately 250 seconds and the ACT of the blood returning to the patient at the predialysis baseline.[32]

Protamine is a strongly basic low-molecular-weight protein that binds to and neutralizes the anticoagulant activity of UF heparin. Although precise dosing must be based on the results of clotting times, in general, 1 mg of protamine will antagonize 100 U of heparin. When protamine is used to counter the effects of heparin, there is a risk of rebound anticoagulation. This risk occurs because heparin is metabolized more slowly than protamine, thus free heparin is released from the protamine-heparin complex back into general circulation.[33] Compounding this effect is the fact that doses of heparin used in regional anticoagulation are typically higher than those used in routine heparin hemodialysis, thereby exacerbating the bleeding risk from rebound anticoagulation. Protamine may also cause dyspnea, bradycardia, and hypotension when administered rapidly. Because of the adverse effects described, the need for diligent monitoring, and the lack of proved benefit over other alternative methods of anticoagulation, regional heparinization is rarely used in routine practice.

Regional Citrate Anticoagulation

Another method of regional anticoagulation involves the continuous infusion of trisodium citrate solution into the arterial limb of the extracorporeal circuit.[34] Regional citrate anticoagulation has been shown to reduce the incidence of bleeding in high-risk patients compared with standard heparin protocols.[35] Citrate binds to ionized calcium in the blood and is a potent inhibitor of coagulation. The citrate-calcium complex is partially removed by the dialyzer. This removal is enhanced when calcium-free dialysate is used. To neutralize the effects of any remaining citrate, calcium chloride is infused into the venous return line. The citrate infusion rate is adjusted to keep the ACT at approximately 200 seconds in the arterial limb. Plasma calcium levels must be measured frequently and the calcium chloride infusion must be constantly adjusted accordingly to prevent hypocalcemia or hypercalcemia.

Another approach, proposed to minimize the amount of calcium infused and complications caused by a calcium-free dialysate, uses hypertonic trisodium citrate and a dialysate containing a calcium concentration of 3 mEq/L.[36] Complications associated with regional citrate anticoagulation are generally related to the patient calcium level, but metabolic acidosis because of the bicarbonate generated during citrate metabolism and hypernatremia from the citrate solution may occur as well. Careful monitoring of the electrolytes levels and acid-base status of the patient helps to prevent these complications.

ALTERNATE METHODS OF ANTICOAGULATION

In human medicine, UF heparin has been associated with significant adverse effects in some patients, most notably, HIT type II. In these cases, alternative strategies to prevent clotting in the extracorporeal circuit must be used.[37] Although some of these methods have been used extensively in human medicine, their use has not been reported in veterinary medicine. A brief description of some of the more common alternate methods of anticoagulation is outlined in the following sections. In general, these anticoagulants are significantly more expensive than UF heparin, thus limiting their use in veterinary medicine.

LMWH

LMWH has been used as an alternative to UF heparin for anticoagulation in hemodialysis.[38] LMWHs have average molecular weights ranging from 4 to 9 kDa and are produced from the controlled fractionation of heparin. Their smaller size produces more predictable pharmacokinetics, which makes their dosing simpler than UF heparin. LMWH binds antithrombin and inhibits factor Xa. The anticoagulant effect of LMWH can be monitored by determining the antifactor Xa activity in the patient's plasma.

LMWHs are expensive and have generally not been found to be superior to heparin in terms of dialysis-related bleeding or other complications.[39,40]

Direct Thrombin Inhibitors

Hirudins are polypeptides originally derived from the saliva of leeches. Hirudins act as potent direct thrombin inhibitors and do not require endogenous cofactors. Recombinant hirudins, such as lepirudin, have been investigated as anticoagulants for hemodialysis.[41] Typically, they are administered as a single dose at the beginning of the treatment. Use of hirudins in patients with kidney disease can be complicated because these substances are excreted via the kidneys and are not removed by conventional hemodialysis. In patients with renal disease, the half-life of hirudins may be significantly prolonged, sometimes for days. Hirudins are seldom used in clinical practice because of the significant risk of bleeding.

Synthetic thrombin inhibitors, such as argatroban, have been investigated as an alternative to heparin for anticoagulation during dialysis. Argatroban is metabolized in the liver and therefore may be used in patients with significant kidney disease, with some dose adjustment. With careful monitoring, argatroban has been used in dialysis of human patients who are intolerant to UF heparin due to HIT syndrome. Argatroban has been shown to provide acceptable anticoagulation with tolerable side effects.[42]

Prostacyclin Anticoagulation

Prostacyclin is a vasodilator and potent inhibitor of platelet aggregation.[43] Prostacyclin is administered as a continuous infusion into the arterial limb of the extracorporeal circuit to prevent clotting. It has a relatively short half-life (approximately 4 minutes) and is rapidly metabolized by the endothelium, allowing for rapid adjustment of dose and tight control of coagulation. Hypotension from vasodilatation is a common and often serious side effect. In addition, human patients often report headache and dizziness. Because these side effects limit the clinical usage of prostacyclin, current efforts are directed toward the development of analogues without the hypotensive effects.

SUMMARY

Several methods to prevent extracorporeal circuit clotting during hemodialysis have been used in human medicine. UF heparin remains the mainstay of anticoagulant therapy in both human and veterinary intermittent hemodialysis. Different UF heparin regimes may be used depending on the bleeding risk of the patient. In patients with active bleeding or with a recent history of surgery or hemorrhagic episodes, hemodialysis may be performed without any anticoagulation or with regional anticoagulation.

REFERENCES

1. Suranyi M, Chow JS. Review: anticoagulation for haemodialysis. Nephrology (Carlton) 2010;15:386–92.
2. MacFarlane RG. An enzyme cascade in the blood clotting mechanism, and its function as a biochemical amplifier. Nature 1964;202:498–9.
3. Luchtman-Jones L, Broze J. The current status of coagulation. Ann Med 1995; 27(1):47–52.
4. Smith SA. The cell-based model of coagulation. J Vet Emerg Crit Care (San Antonio) 2009;19(1):3–10.
5. Hoffman M, Munroe D. Rethinking the coagulation cascade. Curr Hematol Rep 2005;4:391–6.
6. Osterud B, Bjorklid E. Sources of tissue factor. Semin Thromb Hemost 2006;32: 11–23.
7. Amabile N, Guerin AP, Leroyer A, et al. Circulating endothelial microparticles are associated with vascular dysfunction in patients with end stage renal failure. J Am Soc Nephrol 2005;16:3381–8.
8. Daniel L, Fakhouri F, Joly D, et al. Increase of circulating neutrophil and platelet microparticles during acute vasculitis and hemodialysis. Kidney Int 2006;69: 1416–23.
9. Deykin D. Uremic bleeding. Kidney Int 1983;24:698–705.
10. Galbusera M, Remuzzi G, Boccardo P. Treatment of bleeding in dialysis patients. Semin Dial 2009;22(3):279–86.
11. Rabolink TJ, Zwaginga JJ, Koomas HA, et al. Thrombosis and hemostasis in renal disease. Kidney Int 1994;46:287–96.
12. Noris M, Benigni A, Boccardo P, et al. Enhanced nitric oxide synthesis in uremia: implications for platelet dysfunction and dialysis hypotension. Kidney Int 1993;44: 445–50.
13. Zwaginga JJ, Ijsseldijk MJ, Beeser N, et al. High von Willebrand factor concentration compensates a relative adhesion defect in uremic blood. Blood 1990; 75:1498–508.
14. Noris M, Remuzzi G. Uremic bleeding: closing the circle after 30 years of controversy? Blood 1999;94:2569–74.
15. Fischer KG. Essentials of anticoagulation in hemodialysis. Hemodial Int 2007;11: 178–89.
16. Gawaz MP, Mujaos SK, Schmidt B, et al. Platelet-leukocyte aggregates during hemodialysis: effect of membrane type. Artif Organs 1999;23:29–36.
17. Krivitski NM, Kislukhin VV, Snyder J, et al. In vivo measurement of hemodialyzer fiber bundle volume: theory and validation. Kidney Int 1998;54:1751–8.
18. Brunet P, Simon N, Opris A, et al. Pharmacodynamics of unfractionated heparin during and after a hemodialysis session. Am J Kidney Dis 2008;51(5):789–95.
19. Chuang YJ, Swanson R, Raja SM, et al. Heparin enhances the specificity of antithrombin for thrombin and factor Xa independent of the reactive center loop

sequence. Evidence for an exosite determinant of factor Xa specificity in heparin-activated antithrombin. J Biol Chem 2001;276(18):14961–71.

20. Charif R, Davenport A. Heparin induced thrombocytopenia: an uncommon but serious complication of heparin use in renal replacement therapy. Hemodial Int 2006;10:235–40.

21. Warkentin TE, Levine MN, Hirsh J, et al. Heparin induced thrombocytopenia in patients treated with low molecular weight heparin or unfractionated heparin. N Engl J Med 1995;332:1330–5.

22. Smythe MA, Koerber JM, Westley SJ, et al. Use of the activated partial thromboplastin time for heparin monitoring. Am J Clin Pathol 2001;115:148–55.

23. Hattersley PG. Activated coagulation time. JAMA 1966;196:436–40.

24. Hattersley PG, Mitsuoka JC, King JH. Heparin therapy for thromboembolic disorders: a prospective evaluation of 134 cases monitored by the activated clotting time. JAMA 1982;250:1413–6.

25. Congdon JE, Kardinal CG, Wallin JD. Monitoring heparin therapy in hemodialysis. JAMA 1973;226:1529.

26. Hattersley PG, Mitsuoka JC, Ignoffo RJ, et al. Adjusting heparin infusion rates from the initial response to activated coagulation time. Drug Intell Clin Pharm 1983;17:632–4.

27. Mehta RL. Anticoagulation during continuous renal replacement therapy. ASAIO J 1994;40:931–5.

28. Wilhelmsson S, Lins LE. Whole blood activated coagulation time for evaluation of heparin activity during hemodialysis: a comparison of administration by single-dose and by infusion. Clin Nephrol 1983;19:82–6.

29. Sanders PW, Taylor H, Curtis JJ. Hemodialysis without anticoagulation. Am J Kidney Dis 1985;5:32.

30. Schwab SJ, Onorato JJ, Sharar LR, et al. Hemodialysis without anticoagulation. One-year prospective trial in hospitalized patients at risk for bleeding. Am J Med 1987;83:405.

31. Gorden LA, Simon ER, Rukes JM, et al. Studies in regional heparinization. N Engl J Med 1956;255:1063.

32. Maher JF, Lapierre L, Schreiner GE, et al. Regional heparinization for hemodialysis. N Engl J Med 1963;268:451.

33. Blaufox MD, Hampers CL, Merrill JP. Rebound anticoagulation occurring after regional heparinization for hemodialysis. Trans Am Soc Artif Intern Organs 1966;12:207–9.

34. Pinnick RV, Wiegmann TB, Diederich DA. Regional citrate anticoagulation for hemodialysis in the patient at high risk for bleeding. N Engl J Med 1983; 308(5):258–61.

35. Janssen MJ, Huijgens PC, Bouman AA, et al. Citrate versus heparin anticoagulation in chronic haemodialysis patients. Nephrol Dial Transplant 1993;8:1228.

36. von Brecht JH, Flanigan MJ, Freeman RM, et al. Regional anticoagulation-hemodialysis with hypertonic sodium tricitrate. Am J Kidney Dis 1986;8:196.

37. Lohr JW, Schwab SJ. Minimizing hemorrhagic complications in dialysis patients. J Am Soc Nephrol 1991;2:961.

38. Schrader J, Stibbe W, Armstrong VW, et al. Comparison of low molecular weight heparin and standard heparin in hemodialysis/hemofiltration. Kidney Int 1988; 33:890.

39. Davenport A. Review article: low molecular weight heparin as an alternative anticoagulant to unfractionated heparin for routine outpatient hemodialysis treatments. Nephrology 2009;14:455–61.

40. Schrader J, Stibbe W, Kandt M, et al. Low molecular weight heparin versus standard heparin: a long-term study in hemodialysis and hemofiltration patients. ASAIO Trans 1990;36:28.
41. Van Wyk V, Bandebhorst PN, Luus HG, et al. A comparison between the use of recombinant hirudin and heparin during hemodialysis. Kidney Int 1995;48:1338.
42. Reddy BV, Grossman EJ, Trevino SA, et al. Argatroban anticoagulation in patients with heparin-induced thrombocytopenia requiring renal replacement therapy. Ann Pharmacother 2005;39:1601–5.
43. Caruana RJ, Smith MC, Clyne D, et al. Controlled study of heparin versus epoprostenol sodium (prostacyclin) as the sole anticoagulant for chronic hemodialysis. Blood Purif 1991;9(5–6):296–304.

Equipment Commonly Used in Veterinary Renal Replacement Therapy

Karen Poeppel, LVT, Cathy E. Langston, DVM*,
Serge Chalhoub, DVM

KEYWORDS

- Dialysis machine • Monitor • Water treatment system
- Intermittent hemodialysis
- Continuous renal replacement therapy

INTERMITTENT HEMODIALYSIS MACHINES

There are several basic types of dialysis machines. In general, dialysis machines are designed to be used either for intermittent hemodialysis (IHD) or for continuous renal replacement therapy (CRRT), although "hybrid" machines, which are able to perform both types of therapies, have recently become available. Intermittent hemodialysis machines can be also used to provide sustained low-efficiency dialysis (SLED) treatments in addition to highly efficient intermittent treatments. Specific details of operation vary among machines (eg, minimum and maximum ranges for blood or dialysate flow and dialysate component concentrations); general ranges of commonly available machines are listed and illustrated here.

In the United States, most veterinary units performing intermittent hemodialysis use either Gambro (Phoenix or CentrySystem 3 models) **(Figs. 1** and **2)** or Fresenius machines **(Fig. 3)**. The Gambro machines have a cartridge system for the extracorporeal circuit that includes all of the necessary tubing. The dialyzer is separate. The snap-in cartridge simplifies machine set-up, but limits tubing choices. The Fresenius machines incorporate several tubing components that are selected separately during machine set-up. This arrangement provides more flexibility with tubing size, volume, and manufacturers, but lacks the simplicity of the Gambro cartridge. There are several other types of dialysis machines that are approved for use in Europe or Canada but not in the United States. Many of these machines have the capability of on-line

Renal Medicine Service, The Animal Medical Center, 510 East 62nd Street, New York, NY 10065, USA
* Corresponding author.
E-mail address: Cathy.langston@amcny.org

Vet Clin Small Anim 41 (2011) 177–191
doi:10.1016/j.cvsm.2010.09.002   **vetsmall.theclinics.com**

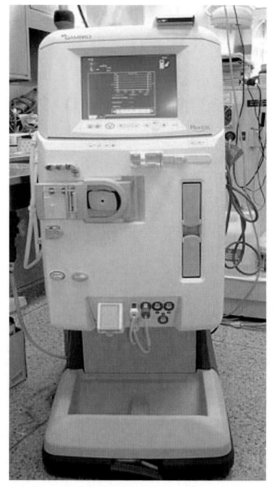

Fig. 1. Gambro Phoenix Intermittent Hemodialysis machine.

hemodiafiltration, which means they can provide large volumes of solutions to infuse into the patient as replacement fluid, in addition to producing large volumes of dialysate.

Regardless of the model or manufacturer, all modern IHD machines have certain common characteristics. First, they all contain a display screen, which may be a touch screen on newer models. This screen displays the current dialysis treatment mode, all options available in that mode, treatment parameters, alarm conditions, and any necessary instructions. During the dialysis treatment, the screen also displays treatment status (ie, time left, amount of fluid removed, catheter pressures, and so forth).

IHD machines house a dialysate proportioning system. This system takes incoming purified water and mixes it with the appropriate amount of electrolyte and bicarbonate concentrates to create dialysate at a rate of 300 to 800 mL/min. The electrolyte solution is a highly concentrated salt solution containing sodium, chloride, glucose, and other components as desired (potassium, calcium, magnesium). The machine operator sets the desired sodium concentration of the dialysate (within the limits of the

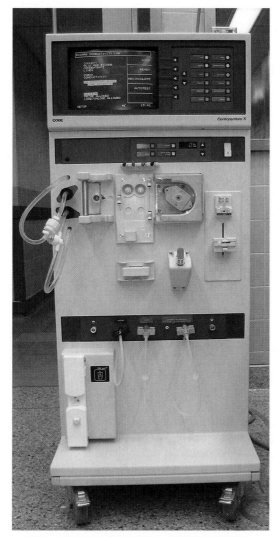

Fig. 2. Gambro CenturySystem3 Intermittent Hemodialysis machine.

machine of between 130 and 155 mEq/L) based on patient parameters. The sodium concentration can be readily adjusted to avoid large or rapid changes in the patient's serum sodium concentration, thus avoiding dramatic fluid shifts. Sodium profiling is a feature of most machines that allows the dialysate sodium concentration to automatically adjust throughout the treatment to match a preset pattern. The dialysate sodium may be set slightly higher than the patient's serum concentration at the start of the treatment and gradually decrease to normal over the course of the treatment. This profile enhances diffusion of sodium into the patient early in the course of treatment when urea removal is most rapid, and helps maintain a stable patient osmolality. This process decreases the risk of cerebral edema and the related neurologic symptoms known as dialysis disequilibrium syndrome. The sodium concentration is lowered by the end of the treatment to avoid loading the patient with sodium, which

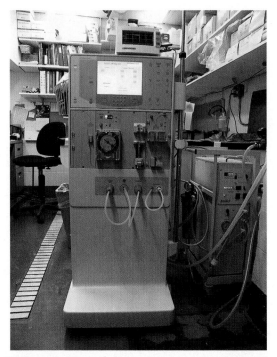

Fig. 3. Fresenius 2008H Intermitttent Hemodialysis machine. (*Courtesy of* Mary Anna Labato, Tufts University, North Grafton, MA.)

can enhance thirst and water retention in the interdialysis interval.[1] The concentration of other dialysate components will be proportional to the sodium concentration and cannot be individually adjusted. However, different salt solutions can be used, such as potassium-free or calcium-free solutions.

Bicarbonate is incorporated separately because bicarbonate and calcium from the electrolyte concentrate are incompatible in a concentrated form without inducing precipitation, thus allowing the bicarbonate concentration to be adjusted independently from sodium concentration, generally within the range of 25 to 40 mEq/L. To combat metabolic acidosis that is commonly present, the dialysate bicarbonate concentration is usually higher than that of the patient, allowing diffusion of bicarbonate from the dialysate into the patient. The typical dialysate bicarbonate concentration used in people (35 mEq/L) leads to panting in dogs; a slightly lower concentration (30 mEq/L) is typically used in veterinary hemodialysis. If acidosis is severe, a high dialysate bicarbonate concentration may cause paradoxic central nervous system acidosis and dialysis disequilibrium syndrome.

An alternative method of producing dialysate involves mixing the salt and buffer solutions with water in a large bulk tank, where it is stored until being piped to the individual dialysis machines in the unit. Every patient in the unit would use the same dialysate composition. This method is rarely used in veterinary medicine.

Each machine has a blood pump to draw blood from the catheter and return it to the patient. The blood pump speed ranges from 10 to 600 mL/min in most machines. The vast majority of patients are heparinized to prevent blood clotting in the extracorporeal circuit, so all modern dialysis machines have a built-in syringe pump for heparin administration.

In addition to removing uremic toxins, one of the main goals of dialysis is to control the patient's fluid volume. To this end, dialysis machines are able to remove fluid from the blood via a process called ultrafiltration. A vacuum is applied to the outgoing dialysate flow to create hydrostatic pressure. The result is that pressure within the straw-like semipermeable membrane in which the blood is traveling is positive in relation to the dialysate. The pressure forces fluid out of the blood and into the dialysate. The volume of fluid to be removed is programmed by the technician, and the dialysis machine will then automatically set the removal rate based on the intended duration of the treatment. Ultrafiltration rates vary from 0 to 4 kg/h (4 L/h). In older machines, the smallest increment of fluid removal is 100 mL/h, which can be excessive for small patients. As a safety feature of some new machines, such as the Gambro Phoenix, some degree of ultrafiltration must be used to maintain a positive pressure gradient across the entire dialyzer. The ultrafiltration prevents any back leakage of dialysate into the bloodstream, thus decreasing risk to the patient in the event the dialysate has any bacterial contamination. If this degree of fluid removal (100 mL/h) is not desired in a smaller patient, intravenous fluid administration may be necessary to avoid causing hypovolemia. Dialysate sodium concentration can also be profiled in such a way to maximize fluid removal from the patient, following osmotic gradients.

Some newer machines can be set to remove fluid at variable rates during the dialysis treatment. A common profile involves a faster rate of fluid removal at the beginning of the treatment, when the extra fluid is readily accessible in the bloodstream, and a slower rate toward the end, to account for a slower transfer from the interstitium to the bloodstream as the patient nears the optimal fluid status.[1] In intermittent hemodialysis, with its high dialysate flow rate, ultrafiltration contributes relatively little to the overall solute clearance.[2]

Most newer dialysis machines also incorporate ionic dialysance measurement. Dialysance is a measure of solute mass transfer from blood to dialysate. The collective dialysance of small molecular weight ions is considered equivalent to the urea dialysance. For conventional single-pass hemodialysis circuits, urea dialysance is equal to urea clearance. By programmed alterations in dialysate conductivity and measurement of conductivity at the dialysate inlet and outlet, the dialysis machine can calculate the dialyzer ionic dialysance and thus urea clearance. Repeated measurements are made throughout the treatment, allowing calculation of urea clearance over time (Kt) for each dialysis treatment. By entering the patient weight and volume of distribution, the machine will calculate the dialysis adequacy (Kt/V) throughout the dialysis treatment.[3]

Because of the difficulties associated with maintaining an adequately functioning vascular access, most dialysis machines can be programmed for blood removal and return through a single lumen of a catheter, referred to as single-needle dialysis. Such dialysis involves a discontinuous flow of blood, therefore single-needle dialysis is less efficient than standard dialysis.

A therapeutic plasma exchange cartridge can be used to separate plasma from the cellular blood components. Thus, plasma can be removed from the patient and replaced with a colloid solution while preserving the patient's red cells, white cells, and platelets. Therapeutic plasma exchange may be helpful in the treatment of autoimmune disease such as myasthenia gravis, as the offending antibodies are discarded. A charcoal hemoperfusion cartridge can be placed in the extracorporeal circuit to allow treatment of certain toxicities.

It is essential for patient safety that the dialysate is proportioned consistently and accurately to the technician's specifications. To that end, the machines have many built-in sensors and alarms to ensure patient safety. There are sensors that monitor pressure changes in the extracorporeal circuit, air in the return line, blood leaks in the dialyzer, or other unsafe conditions. Sensors constantly monitor dialysate composition and temperature. The machine does not monitor specific dialysate components; rather, the system monitors total electrical conductivity, which is dependent on solute concentration. If any unsafe or potentially unsafe conditions are detected in the dialysate, its flow is diverted from the dialyzer while blood continues to circulate; this minimizes the likelihood of clotting while the dialysate error is corrected. If blood path conditions are potentially compromised, as indicated by excessively high or low pressures in the circuit, the blood pump stops and the blood lines are automatically clamped to prevent further removal of blood from the patient or unsafe return of patient's blood. On-screen instructions notify the operator of the specific alarm, which must be remedied to restart the treatment. In extreme situations, the machine will require the operator to perform an emergency stop treatment procedure. Despite the myriad safeguards and in many cases, duplicate monitors installed in the machine, technician error can still occur. Only personnel specifically trained to use and troubleshoot the specific machine should perform IHD treatments.

Machine maintenance involves routine internal cleaning and intermittent machine calibration. At the end of each treatment day, the technician may be required to put the machine in a rinse cycle to flush bicarbonate out of the tubing to avoid precipitation. A cleaning cycle involving bleach removes any protein deposits from the dialysate tubing. Some of the newer machines automatically perform these cleaning steps without technician input. Weekly disinfection should be part of the dialysis unit routine. Chemical disinfection can be performed using a variety of cleaners. A blend of peroxyacetic acid and hydrogen peroxide (Actril; Minntech, Minneapolis, MN, USA) is popular. The cleaning solution is distributed throughout the internal tubing of the machine via the acid and bicarbonate ports and is allowed to dwell for several minutes to hours. In many units, the disinfect cycle is started at the end of the day, so the dwell period occurs overnight. There is a mandatory rinse cycle afterwards, and the technician should then check that no residual disinfectant is in the dialysate (generally using a simple dipstick test). Some machines can also perform a heat disinfect cycle, which heats water in the tubing for several hours to destroy any bacterial contaminants. In machines that are capable of both chemical and heat disinfection, alternating weekly is recommended.

Water Treatment System

A well-maintained water treatment system is essential to provide a safe hemodialysis treatment. The patient is exposed to roughly 20 gallons (76 L) of water in an average dialysis treatment, so even trace amounts of impurities can have detrimental effects.[4–6] Water treatment systems vary in size and water output, from a small portable unit that fits on the back of a dialysis machine to an entire room full of equipment that provides water for up to 30 dialysis machines (**Fig. 4**), but they all have certain common features. A typical system contains a hot and cold water mixing valve, a sediment filter (to remove debris), an ion exchange tank (to remove calcium and magnesium), carbon tanks (to remove organic components), and a reverse osmosis or deionization filter (to remove any remaining contaminants and ions). Daily monitoring of the product water is required to ensure patient safety. The technician performing the hemodialysis treatment generally performs this task. The water treatment system is so essential to performing a safe hemodialysis treatment that it

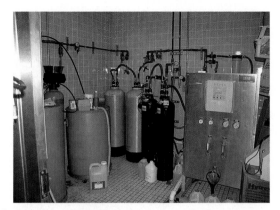

Fig. 4. Example of a water treatment system.

is highly recommended to have a backup system that can be placed in-line almost immediately.

Newer dialysis machines are capable of producing "ultrapure" dialysate. The dialysate made from purified water is filtered through a special membrane before it is passed into the dialyzer. Water and electrolytes are able to pass through the membrane, but any bacterial contaminants are excluded. The ultrapure dialysate is then delivered to the dialyzer that contains the patient's blood. Ultrapure dialysate is thought to decrease systemic inflammation that can occur when patients are exposed to small amounts of endotoxins present in dialysate; however, this has not yet been proved.[7]

On every day that dialysis is performed, the water treatment system needs to be checked to ensure proper performance. Inadequate water treatment can expose the patient to harmful contaminants in the water. The specific testing necessary depends on the unit. In addition to daily monitoring, scheduled weekly or biweekly cultures of water and dialysate should be performed for surveillance of bacterial contamination, and water samples should be analyzed biannually for chemical composition to ensure safe levels of various other compounds (heavy metals, nitrates, and so forth).

CONTINUOUS RENAL REPLACEMENT THERAPY MACHINES

Most veterinarians in the United States who offer CRRT use one of the Gambro machines, either the older Prisma (**Fig. 5**), or the newer PrismaFlex (**Fig. 6**). Although the basic premise of clearance across a semipermeable membrane housed in a dialyzer is the same with intermittent and continuous dialysis, the machines used have several key features that differ. The Gambro CRRT machines, like the IHD machines, use a dialyzer (frequently referred to as a hemofilter) and tubing incorporated into a cartridge system that easily snaps onto the machine for easy set-up.

CRRT involves a much slower dialysate flow rate than IHD. Rather than having the CRRT machine create dialysate from purified water and an electrolyte concentrate, CRRT uses prepared sterile dialysate, which is prepackaged in bags similar to intravenous fluids. Several formulations are available with different components or concentrations, such as potassium-free or calcium-free, to allow prescriptions to be tailored to the individual patient's needs. The sodium concentration cannot be varied during treatment as it can with IHD. It is possible to modify intravenous fluid solutions to

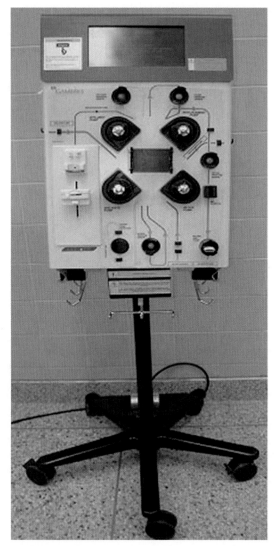

Fig. 5. Gambro Prisma CRRT machine.

function as dialysate, although this introduces more chances for formulation errors and bacterial contamination. The Prisma machine dialysate flow rate varies from 0 to 2500 mL/h in 50-mL increments; the PrismaFlex can deliver up to 8000 mL/h.

While both IHD and CRRT use diffusive and convective clearance, CRRT uses convective clearance to a greater degree than IHD. The fluid removal rate to control overhydration is prescribed based on the patient's volume status and the excess fluid is removed by ultrafiltration. Ultrafiltration rates range from 0 to 1000 mL/h in 10-mL increments with the Prisma, and up to 2000 mL/h with the PrismaFlex. While both IHD and CRRT use diffusive and convective clearance, CRRT uses convective clearance to a greater degree than IHD. By employing additional fluid removal, plasma fluid and small to moderately sized molecules (eg, urea) are drawn out of the blood and discarded, a process called convective clearance. This fluid is then replaced with

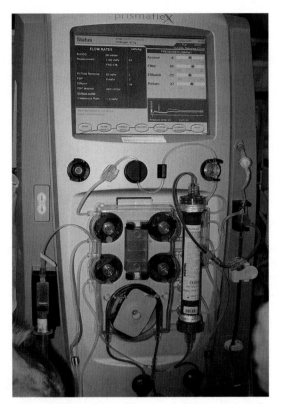

Fig. 6. Gambro PrismaFlex CRRT machine. (*Courtesy of* Mary Anna Labato, Tufts University, North Grafton, MA.)

a balanced electrolyte solution. The dialysis technician sets the replacement fluid rate; the CRRT machine then simultaneously removes fluid from the patient via the effluent pump and replaces the same volume of fluid via the replacement fluid pump. Replacement fluid rates range from 0 to 4500 mL/h in 100-mL increments for the Prisma, and up to 8000 mL/h with the PrismaFlex. The dialysis technician sets the replacement fluid rate; the CRRT machine then simultaneously removes fluid from the patient via the effluent pump and replaces the same volume of fluid via the replacement fluid pump. Replacement fluid rates range from 0 to 4500 mL/h in 100-mL increments for the Prisma, and up to 8000 mL/h with the PrismaFlex.

The Gambro Prisma and PrismaFlex systems determine these various fluid rates by weight. The bags of dialysate, replacement fluid, and effluent (the combined spent dialysate and ultrafiltrate from patient fluid removal and fluid used for convective clearance) are placed on scales built into the machine. Excessive motion of the machine will cause the bags to sway, interfering with accurate weight measurement and thus causing a machine alarm until the problem is corrected. The total rate of effluent production that is possible with the Prisma machine is 5500 mL/h, compared with 10 L/h with the PrismaFlex.

Because CRRT is intended to be provided over a longer treatment period (ie, 24 hours a day compared with 4–5 hours a day for IHD), a slower blood flow rate is generally selected. In addition, clearance with CRRT is influenced more by effluent rate than by blood flow rate, making a rapid blood flow rate unnecessary in most cases. The

Prisma machine can provide a blood flow rate from 10 to 180 mL/min in 5-mL increments. The PrismaFlex machine provides a blood flow rate from 10 to 450 mL/min in 10-mL increments.

Both the Prisma and PrismaFlex have an incorporated syringe pump to allow infusion of heparin. The PrismaFlex has an additional pump system to allow infusion of an additional fluid if desired. Attachments to externally warm the bloodlines are available for both machines.

Because the CRRT machines do not prepare dialysate, there is no need for internal conductivity meters. At the end of treatment, all of the fluid bags and blood lines are discarded, so there is no need for disinfecting or cleaning cycles for CRRT machines. The scales should be calibrated by the dialysis technician on a scheduled basis.

Therapeutic plasma exchange cartridges are available for the Prisma and Prisma-Flex. Charcoal hemoperfusion cartridges are available for the PrismaFlex.

ANCILLARY EQUIPMENT

Patients undergoing IHD require a significant amount of monitoring in the course of a treatment. One device specifically used during hemodialysis treatments is the Crit-Line in-line hematocrit monitor (CLM III TQA; Hema Metrics, Kaysville, UT, USA). This monitor measures real-time hematocrit, venous oxygen saturation, and percent change in blood volume (**Fig. 7**). A sterile, disposable Crit-Line blood chamber is placed in the patient's extracorporeal circuit during priming (**Fig. 8**). This chamber fills with the patient's blood during treatment, and an optical sensor placed on the chamber reads the hematocrit of the blood as it flows through the chamber and detects changes instantaneously. While it is useful to know the patient's hematocrit throughout the treatment, the real value of this is the ability to concurrently appreciate changes in the patient's intravascular volume. Presuming there is no ongoing bleeding or transfusion, any changes in hematocrit reflect changes in intravascular volume. A rapid decrease in intravascular volume (10% per hour) from an excessively rapid ultrafiltration rate may precipitate symptomatic hypotension.

The Crit-Line also monitors the oxygen saturation (SvO_2) of the blood in the extracorporeal circuit, which is considered mixed venous blood. SvO_2 is the balance between oxygen delivery and oxygen consumption (metabolic rate). Mixed venous oxygen saturation is affected by cardiac output, blood pressure, oxygenation, and hemoglobin. An SvO_2 of more than 70% is considered normal, however, many patients with values around 50% show no noticeable ill effects during IHD treatments.[8] A significant decrease in SvO_2 may be an indicator of an impending hypotensive episode. The ability to see changes in blood volume and predict a hypotensive

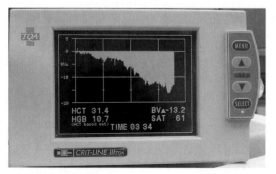

Fig. 7. Crit-Line Blood Volume Monitor.

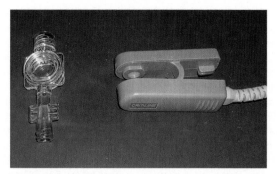

Fig. 8. A Crit-Line blood chamber (*left*) and the Crit-Line sensor (*right*) that is attached to the blood chamber to detect hemoglobin and oxygen saturation.

episode is important because it is sometimes necessary to remove large volumes of extra fluid from a patient. The Crit-Line monitor has become a valuable tool in helping to assess how quickly and how much fluid can safely be removed.

The Crit-Line monitor can be used to measure access recirculation in dialysis catheters by sequential injections of a small volume of saline into the extracorporeal circuit.[9] Access recirculation is the reuptake of blood into the arterial lumen that has just been returned through the venous lumen (ie, reuptake of clean blood). Recirculation will decrease the efficiency of the dialysis treatment, so it is important that it be monitored. An increase in the measured amount of recirculation over several treatments is also an indication that the access is beginning to fail, so early detection will help guide intervention. An additional function of the Crit-Line monitor in human hemodialysis patients is to measure access recirculation in arteriovenous fistulas and grafts. In veterinary medicine, catheters are used almost exclusively for vascular access, so this function of the machine is not used.

Another method of monitoring for access recirculation is the Transonics Flow Monitor (Transonics Systems, Ithaca, NY, USA). These machines measure access recirculation in all types of hemodialysis vascular access, and they seem to have a greater sensitivity and more accuracy than the Crit-Line device.[10] The Transonics device can also be used to measure actual, in-line blood flow through the dialysis circuit. At lower blood pump speeds the blood flow should equal the blood pump speed, and therefore the Transonics machine acts as a calibration device. At higher blood pump speeds the actual blood flow will be less than the blood pump speed, therefore knowing the actual blood flow allows for more accurate prediction of the dialysis treatment efficacy. Some of the newer hemodialysis machines have built-in sensors to measure actual blood flow.

Blood pressure monitors are a very important monitoring tool in hemodialysis. Renal failure patients often have blood pressure abnormalities before institution of dialytic therapy. Dialysis itself involves removing anywhere from 47 to 150 mL of blood from the patient just to fill the extracorporeal circuit, which can lead to a noticeable drop in blood pressure at the start of treatment. Anuric and oliguric patients are often overhydrated and require fluid removal during a dialysis treatment. A fluid removal rate in excess of the rate of intravascular refilling from the interstitium can cause hypotension, therefore blood pressure must be monitored. Noninvasive blood pressure monitors are most commonly used. For cats and small dogs, an Ultrasonic Doppler Monitor (Parks Medical Electronics, Inc, Aloha, OR, USA) works very well. Oscillometric monitors are used on medium- to large-sized patients because they measure diastolic and mean blood pressures. These monitors can also be set to cycle on a regular basis, usually every 15 minutes. In a dialysis unit, it is essential to have access to one blood pressure machine for each dialysis machine because every patient on dialysis will require frequent blood pressure monitoring.

When patients undergo IHD, their blood is removed from their bodies and run through an extracorporeal circuit. The blood is exposed to foreign material that may activate the clotting cascade. Therefore, anticoagulant therapy is often required during a dialysis treatment, and equipment is necessary for monitoring the level of anticoagulation. The most common anticoagulant used in veterinary IHD is unfractionated heparin. Previously, the most practical method of measuring the level of anticoagulation was to measure activated clotting time (ACT), generally accomplished using an ACT II monitor (Medtronic, Minneapolis, MN, USA; **Fig. 9**). The sample required is fresh whole blood, and sampling is done anywhere from 15 to 60 minutes apart, so it is essential to have at least one dedicated ACT machine for the dialysis unit. If newer cage-side anticoagulation monitors are validated for measuring partial thromboplastin time on whole blood, they may supplant ACT measurement.

Another method of anticoagulation is regional anticoagulation with citrate. Citrate is infused into the patient's blood as it enters the extracorporeal circuit, and chelates calcium in the blood rendering it incapable of clotting. To prevent the patient from becoming hypocalcemic, calcium is restored as an infusion. Citrate is not used as often in IHD as in continuous therapies, but it may be useful in certain patients. When using citrate regional anticoagulation, the level of anticoagulation is assessed by measuring the ionized calcium concentration in the extracorporeal circuit. The patient's ionized calcium is also measured to ensure proper infusion rates. Once in the body, citrate is converted into bicarbonate; therefore, a chemistry analyzer capable of measuring both ionized calcium and pH becomes essential. Most specialty veterinary practices will have at least one in-house analyzer that runs ionized calcium, so it might not be absolutely necessary to install a separate one in the dialysis unit. However, this increases the personnel needs because then a second person must be available at times to take the blood sample to the machine to run the ionized calcium. Handheld analyzers, such as the iStat (Abaxis, Union City, CA, USA), are convenient because they can be moved to the dialysis treatment area when necessary, and they are a quick method of performing the needed assays (**Fig. 10**).

Even with a handheld chemistry analyzer, it is useful to have a tabletop analyzer. The level of azotemia is evaluated often in hemodialysis patients, and it useful to evaluate individual blood urea nitrogen and creatinine concentrations. Tabletop analyzers

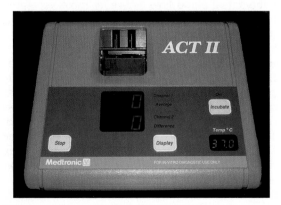

Fig. 9. ACT II monitor to measure activated clotting time.

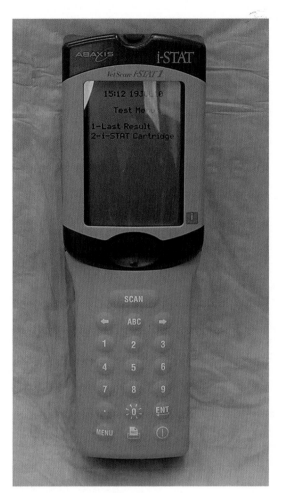

Fig. 10. iStat Handheld chemistry monitor.

usually offer more flexibility in choosing exactly which chemistries to run, as opposed to handheld monitors that run only predetermined panels.

One additional piece of equipment that should not be overlooked is a heat source. Patients undergoing IHD tend to be hypothermic due to their azotemia and hypotension. These patients tend to lose some heat in the blood tubing because their blood is exposed to room air. The temperature of the dialysate can be adjusted so that the patient's blood can be warmed (or cooled) as it passes through the dialyzer, but because IHD machines are manufactured solely for human use, the temperature range is such that animal blood is often cooled even at the highest temperature setting. Circulating water heating pads provide some heat, but to combat the cooling effects of the dialysate, the patient needs to be surrounded by heat. A second pad could be placed over the patient, or a heat lamp could be placed on the patient. A method that has proven effective in the authors' unit is to use a hot air machine (Bair Hugger, Augustine Medical, Eden Prairie, MN, USA) to create a microenvironment that is much warmer than the surrounding room (**Fig. 11**). As with anesthetized patients, small and obtunded patients undergoing IHD can lose a significant amount of body heat if not properly monitored.

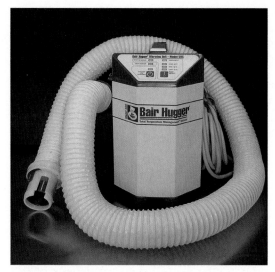

Fig. 11. Bair Hugger warm air heater.

Bioimpedance analyzers are used in human medicine to measure total body fat and water. The distribution of water is of importance when trying to remove fluid from a hemodialysis patient. Extra water can only be removed from the vascular space, so an overhydrated patient can become hypotensive if the extra water is not distributed appropriately. Patients can also become hypotensive if too much water is removed from the entire body and they become dehydrated. Bioimpedance analyzers help the clinician determine if a patient is becoming hypotensive because the vascular space is not refilling or because the patient truly is no longer overhydrated. These analyzers are expensive and are not manufactured for veterinary patients, so their use in veterinary hemodialysis is still being studied.

SUMMARY

There are several different machines available for the performance of renal replacement therapy in veterinary medicine. Extracorporeal renal replacement therapies (IHD and CRRT) involve dedicated personnel who are familiar with the operations and maintenance of the equipment. The availability of such equipment has resulted in the ability to treat both acute kidney injury and chronic kidney disease.

ACKNOWLEDGMENTS

The authors would like to thank Eleanora Mitelberg, LVT, for assistance in manuscript preparation and image acquisition.

REFERENCES

1. Stiller S, Bonnie-Schorn E, Grassmann A, et al. A critical review of sodium profiling for hemodialysis. Semin Dial 2001;14(5):337–47.
2. Yeun JY, Depner TA. Principles of hemodialysis. In: Pereira BJG, Sayegh MH, Blake P, editors. Chronic kidney disease, dialysis, transplantation. 2nd edition. Philadelphia: Elsevier Saunders; 2005. p. 307–40.

3. Gross M, Maierhofer A, Tetta C, et al. Online clearance measurement in high-efficiency hemodiafiltration. Kidney Int 2007;72(12):1550–3.
4. Ward RA. Water treatment for in-center hemodialysis including verification of water quality and disinfection. In: Nissenson AR, Fine RN, editors. Dialysis therapy. Philadelphia: Hanley & Belfus, Inc; 2002. p. 55–60.
5. Van Stone JC. Hemodialysis apparatus. In: Daugirdas JT, Ing TS, editors. Handbook of dialysis. Boston: Little, Brown and Company; 1994. p. 30–52.
6. Ward RA. Water treatment equipment for in-center hemodialysis: including verification of water quality and disinfection. In: Nissenson AR, Fine RN, editors. Handbook of dialysis therapy. 4th edition. Philadelphia: Saunders Elsevier; 2008. p. 143–56.
7. Bommer J, Jaber BL. Ultrapure dialysate: facts and myths. Semin Dial 2006; 19(2):115–9.
8. Marino PL. Oximetry and capnography. The ICU book. 2nd edition. Baltimore (MD): Williams & Wilkins; 1998. p. 355–70.
9. Sherman RA, Kapoian T. Dialysis access recirculation. In: Nissenson AR, Fine RN, editors. Handbook of dialysis therapy. 4th edition. Philadelphia: Saunders Elsevier; 2008. p. 102–8.
10. Lopot F, Nejedly B, Sulkova S, et al. Comparison of different techniques of hemodialysis vascular access flow evaluation. Int J Artif Organs 2003;26(12):1056–63.

Urea Kinetics and Intermittent Dialysis Prescription in Small Animals

Larry D. Cowgill, DVM, PhD

KEYWORDS

- Hemodialysis • Kt/V • $_{sp}$Kt/V • $_{dp}$Kt/V • $_{e}$Kt/V • $_{std}$Kt/V
- Urea clearance • Urea generation

Intermittent hemodialysis is an extracorporeal renal replacement therapy with a 40-year foundation in veterinary therapeutics, but only recently has it transitioned from a clinical curiosity to the advanced standard for the management of acute renal failure in dogs and cats.[1–7] No conventional medical therapies can reproduce the efficacy of hemodialysis for correction of the cumulative biochemical, acid-base, endocrine, and fluid disorders associated with kidney failure. Acute kidney injury (AKI) is the most common indication for intermittent hemodialysis in dogs and cats. Delay in instituting dialysis leads to greater uremic symptomology, morbidity, and recruitment of additional organ dysfunction.[5,7,8] Indefinite use of intermittent hemodialysis in animals with chronic kidney disease is equally indicated, but cost and logistic realities have limited its routine use for this indication. Hemodialysis alone or in combination with hemoperfusion is an important therapy to clear toxins and toxic metabolites from animals after accidental poisoning or drug overdosage or to relieve excessive iatrogenic or pathologic fluid loads.[5,9–11] The dog and cat equally share the demand and use of therapeutic hemodialysis, but the techniques and equipment for the delivery of intermittent hemodialysis are safe and effective for animals as small as 1.5 kg or as large as 600 kg. Diverse creatures from tortoises and rabbits to sheep and horses have been managed with creative modifications of the procedures and equipment devised for human application.[6]

THERAPEUTIC PRINCIPLES OF HEMODIALYSIS

The therapeutic role of hemodialysis is to eliminate (clear) accumulated uremia retention solutes (uremia toxins) and water from the body and alleviate the morbidity and clinical features they impart to animals with uremia. Uremia retention solutes are

Department of Medicine and Epidemiology, School of Veterinary Medicine, University of California-Davis, 2108 Tupper Hall, Davis, CA 95616, USA
E-mail address: ldcowgill@ucdavis.edu

Vet Clin Small Anim 41 (2011) 193–225
doi:10.1016/j.cvsm.2010.12.002
vetsmall.theclinics.com
0195-5616/11/$ – see front matter © 2011 Elsevier Inc. All rights reserved.

broadly and arbitrarily classified based on their physicochemical properties as small (water-soluble) solutes (molecular weight [MW] <500 Da), middle molecules (>500 Da), and protein-bound solutes, which, together with their compartmentalization, influence their propensity and accessibility for dialytic removal.[12–14] Hundreds of solutes have demonstrated intrinsic toxicity that mimics or reproduces particular aspects of the uremic syndrome, and thousands of retained solutes have now been demonstrated by mass spectroscopy in subjects with uremia.[13–15] Some retained solutes, like urea, have minimal inherent toxicity but serve as markers for retention of similar but unidentified solutes with greater clinical significance; whereas, others clearly mediate the clinical consequences of uremia.[16–19] Extensive prospective studies in human patients with kidney failure confirm significant outcome benefits associated with the extent of small-molecular-weight solute removal (ie, dialysis dose).[20–23] However, uremic toxicity is more complex than can be explained by retention of small-molecular-weight solutes and attention has refocused on retention of middle molecules and protein-bound solutes that are removed poorly by dialysis.[13–15,24,25]

Urea is a small molecular weight (60 Da) nitrogenous metabolite whose plasma concentration exceeds that of all other uremic solutes. It contributes minimally to the clinical manifestations of uremia but has remained fundamentally associated with the morbidity and outcome of the uremic syndrome because of its abundance and its link to the metabolism of dietary and endogenous nitrogen.[16,26,27] Azotemia must be viewed as a marker for the collective appearance of numerous small water soluble compounds, protein carbamylation, redirected metabolic pathways, or other small-molecular-weight solutes coupled to nitrogen metabolism or bound to body proteins.

The proven correlation of urea removal by hemodialysis with outcomes in renal failure has prompted the designation of urea as a surrogate index for all putative small-molecular-weight retention solutes that remain unidentified or unmeasured.[16,22] Reduction of urea appearance and the extrarenal removal of urea are used to prescribe the therapy for uremia and to monitor the efficiency and adequacy of these therapies.[28–31] This designation is both rational and problematic. Urea is uncharged, present at high concentration, readily detected, and readily diffuses across all body fluid compartments and the dialysis membrane. As such, it serves as an excellent solute to document dialyzer performance and whole-body clearance of low-molecular-weight solutes. However, these unique features and its minimal uremic toxicity question whether it appropriately or accurately reflects the dialytic behavior of other solutes with more profound uremic toxicity and thus may over represent removal of these solutes.[17,19,32]

Dialytic therapies alter the composition of body fluids by exposing blood to a contrived solution, the dialysate, across an interposed semipermeable membrane. The mass transfer of solute and water occurs by diffusive and convective forces across the membrane, and the magnitude of the exchange is predicated on the chemical and physical characteristics of the solute and the ultrastructure of the porous membrane. These principles directly influence the adequacy of hemodialysis and must be integrated into its prescription. Water and low-molecular-weight solutes (<500 Da) pass readily through the membrane pores, but the movement of larger solutes, plasma proteins, and the cellular components of blood are restricted by pore size and physical characteristics of the membrane. Diffusive transfer (dialysis) occurs by the thermal motion of the molecules in each solution (blood and dialysate) causing their random encounter with the membrane and subsequent transfer through porous channels of the appropriate size. These random events are proportional to the respective concentration and thermodynamic potential of the solute on each side of the membrane and the physical properties of the dialysis membrane. The diffusive potential for every solute varies under differing physiologic conditions, but molecular weight is the main determinant of kinetic motion. When there is no concentration gradient for a solute across the membrane, the solute is at filtration equilibrium. At this point, the driving force for diffusion stops and there is no further net change in concentration of the respective solutions despite ongoing bidirectional and equal molecular exchanges between them.

Membrane permeability is determined by its thickness, its effective surface area, and the number, size, and shape of its pores or diffusion channels.[33] In addition to intrinsic solute and membrane characteristics, molecular charge, protein binding, volume of distribution, and cellular seclusion influence the bulk transfer of uremia toxins and solutes from the body independently from their predicted diffusion.

Convective transport of solutes across dialysis membranes is associated with the process of ultrafiltration, in which water is driven through the membrane by hydrostatic pressure gradients. Diffusible solutes dissolved in the water are swept through the membrane by solvent drag.[33] Unlike diffusive transport, convective transport does not require a concentration gradient across the membrane and does not alter diffusive gradients or serum concentrations. The transmembrane hydrostatic pressure gradient between the blood and dialysate compartments, the hydraulic permeability, and the surface area of the membrane determine the rate of ultrafiltration and solute transfer. During hemodialysis, a dialysate-directed transmembrane pressure gradient (dialysate pressure < blood-side pressure) is generated to initiate and control the rate of ultrafiltration. Independent changes in the dialysate and blood-side pressures can influence the rate of ultrafiltration by attendant changes to the transmembrane pressure. The hydraulic permeability of a dialyzer is determined by physical features of the membrane (eg, composition, thickness, pore size) and is rated by its ultrafiltration coefficient, K_{uf}, defined as milliliters of fluid transferred per hour per millimeter mercury of transmembrane pressure. Hemodialyzers are qualified as low flux or high flux according to their K_{uf}. A minimal transmembrane pressure of 25 mm Hg is required for ultrafiltration to offset the oncotic pressure of plasma proteins, which favors fluid reabsorption and opposes ultrafiltration. Convective transport can contribute to total solute removal, especially for large solutes with limited diffusibility. However, for standard hemodialysis, ultrafiltration primarily is targeted at fluid removal, and convective clearance contributes less than 5% to total solute removal.

PRESCRIBING INTERMITTENT HEMODIALYSIS

The hemodialysis session is defined by the dialysis prescription, which is an interactive procedure involving the patient, the attending clinician, and the dialysis delivery system. For the prescription to be effective, the clinician must understand the clinical and biochemical status of patients, the principals of dialysis, and the operational capabilities of the dialysis delivery system. It also is necessary to have a clear understanding of the therapeutic goals for the dialysis session and insure that the goals are achieved (**Box 1**). The effects of hemodialysis may be permanent in the case of intoxications or overhydration or transient if there is ongoing generation of toxic metabolites as in renal failure or accumulation of fluid as in heart failure. The dialysis prescription attempts to correct all disordered solutes, but for most it represents a blind projection to achieve a theoretically forecasted outcome. Most uremia toxins are not known with precision and not measured routinely. Urea has been designated the surrogate index for all putative small-molecular-weight uremic toxins, and

---

Box 1
Clinical considerations influencing the hemodialysis prescription

1. Patient characteristics (species, size, age, body condition)

2. Severity of the azotemia and retained uremic toxins

3. Degree of anemia

4. Electrolyte and mineral disorders: sodium, potassium, chloride, bicarbonate calcium, magnesium, and phosphate

5. Acid-base imbalances and depleted or deficient solutes: bicarbonate, calcium, glucose

6. Exogenous intoxications (eg, ethylene glycol)

7. Hydration status and fluid balance

8. Physiologic disturbances: blood pressure, hematocrit, body temperature, oxygenation, change in body weight, mental state

9. Coagulation status

10. Medications, surgical history, and comorbid clinical conditions

11. Dialysis treatment history

---

reduction of urea appearance and extra-renal removal of urea are used both to prescribe and to monitor the efficiency and adequacy of dialytic therapy.

Hemodialysis Prescription for Acute Uremia

The major application of intermittent hemodialysis is for the transient elimination of innumerable and unspecified solutes and fluid retained during AKI that otherwise would be cleared by healthy kidneys. The benefits of intermittent dialysis are transient, and with cessation of dialysis, the concentrations of urea and all retained uremia solutes with continued generation increase immediately until a new steady state is achieved or until the next dialysis session (**Fig. 1**). It is firmly established that dialytic removal of these solutes to minimize the time-average urea concentrations mitigates the associated morbidity and mortality of uremia but does not resolve all uremic symptomatology.[16,21,22,34] It is equally established that additional classes of retention solutes are poorly dialyzed by conventional high-flux diffusive and hemofiltration techniques limiting the efficacy of extracorporeal therapy.[13–15,34–36] The diffusive removal of urea and small-molecular-weight solutes is exceptionally efficient in animals, but clinical sequelae associated with abrupt excursions in the solute and fluid content of patients often limit the rate and magnitude that they can be altered. The intensity of the dialysis treatment can be adjusted by altering blood flow rate (Q_b), dialysate flow rate (Q_d), clearance of the hemodialyzer (K_d), rate of ultrafiltration, or length of the dialysis session (T_d) to accommodate the size and therapeutic needs of the animal. After dialysis, blood urea nitrogen (BUN), and other retained uremia solutes, increases in proportion to urea generation from dietary nitrogen and endogenous protein catabolism (G) and inversely with residual renal function (K_r) (see **Fig. 1**). Higher dietary protein intake, increased catabolism, and lower residual renal function will produce a steeper increase and higher steady-state concentration of urea after dialysis unless interrupted by an intervening dialysis treatment before achieving steady state. The peak predialysis urea, time-averaged urea concentrations, and the exposure to urea and other uremic toxins will be lower the more frequently and effectively patients are dialyzed.[29,30,37,38]

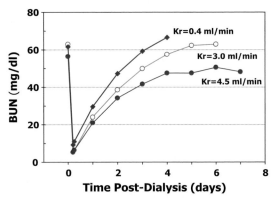

Fig. 1. Changes in BUN during and after 5-hour hemodialysis treatments in a 33-kg dog presented for AKI at varying degrees of residual urea clearance during recovery. The predialysis and immediate postdialysis BUN concentrations reflect a simple assessment of treatment intensity (dose). The $_eKt/V$ (~2.9 per session) for the dialysis treatments was identical for each level of urea clearance, and the BUN increases immediately following dialysis to its steady state (3–6 days). The rate of increase and the steady-state BUN concentration following dialysis is influenced by the patient's residual urea clearance (Kr). (*From* Cowgill LD, Francey T. Hemodialysis. In: DiBartola SP, editor. Fluid therapy in small animal practice. St Louis (MO): Elsevier; 2006. p. 650–77; with permission.)

The dialysis prescription must accommodate the physiologic, hematologic, and biochemical status of patients before dialysis and target the desired modifications at the end of the session (see **Box 1**). The prescription is individualized for each patient and every dialysis session by selecting dialytic options that best achieve the solute removal and ultrafiltration goals of the session without predisposing therapeutic risk (**Box 2**). Hemodialysis prescriptions for animals with acute uremia have been derived empirically as consensus-based guidelines for a diverse array of animal types and clinical conditions. There has been little validation or standardization of dialysis therapy based on outcome assessment.

The hemodialysis prescription for animals with AKI is prioritized to resolve hyperkalemia, profound azotemia, fluid imbalance, metabolic acidosis, and persisting nephrotoxins as well as to accommodate ongoing therapies (eg, parenteral feeding). The initial treatments must be prescribed judiciously to prevent overtreatment when the risks of dialysis-related complications (disequilibrium), hypovolemia and hypotension, and bleeding are high. Consequently, dialysis goals for initial treatments in animals with AKI differ considerably from the goals and prescription for later dialysis treatments.

Hemodialyzers

For small animals, the hemodialyzer is selected initially on its contribution to the extracorporeal volume and secondarily on its diffusive, convective, and biocompatibility properties. **Table 1** provides guidelines for dialyzer selection based on the size of patients and the expected compromise to vascular volume. For cats and dogs weighing less than 6 kg, a dialyzer with a surface area between 0.2 m^2 and 0.4 m^2 and a priming volume less than 30 mL is generally tolerated but may represent up to 40% of vascular volume. A synthetic dialyzer (neonatal or pediatric) with a surface area between 0.4 m^2 and 0.8 m^2 and a priming volume less than 45 mL is appropriate for use in dogs weighing between 6 and 12 kg. Dialyzers with surface areas up to

---

Box 2
Components of the hemodialysis prescription

1. Selection of the hemodialyzer (surface area, fiber bundle volume, solute and ultrafiltration characteristics, hemocompatibility, and biocompatibility)

2. Selection of extracorporeal circuit and priming solution

3. Blood flow rate (Qb)

4. Dialysis time (Td) and scheduled bypass time

5. Dialysate composition or modeling

6. Dialysate flow rate and direction (Qd)

7. Treatment schedule

8. Access connection (single needle reversed direction)

9. Anticoagulation (anticoagulant, target activated clotting time, protocol)

10. Ultrafiltration (volume target, rate)

11. Ancillary medications

12. Monitoring schedule

13. Rinse back (solution, volume, air)

14. Catheter locking solution

15. After treatment (medications, monitoring)

1.5 m^2 and priming volumes up to 80 mL can be used on dogs between 12 and 20 kg. Larger dialyzers with surface areas greater than 2.0 m^2 and priming volumes greater than 100 mL can be used in dogs weighing more than 30 kg.

Purposeful selection of a dialyzer with a smaller surface area and priming volume than recommended is warranted in patients who are markedly azotemic to reduce the intensity of the treatment and risk of clotting at slow blood-flow rates. Solute removal follows first-order kinetics, and animals with marked azotemia (BUN, >250 mg/dL) will experience quantitatively greater urea removal per unit of time and blood flow than those with lesser degrees of azotemia. The smaller the volume of the dialyzer, the shorter will be the resident time for blood in the dialyzer. At a blood flow rate of 20 mL/min, the resident time of blood in a 28 mL dialyzer is only 1.4 minutes; whereas, the resident time would be 9 minutes in a 1.5 m^2 dialyzer with

---

Table 1
Recommended extracorporeal volumes used for hemodialysis in dogs and cats

	Body Weight (kg)	Dialyzer Volume (mL)	Total Extracorporeal Volume (mL)	% Blood Volume
Cats, dogs	<6	<30	<70	13–40
Cats	>6	<30	<70	<23
Dogs	6–12	<45	<90	9–19
Dogs	12–20	<80	100–160	6–17
Dogs	20–30	<120	150–200	6–13
Dogs	>30	>80	150–250	6–10

a blood volume of 180 mL. At 20 mL/min, both dialyzers would deliver the same clearance, approximately 20 mL/min.

Treatment intensity
Initial dialysis treatments typically are less intensive (less solute removal, slower blood flow rate, smaller dialyzer surface area, and possibly shorter treatment time) than those prescribed for subsequent treatments. At slow blood flow rates, urea extraction across the dialyzer approaches 100%, and urea clearance (K_{d-urea}, in mL/min) is approximately equal to extracorporeal blood flow (Q_b, in mL/min) regardless of the size of the dialyzer. When large surface area, high-flux dialyzers are used, K_{d-urea} increases quantitatively with Q_b until blood flow exceeds 200 mL/min.[30] At blood flow rates higher than 200 mL/min, the relationship flattens as urea clearance is influenced by membrane characteristics and dialysate flow in addition to Q_b.[30] At blood flow rates greater than 300 mL/min, dialyzer performance is influenced minimally by increased single-pass flow, and total solute removal increases in proportion to the cumulative flow through the dialyzer. The total volume of blood passed through the dialyzer during the treatment ($Q_b \cdot t$, where t is the dialysis treatment time) has been established as a reasonable predictor of the intensity of the treatment as estimated by the urea reduction ratio (URR) (**Figs. 2** and **3**).[4,5,8] This relationship can be used as an operational parameter to guide the prescription and delivery of dialysis by targeting the URR to differing severities of uremia and phases of management (**Table 2**).

Dialysis time
The treatment interval is determined in sequence once the target URR and approximate volume of blood requiring dialytic processing are defined for the treatment (see **Figs. 2** and **3**). From this volume ($Q_b \cdot t$), appropriate combinations of blood flow rate (Q_b) and dialysis time (t) can be derived. A long dialysis session time (slow Q_b)

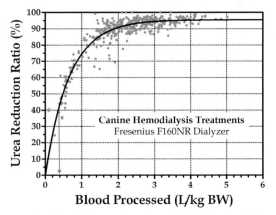

Fig. 2. Predicted urea reduction ratio as a function of the volume of blood processed in 413 hemodialysis sessions with a Fresenius F160NR hemodialyzer (Fresenius Medical Care, Waltham, MA, USA) in dogs. URR was computed from predialysis and immediate postdialysis BUN concentration (Appendix 1, Equation 1). The volume of blood processed ($Q_b \times t$) was indexed to body weight to compare dogs of different sizes. The solid line represents the exponential regression of all treatments. To achieve a low-intensity treatment with URR equal to 40%, a volume of 0.4 L of blood/kg body weight (*arrows*) must be dialyzed during the treatment. Similarly, a URR treatment goal of 90% requires approximately 1.8 L/kg of blood to be dialyzed.

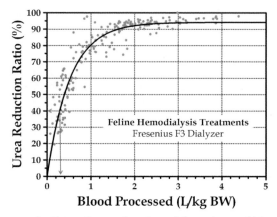

Fig. 3. Predicted urea reduction ratio as a function of the volume of blood processed in 200 hemodialysis sessions with a Fresenius F3 hemodialyzer (Fresenius Medical Care, Waltham, MA, USA) in cats. URR was computed from predialysis and immediate postdialysis BUN concentration (see Appendix 1, Equation 1). The solid line represents the exponential regression of all treatments. To achieve a low-intensity treatment with URR equal to 40%, a volume of 0.3 L of blood/kg body weight (*arrows*) must be dialyzed during the treatment. Treatment predictions are specific to each dialyzer and should be established independently in ever dialysis program.

is preferable to a short session time (fast Q_b) for patients with moderate to severe azotemia. A dialysis session time less than 180 minutes generally dictates faster and perhaps inappropriate blood flow rates that induce rapid changes in BUN and life-threatening dialysis complications. Short treatments usually cause inadequate URR outcomes that delay resolution of the azotemia.

The hourly URR can be used as an additional guide to select an appropriate treatment time. An excessive hourly URR is more likely to cause intradialytic complications than the absolute decrease in BUN over the dialysis session.[4] The risk of dialysis disequilibrium syndrome can be minimized by adherence to the hourly URR recommendations as indexed to the degree of azotemia in **Table 2**. An appropriate treatment

Table 2 Treatment intensity prescription	
Initial Treatment	
BUN <200 mg/dL	URR <0.5 @ no >0.1 URR/h
200–300 mg/dL	URR 0.5–0.3 @ no >0.1 URR/h
>300 mg/dL	URR ≤0.4 @ no >0.05–0.07 URR/h
Second treatment	
BUN <200 mg/dL	URR 0.6–0.7 @ 0.12–0.15 URR/h
200–300 mg/dL	URR 0.6–0.4 @ no >0.05–0.1 URR/h
>300 mg/dL	URR ≤0.4 @ no >0.05–0.1 URR/h
Third and subsequent treatments	
BUN <150 mg/dL	URR >0.8 @ >0.15 URR/h
150–300 mg/dL	URR 0.5–0.6 @ 0.15–0.1 URR/h
>300 mg/dL	URR 0.5–0.6 @ <0.1 URR/h

time can be determined by dividing the URR goal for the treatment by the recommended hourly URR. URR is determined cumulatively over the entire dialysis treatment, but the rate and absolute change in serum urea and osmolality will be highest at the beginning of the treatment. Hourly URR recommendations could exceed safe guidelines at the beginning of the treatment in extremely azotemic animals if the URR goal is too high or the treatment time is short despite appropriate URR prescription for the entire treatment.

Use of extended, slow dialysis treatments also facilitates removal of large volumes of fluid that risk volume contraction and hypotension during shorter treatments. Treatment intensity is indexed conventionally to urea transfer, which occurs faster than other solutes (eg, potassium, phosphate, and creatinine) that are less diffusible or compartmentalized and poorly transferable. Longer treatments enhance removal of urea in addition to secluded solutes that do not behave like urea.[31,38,39]

Extracoporeal blood flow

Blood flow is the last parameter determining treatment intensity as the URR goal, required volume of processed blood, and treatment time are determined. For a 20 kg dog presenting with AKI and a BUN of 295 mg/dL, a URR of 0.4 (40%) might be prescribed. The requisite treatment volume for this target would be 0.4 L/kg or 8.0 L of total treatment (see **Fig. 2**). Appropriate combinations of dialysis time and blood flow rate are next computed to achieve the 8.0 L goal. For a 240-minute dialysis session time (0.1 URR/h), the required Q_b would be 33 mL/min (ie, 8000 mL/240 min; 1.7 mL/kg/min); whereas, for a 360-minute session time (0.06 URR/h), the required Q_b would be 22 mL/min (1.1 mL/kg/min). A higher first-treatment URR target could be selected with appropriate extension of the treatment time to maintain a safe hourly URR.

Without URR-derived estimates for Q_b, blood flow must be determined empirically. When the initial BUN concentration is greater than 300 mg/dL, the blood flow rate should be limited to 1.0 to 1.5 mL/kg/min or less to prevent overly intense or rapid treatments. If the BUN concentration is between 150 and 300 mg/dL, blood flow should be limited to 1.5 to 2.0 mL/kg/min for initial treatments. By the third and subsequent treatments, the BUN is usually less than 150 mg/dL, and blood flow can be increased cautiously to 5 mL/kg/min. For intense treatments during the maintenance phase of management, blood flow rates between 10 and 20 mL/kg/min or the maximal flow achieved by the vascular access can be used.

For severely uremic cats or small dogs with BUN concentrations greater than 250 mg/dL, it is preferable to extend the treatment time to greater than 5 hours while providing exceptionally slow blood flow and urea clearance rates to deliver URR target less than 0.1 URR/hr. In some cases, it may not be possible to adjust the pump speed sufficiently to deliver a blood flow rate slow enough to correct the azotemia safely. For example, a 4 kg cat with an initial BUN of 330 mg/dL would require approximately 1.2 L of blood processing to achieve a treatment URR of 0.4 (or 40%) (see **Fig. 3**). If the treatment were delivered safely over 360 minutes (0.07 URR/hr), the required Q_b would be 3.3 mL/min. The dilemma is that most dialysis machines cannot accurately deliver a blood flow at this low rate. A faster Q_b will intensify the treatment and shorten the time-to-treatment goal unacceptably. At a Q_b of 10 mL/min (which is still too slow for many machines), the treatment time would be only 120 minutes (0.2 URR/hr) and unsafe for the target URR. In these circumstances, it is possible to extend the treatment time and lower the effective Q_b by alternating periods of active dialysis with deliberate intervals of bypass in which blood flow continues but dialysate flow (and hence dialysis) is stopped. By alternating 5 to 10 minutes of dialysis with 5 to 20 minutes of bypass, the effective Q_b and hourly URR is decreased and the time-to-treatment goal is extended by 2-fold to 4-fold. Ultrafiltration continues during bypass facilitating fluid removal during the extended treatment time. Blood flow can be increased during the bypass intervals to minimize clotting in the extracorporeal circuit without the risk of excessive dialysis.

Dialysate composition

Dialysate is formulated to maximize removal of uremia toxins, prevent depletion of normal blood solutes, replenish depleted solutes, and minimize physiologic and metabolic perturbations during and after the dialysis sessions. Conventional dialysate formulations for dogs and cats include sodium, approximately 145 mmol/L (dogs) and 150 mmol/L (cats); potassium, 0.0 to 3.0 mmol/L, bicarbonate, 25 to 40 mmol/L; chloride, approximately 113 mmol/L (dogs) and approximately 117 mmol/L (cats); calcium, 1.5 mmol/L; magnesium, 1.0 mmol/L; and dextrose, 200 mg/dL. The conventional dialysate flow is 500 mL/min counter current to the blood flow, and for practical purposes there is little advantage to decrease or increase dialysis flow to modify solute clearance unless Qb is greater than 300 mL/min.

Rapid solute removal exposes patients to nonphysiologic osmotic shifts that can cause osmotic disequilibrium between the vasculature, the interstitium, and cells. The accompanying shifts of fluid out of the vasculature and interstitium can cause signs of hypovolemia, hypotension, cramping, nausea, vomiting, and neurologic manifestations of dialysis disequilibrium syndrome. Patients may experience additional hypovolemia, hypotension, and poor catheter performance when ultrafiltration is superimposed on these effects. These signs are especially likely to develop early in the treatment when solute removal is greatest. To offset these trends, the sodium composition of the dialysate can be modeled (or profiled) so that dialysate sodium is adjusted systematically during the treatment to counteract solute disequilibrium, promote vascular refilling, and lessen or prevent these adverse signs.[40–43]

Dialysate sodium can be programmed to change in stepped or linear adjustments from hypernatremic (155–160 mmol/L) during the initial stages of the dialysis treatment to isonatremic or hyponatremic (150–140 mmol/L) at the termination of the treatment to offset the shifting of fluid out of the vasculature during the beginning of the treatment. During the hypernatremic phase of the profile, the sodium gradient from dialysate to plasma causes sodium loading and expansion of intravascular volume during this critical time when the extracorporeal circuit has filled, ultrafiltration has started, and solute removal and fluid shifts are greatest.[41–48] A modeled dialysate with a sodium concentration of 155 mmol/L for the initial 20% to 25% of the treatment, 150 mmol/L for the next 40% of the treatment, and 140 to 145 mmol/L for the remainder of the treatment has been is used for small dogs that are not hypertensive and predisposed to hypovolemia.[5] A respective sodium profile for cats of 160 mmol/L, 155 mmol/L, and 145 to 150 mmol/L appears to prevent hypotension in the face of the large extracorporeal volume required for hemodialysis.

Modeling dialysate sodium from isonatremic or hyponatremic to hypernatremic (dogs: 145 mmol/L for the initial 20% to 25% of the treatment, 150 mmol/L for the next 40% of the treatment, and 155 mmol/L for the remainder of the treatment; cats: 150 mmol/L, 155 mmol/L, and 160 mmol/L, respectively) has been used preventively to forestall neurologic manifestations of dialysis disequilibrium in severely azotemic animals. This sodium profile promotes osmotic (sodium) loading of the extracellular fluid at a time when urea disequilibrium can cause intracellular fluid shifts exacerbating cerebral edema and increased intracranial pressure.[5,7] Although this profile has been derived empirically and has not validated prospectively, it appears to offer protection in animals with BUN concentrations greater than 200 mg/dL. Sodium profiling will alter patients' sodium balance if not programmed to provide a neutral balance in which sodium loads are offset by sodium removal. A transient positive sodium balance is accepted in patients at risk for dialysis disequilibrium, but a positive sodium balance, postdialysis thirst, interdialysis weight gain, hyperkalemia, and hypertension may develop with sodium modeling.[7,49,50]

The dialysate potassium concentration is generally set at 3 mmol/L. This concentration can be used for most animals with acute or chronic renal failure. The bulk of potassium is sequestered in intracellular pools accessible to dialysis only following transfer to the vascular compartment. Dialysate potassium may be set to a lower concentration or 0 mmol/L to promote potassium transference during short dialysis sessions in animals with severe hyperkalemia or during treatments using slow blood-flow rates. Life-threatening electrocardiographic abnormalities resulting from hyperkalemia can be reversed completely within minutes of initiating hemodialysis using a dialysate containing 0 mmol/L of potassium.[5,7] Consequently, for dialysis sessions in which the predialysis serum potassium is greater than 6.0 mmol/L, a dialysate containing 0 mmol/L of potassium has been recommended.[1,3,5,8] Transfer of potassium from secluded intracellular pools may lag behind its rate of removal from the extracellular compartment causing transient hypokalemia at the end of dialysis sessions.[51] A rebound hyperkalemia may occur following the delayed transfer within hours of ending dialysis that extends to the next dialysis treatment. Daily dialysis may be required until the bulk of the potassium burden is corrected.

The use of dialysate potassium concentrations less than 1.0 mmol/L can generate large gradients or rapid changes in serum potassium concentration and potentially alter the intracellular/extracellular potassium ratio, the resting cell membrane potential, and increase the risk for ventricular arrhythmias and sudden cardiovascular death.[52–54] Sudden intradialytic cardiovascular death is uncommon in animal patients undergoing acute dialysis; however, these risks should be considered in the potassium prescription. For safety, the dialysate should be changed to 2 or 3 mmol/L of potassium with the appearance of ventricular arrhythmias during treatments employing a dialysate potassium less than 1.0 mmol/L.

Buffer formulation
The acid load in patients is buffered by base equivalents supplied by bicarbonate in the dialysate. Bicarbonate is formulated to a concentration between 25 and 40 mmol/L to promote accrual of new buffer by patients and to replenish deficits caused by uremia. A low dialysate bicarbonate concentration (25 mmol/L) has been suggested for patients with severe metabolic acidosis (serum bicarbonate, <12 mmol/L) to prevent rapid correction of the bicarbonate, increased cerebrospinal fluid (CSF) P_{CO_2}, and decreased CSF pH, that could precipitate paradoxic cerebral acidosis, cerebral edema, and dialysis disequilibrium syndrome.[1,5,55,56] In practice, it is difficult to change the serum bicarbonate concentration during short treatments at low blood flow rates even with high dialysate bicarbonate concentrations.[57] Dialysate bicarbonate can be set to 30 to 32 mmol/L with little likelihood of neurologic complication but should be decreased if the animal shows signs of tachypnea, restlessness, stupor, blindness, or other clinical evidence of impending dialysis disequilibrium syndrome.

Serum bicarbonate will increase more rapidly in animals with severe metabolic acidosis undergoing intensive dialysis (as in antifreeze intoxication), and dialysate bicarbonate concentration should be set between 20 and 25 mmol/L. A low dialysate bicarbonate concentration also should be selected for treatment of animals with metabolic or respiratory alkalosis. For maintenance hemodialysis treatments of greater than 4 hours, a dialysate bicarbonate concentration of 30 mmol/L will produce a postdialysis serum bicarbonate concentration of approximately 23 mmol/L. A dialysate concentration of 35 to 40 mmol/L yields greater accrual of buffer but often is associated with relentless panting during the treatment.

Dialysate additions

Hyperphosphatemia is a common feature of acute and chronic uremia,[58–60] and for both conditions the dialysate is formulated to contain no phosphate to facilitate phosphate removal. The dialysance of phosphate is more complex than for either urea or creatinine with 4 contributory pools possibly participating in its removal.[61] These interactive extracellular, intracellular, and reserve pools of phosphate are large, compartmentalized, poorly exchangeable with the serum pool, and subject to regulatory control. Consequently, the amount of phosphate eliminated during a dialysis treatment may be small compared with the overall phosphate load.[62,63] Hyperphosphatemia usually is not corrected during short and less intensive treatments, but it can be normalized or transient hypophosphatemia can develop with daily hemodialysis schedules or treatments longer than 4 or 5 hours.[5,61,63] Postdialysis hypophosphatemia quickly rebounds after treatment without development of clinical signs in uremic animals. In contrast, persistent hypophosphatemia and the risks of hemolysis, decreased oxygen delivery, or central nervous system and neuromuscular disturbances can develop in animals with normal predialysis serum phosphate concentrations when dialyzed with a standard (no phosphate) dialysate. For these conditions (ie, hemodialysis for toxin or fluid removal or well-managed patients with chronic kidney disease [CKD]), the dialysate phosphate concentration can be adjusted to physiologic ranges by addition of a neutral sodium phosphate solution (Fleet Enema, Fleet Brand Pharmaceuticals, C. B. Fleet Company, Inc, Lynchberg, VA, USA) to the dialysate concentrate. The required additive will vary with the proportioning ratio of the delivery system, but 67 mL (2.2 oz) or 133 mL (4.5 oz) of Fleet Enema solution per gallon of concentrate solution produces a dialysate phosphate concentration that is approximately 2 mg/dL or 4 mg/dL, respectively, when proportioned at roughly 1:40.[7]

Ethyl alcohol is an important additive to bicarbonate-based dialysate for the treatment of acute ethylene glycol or methanol intoxications.[64] Alcohol is added directly to the acid concentrate in sufficient volume to produce an enriched dialysate with a proportioned concentration of approximately 0.1% ethanol. The alcohol achieves a steady-state blood concentration that competitively inhibits alcohol dehydrogenase and minimizes further metabolism of the ethylene glycol during the treatment.[65]

Dialysate temperature

Dialysate temperature is an integral and functional component of the dialysis prescription. The temperature generally is set to the upper temperature limit of 38°C to 40°C for human delivery systems. Signs of chills at these temperatures can be controlled with heated blankets or heat lamps. Dialysate temperature also can influences the hemodynamic stability of patients during routine dialysis treatments and patients predisposed to hypotension during hemodialysis.[46,52,66–71] Heat accumulation from a dialysate temperature higher than body temperature can trigger a thermal homeostatic reflex causing peripheral vasodilatation, decreased peripheral vascular resistance, and symptomatic hypotension in animals undergoing ultrafiltration.[46,52,67,68,72] Animal patients may be protected inadvertently from moderate or overt hemodynamic events by the imposed lower temperature limits of human dialysis delivery systems. Hemodynamic tolerance during hemodialysis may be improved when patients maintain isothermic balance or are slightly cooled.[67–71] If core temperature increases greater than normal during the dialysis session, the dialysate temperature should be adjusted to maintain an isothermic core temperature throughout the treatment.[73] For animals predisposed or symptomatic for hypotension during dialysis, decreasing the dialysate temperature by 0.5°C to 1.5°C could induce peripheral vasoconstriction, central redistribution of blood, increase vascular resistance, and improve oxygenation during the treatment.[71]

Anticoagulation

The interaction of blood with the materials and irregularities of the dialysis membrane and extracorporeal circuit activates all triggers and components of the coagulation cascade and aggregation of platelets to promote thrombosis in the extracorporeal circuit. The predisposition to clotting necessitates routine anticoagulation of patients during the dialysis session.[74] Inadequate anticoagulation promotes thrombosis of the dialyzer, inefficient treatment, blood loss in the extracorporeal circuit, and potential for an abrupt cessation of the treatment. Excessive anticoagulation can cause serious bleeding, although this is infrequent. Unfractionated heparin has been used as the standard anticoagulant for intermittent hemodialysis for 40 years, but coagulation remains variable from animal to animal and treatment to treatment and requires individualized prescription.[7] See the section on heparin and anticoagulation in this edition for a detailed review of anticoagulation and its prescription in hemodialysis.

HEMODIALYSIS PRESCRIPTION FOR CHRONIC KIDNEY DISEASE

Experience with long-term intermittent hemodialysis for animals with chronic kidney disease is less than for acute uremia, yet hemodialysis is clearly indicated, effective, and affords a good quality of life for these animals. Many of the considerations used to prescribe acute hemodialysis are equally valid for chronic dialytic therapy; however, chronic malnutrition, fluid overload, hyperkalemia, hyperparathyroidism, metabolic bone disease, refractory hypertension, progressive anemia, infection, and drug interactions and toxicities replace concerns of hyperkalemia, hypothermia, hypovolemia, and dialysis disequilibrium syndrome so prevalent in animals with AKI. Adequacy standards for animals with CKD await future definition, but intensive hemodialysis provided every 2 to 3 days can augment the medical management of CKD.

The dialysis prescription for CKD is targeted to reduce the azotemia maximally during each session. Animals starting hemodialysis with severe uremia should be approached similarly to those with acute uremia until the predialysis BUN is less than 100 mg/dL. Thereafter, high-intensity dialysis schedules are well tolerated. Chronic dialysis prescriptions have been derived empirically but should promote a predialysis BUN less than 70 mg/dL, a postdialysis BUN less than 10 mg/dL, and a time-averaged BUN less than 50 mg/dL. The targeted $_{sp}Kt/V$ should be greater than 2.0 per session to provide an equivalent renal clearance (EKR) at least 10% of normal renal function (see later discussion). The choice of dialyzer and dialysate composition generally are the same as for maintenance treatments in animals with AKI. Blood flow rate can be increased cautiously to 15 to 25 mL/kg/min or to the performance limits of the vascular access, and dialysis time lengthened to 300 minutes or longer. The temptation to reduce dialysis time with opportunities to use higher-efficiency dialyzers and faster blood and dialysate flow rates should be avoided. Longer treatment times facilitate the removal of many solutes, including creatinine, phosphate, potassium, and middle-molecular-weight solutes that have different kinetic profiles and are slower to dialyze or have delayed transference from cellular or sequestered compartments than urea.[29,30,38,39,66]

Three treatments per week is the traditional schedule for human patients with end-stage CKD and is used for animal patients with serum creatinine concentrations greater than 8 mg/dL. A twice-weekly dialysis schedule has been used for animals with serum creatinine concentrations between 5 mg/dL and 8 mg/dL before starting dialysis therapy but likely represents the minimum schedule that will be beneficial.[27,30,38,39,66] The benefits of hemodialysis can only be improved with more frequent and longer dialysis schedules that impart greater efficiency to this intermittent clearance technique rather than more intensive dialysis provided less often.[27,29,38,39,63,75,76] A twice-weekly dialysis schedule will be effective only if patients have sufficient residual renal function (ie, a continuous clearance) to offset the effects of solute accumulation in the interdialysis interval to maintain predialysis azotemia and the TAC_{urea} within therapeutic guidelines (see **Fig. 1**).

HEMODIALYSIS PRESCRIPTION FOR DISORDERS OF FLUID BALANCE

Animals with oliguric or anuric AKI as well as nonoliguric animals with severe CKD are subject to fluid accumulation and life-threatening overhydration.[2,59] Once established, overhydration may not resolve with cessation of fluid delivery or diuretic administration, leaving no medical therapies to manage these disorders. Restoration of fluid balance is an important indication for hemodialysis and a consistent component of the dialysis prescription.

The volume and rate of fluid removal must be prescribed for each dialysis session based on the estimated fluid burden and deviation from the animal's ideal dry body weight. Ideal dry body weight is a progressively derived value determined as the body weight at which additional fluid removal would produce hypotension or signs of hypovolemia.[77,78] Ideal dry weight is usually predicted from recent historical weight measurements before the onset of illness, or it is estimated from the postdialysis weight when blood pressure was controlled or there was no demonstrated fluid accumulation. Ideal dry weight should not be considered a static parameter but should be redefined regularly to compensate for ongoing changes in lean body mass and body fat. The determination of dry weight can be elusive when based on clinical parameters alone and is facilitated by more objective techniques, including blood volume assessment and bioimpedance spectroscopy.

The rate and volume of ultrafiltration achieved is contingent on the hemodynamic stability of the animal. Ultrafiltration prescription may remove fluid from the vascular space faster than its rate of redistribution (refill) from the interstitium and intracellular compartments. This imbalance can promote hypovolemia, hypotension, and circulatory collapse if ultrafiltration is not prescribed and monitored carefully. Slow rates of ultrafiltration between 5 and 10 mL/kg/h are generally tolerated by dogs and cats, but faster rates must be prescribed cautiously and adjusted according to the animal's vital signs and blood pressure or by use of fluid monitoring equipment (eg, in-line blood volume monitor, venous oxygen saturation, continuous weight, bioimpedance spectroscopy).[7,77–82] In-line blood volume monitors are especially useful to assess the efficacy and the safety of ultrafiltration (**Fig. 4**).[7,83]

Animals often tolerate ultrafiltration better at the beginning of the treatment than at the end, and the rate of fluid removal can be profiled to achieve greater fluid losses at the beginning and scaled back later in the session to achieve the same treatment goal. Sodium profiling can be used to offset the hypovolemic and hypotensive effects of aggressive ultrafiltration to maximize fluid removal. Sodium loading during the hypernatremic stages of the modeling profile expands intravascular volume and facilitates redistribution of fluid from the interstitium and intracellular compartments.[5,7] The administration of small doses of 6% hydroxyethyl starch (hetastarch, at 1–2 mL/kg) helps to achieve ultrafiltration targets by maintaining intravascular volume, supporting

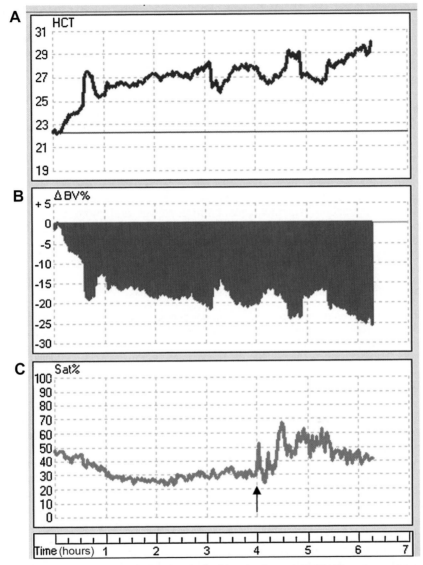

Fig. 4. Change in hematocrit (HCT, *A*), relative blood volume (⊿BV%, *B*), and venous oxygen saturation (Sat%, *C*) assessed by an in-line monitor in a dog with AKI during hemodialysis and continuous ultrafiltration. The figure illustrates the decreases in relative blood volume and venous oxygen saturation associated with hypovolemia induced by ultrafiltration. The late increase in oxygen saturation reflects the supplemental administration of oxygen (*arrow*). (*From* Cowgill LD, Francey T. Hemodialysis. In: DiBartola SP, editor. Fluid therapy in small animal practice. St Louis (MO): Elsevier; 2006. p. 650–77; with permission.)

vascular refilling, and preventing hypotension. The net volume of fluid subsequently removed will far exceed the volume administered and improve the efficiency of the ultrafiltration prescription.

Progressive hypovolemia from excessive ultrafiltration is detectable with in-line blood volume and venous oxygen saturation monitors well before development of hemodynamic signs, permitting adjustment of the ultrafiltration targets to avert hemo-dynamic complications (see **Fig. 4**). Venous oxygen saturation can also be observed visibly as darkening (desaturation) of blood in the extracorporeal circuit. Any decrease in venous oxygen saturation should prompt immediate assessment of patients and possible adjustment to the ultrafiltration goals. Changes in blood pressure and heart rate are rarely sensitive or early predictors of hypovolemia under these conditions.

Ultrafiltration and diffusive solute removal are independent processes controlled by separate functions of the delivery system. Animals with life-threatening fluid overload who do not need dialysis or who would be placed at risk from intensive dialysis can be managed safely by prescribing periods of ultrafiltration without hemodialysis or by scheduling independent periods of ultrafiltration before or after the azotemia has been treated to an appropriate URR. During ultrafiltration without dialysis, the machine is placed in bypass mode to stop dialysate flow to the dialyzer (and diffusive solute removal) while blood flow and transmembrane pressure gradients are maintained to continue ultrafiltration. This technique permits slower and more complete fluid removal without producing unsafe rates of diffusive hemodialysis. Isolated ultrafiltra-tion can be used in patients who are nonuremic to treat fluid congestion associated with heart failure and pulmonary edema refractory to diuretics.[84–90]

HEMODIALYSIS PRESCRIPTION FOR ACUTE INTOXICATIONS

Elimination of toxins and support for the consequences of intoxication are important but overshadowed applications of hemodialysis.[91–94] This use of hemodialysis is especially important if there has been a delay in medical management, there is limited endogenous clearance of the toxin or its metabolites, or there is no specific antidote for the toxicant. The dialytic removal of exogenous toxins is governed by the same molecular characteristics that define dialytic clearance of endogenous toxins. Molec-ular size, concentration in plasma water, distribution volume, degree of protein binding, and lipid solubility significantly influence the potential for a toxin's elimination.[9,10,95] Toxins or drugs with low molecular weights (<1500 Da), small volumes of distribution, and minimal protein binding are excellent candidates for diffusive and convective clearance. Ethylene glycol has a molecular weight of 62 Da, negligible protein binding, and a volume of distribution equivalent to total body water (0.5–0.8 L/kg) and is an excellent candidate for dialytic removal. With timely dialysis, ethylene glycol can be removed from the body before its enzymatic oxidation to more toxic metabolites, including glycoaldehyde, glycolate, glyoxylate, and oxalate.[5,10,92,95] Redistribution (rebound) of a toxin or drug from peripheral tissues or cellular compartments to plasma may limit the efficacy of dialysis to resolve the poisoning. If redistribution of the toxin from extravascular pools is much slower than its dialytic removal, the animal may become reintoxicated within hours after completing dialysis. For these sequestered toxins, the length and frequency of dialysis may need to be increased to facilitate their whole-body elimination.

Hemoperfusion is an adsorptive extracorporeal therapy used to manage endoge-nous and exogenous intoxications that are not cleared efficiently by hemodialysis. Adsorption is the principle of molecular attachment of a solute to a material surface. During hemoperfusion, blood is exposed directly to an adsorbent with the capacity to selectively or nonselectively bind toxins of defined chemical composition within the blood path. Hemoperfusion is more effective, eliminating high-molecular-weight, protein-bound, or lipid-soluble toxins or drugs that are cleared poorly, if at all, by hemodialysis. Toxic indications include mushroom poisoning (amanitin toxins and phalloidin), herbicides, insecticides, overmedication, hepatic failure, and sepsis.[10,91,96] Candidate toxins include barbiturates, salicylates, antimicrobials, antidepressants, chemotherapeutics, as well as nonsteroidal antiinflammatory drugs that historically have been regarded as poorly removed by either hemodialysis or hemoperfusion. Hemoperfusion represents an important extension of the extracorporeal therapies that can be provided when there are no effective or efficient therapeutic alternatives.

Activated charcoal has been the adsorbent used most commonly to eliminate endogenous and exogenous toxins in vivo.[10,96,97] Toxic substances are cleared according to their molecular size and affinity for the charcoal, their concentration in extracellular fluid, distribution volume, degree and affinity of protein binding, and lipid solubility. Activated carbons can remove solutes with a molecular mass ranging from 60 Da to greater than 40,000 Da.[9,97]

The use and established benefits of extracorporeal therapies for known toxins are poorly defined. Extracorporeal therapy is generally indicated if the clinical signs of intoxication are progressive or deteriorating and if the toxin can be cleared faster with the intervention than by endogenous clearance. For an intoxication like ethylene glycol, experience with hemodialysis is extensive, documented, and effective; and treatment decisions are easily justified. It can be recommended and justified above all other treatments. For other toxins, documented efficacy and outcomes are limited, but the window and opportunity for possible benefit is finite and decreases hourly following exposure.

The goals for extracorporeal therapies (hemodialysis or hemoperfusion) are to eliminate the toxin and its metabolites entirely from the animal as quickly as possible and to correct the accompanying fluid, electrolyte, and acid-base disturbances, and attending uremia. For suspected poisonings amenable to extracorporeal elimination hemodialysis or hemodialysis/hemoperfusion should be initiated immediately upon diagnosis to insure rapid elimination of the toxin regardless of previous antidotal therapy or the absence of clinical signs.

Ethylene glycol (antifreeze poisoning) is a common intoxication in companion animal practice.[59,60] It is generally possible to eliminate 90% to 95% or more of the toxin with a single intensive hemodialysis treatment.[5] Guidelines for the URR can be used to predict ethylene glycol reduction and guide the dialytic prescription as urea (MW: 60 Da) is similar in molecular size and distribution volume to ethylene glycol (MW: 62 Da).[5] To achieve a 90% ethylene glycol reduction during the course of treatment, it is necessary to select treatment parameters that would promote the same URR for that patient.

For animals that are nonazotemic, 90% to 100% of the toxin should be removed during the first dialysis treatment. A second treatment is provided if delivery is incomplete during the first session or if there is rebound of ethylene glycol after treatment. The highest volume, high flux hemodialyzer compatible with the extracorporeal volume requirement of the animal should be used to maximize diffusive removal of the toxins. Blood flow rates between 15 and 25 mL/kg/min or faster are tolerated. A standard dialysate flow between 500 and 600 mL/min is used but can be increased if the blood flow rate is greater than 300 mL/min. A dialysate formulated with 3 or 4 mmol/L potassium, 30 to 35 mmol/L bicarbonate, and a physiologic sodium concentration is appropriate unless specific electrolyte, acid-base, or hemodynamic disorders are present. A neutral sodium phosphate additive should be formulated in the dialysate for animals who are nonuremic to prevent hypophosphatemia (see previous discussion of dialysate additives). Ethanol should be added to the dialysate concentrate to achieve a dialysate ethanol concentration of approximately 0.1% in an effort to inhibit ongoing metabolism of ethylene glycol to its toxic metabolites during the extended hours of dialysis (see previous discussion of dialysate additives). Ultrafiltration can be used to correct pulmonary edema or congestive heart failure secondary to the toxin or fluid administration. However, ultrafiltration is minimally effective for pulmonary effusions arising from respiratory distress syndrome or uremic pneumonitis associated with antifreeze poisoning.

In patients who are uremic, the goals for aggressive toxin removal may be constrained by requirements to prevent dialysis disequilibrium syndrome, and dialysis must be delivered carefully to accommodate all of the patients' needs. If the BUN concentration is less than 125 mg/dL, an intensive treatment as used in patients who are nonuremic is suitable. For animals with BUN concentrations greater than 150 mg/dL, the dialysis prescription should targeted a 90% to 100% ethylene glycol reduction, but it must be delivered with a slow-extended treatment tailored to the hourly URR targets appropriate for the degree of azotemia (see **Table 2**). For patients who are severely uremic, safe urea reduction and greater toxin removal is achieved when dialysis is provided over 6 to 10 hours. The remainder of the dialysis prescription should be formulated to specific complications accompanying the uremia, fluid volume status, acid-base and electrolyte disturbances, and hemodynamic stability. Ethanol can be added to the dialysate concentrate as described for nonazotemic animals (previously discussed).

Application of extracorporeal therapies should not be limited to single modalities but should be sequenced and combined to best match the clinical course and kinetics of the toxicant. Continuous versus intermittent therapies should not be considered mutually exclusive but rather complimentary. There is little justification not to include a dialytic device with a hemoperfusion cartridge when contemplating hemoperfusion. For many toxins, hemodialysis has potential to improve toxin clearance in concert with hemoperfusion despite theoretical predictions to the contrary. The dose, blood concentration, changes in protein binding of the toxin, concurrent drugs/toxins, acid-base status, membrane type, and other variables may influence the diffusive potential of a toxin under different clinical conditions.

Hemoperfusion with activated charcoal is generally safe but poses potential disadvantages or complications not generally experienced with hemodialysis. One of the principal concerns is the innate hemocompatibility of the adsorbent. Hemoperfusion with activated charcoal (as well as other sorbent materials) can cause thrombocytopenia and leukopenia as platelets and leukocytes become adhered to the sorbent or entrapped in fibrin films or clots formed on the charcoal. Thrombocytopenia can be especially problematic if daily treatments are required that precludes adequate regeneration of platelets between treatments. If hemoperfusion is not combined with hemodialysis, patients may experience significant cooling because of the duration the extracorporeal blood is exposed to room temperature. The sorbent bed may also become saturated at unpredictable times during the treatment resulting in incomplete removal of the toxin.

HEMODIALYSIS OUTCOME/ADEQUACY AND QUANTIFICATION OF HEMODIALYSIS DELIVERY

Survival is the optimal outcome for animals managed with either acute or chronic hemodialysis. For AKI, survival is until renal function has recovered. For chronic kidney disease it is survival per se as there is no prospect for recovery of renal function. Survival is predicated on more than the adequacy of dialysis delivery and ultimately dependent on the diversity of the underlying etiology, comorbidities, age, chronicity, residual renal function, and economics that may be disassociated from recovery of renal function or adequate delivery of dialysis.[98] Consequently, survival is a difficult outcome parameter to correlate specifically to dialytic interventions, and, in animals, dialysis adequacy may be measured more appropriately by length of survival, owner-perceived quality of life (eg, activity, social interaction, appetite), elimination of uremic symptomatology (hypertension, hyperphosphatemia, anemia), nutritional adequacy, and elimination of dialysis-associated complications.

Nonetheless, the kinetically modeled dose of dialysis (Kt/V) has been shown to correlate independently with survival as an outcome in humans undergoing mainte-nance hemodialysis,[20–22] and it is likely to demonstrate similar links to the success and adequacy of dialysis in animals. The empirical use of proven standards of dialysis adequacy and clinical experience in human patients are useful first approximations for the establishment of veterinary guidelines of adequacy until evidence-based stan-dards are determined for animals.

QUANTIFICATION OF HEMODIALYSIS DELIVERY

The delivery (dose) and efficacy of hemodialysis can be expressed in a variety of ways with differing degrees of complexity and utility. Predialysis and immediate postdialysis concentrations of routine serum chemistries (eg, urea nitrogen, creatinine, phos-phorus, bicarbonate, electrolytes) are the simplest expressions of efficacy and can be interpreted similarly to their use in conventional therapy (see **Fig. 1; Fig. 5**).[28,99] Although useful, these instantaneous assessments do not permit prescription of dial-ysis to animals of differing size or metabolic status or clarify the impact of therapy beyond the dialysis session. The predialysis and postdialysis concentrations of plasma urea (or creatinine) can be expressed further as reduction ratios (URR and CrRR, respectively), which represents the fractional or percent change in urea during the treatment. Urea reduction ratio is the most universally used predictor of adequacy for a dialysis session in animals (see **Figs. 3** and **4**, see **Table 2**; Appendix 1, Equations 1 and 2).[1,3,5,7,22,100–102] Most cats and small dogs will achieve a URR approaching 95%. This level of treatment intensity is considerably higher than achieved in humans where the URR target is 60% to 65%. In large animals (50–70 kg), this degree of treat-ment intensity is often difficult to obtain, and a URR of 80% to 85% is typical.

Reduction ratios are convenient for clinical assessment but do not account for all aspects of solute transfer. Uremic toxicity and patient well-being are not predicted necessarily by the highest or lowest concentration or the intermittent change of specific uremia solutes.[103] The integrated exposure to uremia toxins over time is considered by some a more realistic determinant of well-being and therapeutic adequacy.[21,38,104,105] For urea, the integrated exposure can be expressed as the time-averaged concentration (TAC_{urea}) calculated as the area under the BUN profile (curve) divided by the duration of the dialysis cycle (see **Fig. 5**, Appendix 1; Equation 3). TAC_{urea} has been highly predictive of dialysis adequacy and outcome for survival but fails to distinguish the contributions of dialysis dose, urea generation, nutritional adequacy, residual clearance, and distribution volume to urea metabolism during the dialysis cycle.[22,104,106,107]

At face value, neither predialysis BUN nor TAC_{urea} are adequate surrogates to char-acterize the adequacy of dialytic therapy or urea metabolism. An animal with a low-predialysis BUN or TAC_{urea} can represent effective dialysis (high dialysis delivery), recovering renal function (increased residual renal clearance), inadequate nutrition (low urea generation rate or protein catabolic rate [PCR]), or volume overload (expanded urea distribution volume). Conversely, under dialysis, worsening renal

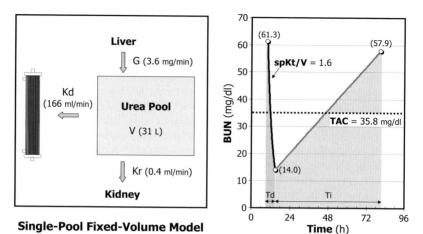

Single-Pool Fixed-Volume Model

Fig. 5. (*Left panel*) Single-pool, fixed-volume kinetic model of the urea metabolism and representative modeled kinetic parameters determined in a 33-kg dog on intermittent maintenance hemodialysis consuming approximately 56 g of dietary protein. Urea is generated in the liver as the major end product of protein metabolism. The urea generation rate, G (mg urea/min), determines the appearance of urea in the urea pool with a volume, V (L). Its removal from the urea pool is determined by the continuous residual renal clearance, Kr (mL/min), and intermittently by hemodialysis via the urea clearance of the dialyzer, Kd (mL/min). (*Right panel*) Graphic illustration of a 3-point BUN profile (before and after hemodialysis values in parentheses) that can be fitted to the single-pool model in the right panel. With direct measurement of renal and dialyzer urea clearances (Kr, see Appendix 1, Equation 5 and Kd Appendix 1, Equation 4, respectively), kinetic modeling allows computation the urea generation rate (G, see Appendix 1, Equation 7), the urea distribution volume (V, see Appendix 1, Equation 8), and the time-average concentration of BUN (TAC$_{urea}$, see Appendix 1, Equation 3). The dose of dialysis expressed as the fractional clearance of the urea distribution volume using single-pool kinetics ($_{sp}$Kt/V, see Appendix 1, Equation 9) can also be calculated. Td is the duration of dialysis, and Ti is the duration of the interdialytic interval. Area-under-the-curve (AUC) is the area under the BUN versus time curve and can be estimated using a trapezoidal method or, ideally, calculated by fitting the changes in BUN to the kinetic model. (*From* Cowgill LD, Francey T. Hemodialysis. In: DiBartola SP, editor. Fluid therapy in small animal practice. St Louis (MO): Elsevier; 2006. p. 650–77; with permission.)

function, high catabolic rate, or volume contraction can all be reflected by a high-predialysis BUN or TAC$_{urea}$.

The dose of dialysis delivered to patients can be defined alternatively by the amount of clearance (solute removal) provided by the hemodialyzer during the dialysis session. Using the instantaneous clearance of the dialyzer for urea (K$_d$, mL/min) and the dialysis session length (t, minutes), the dose of dialysis can be defined as K$_d$ x t, which predicts the volume of the patient cleared of urea during the treatment (mL). The value for the depurated volume can be indexed further to the total reservoir or distribution volume of urea in patients (V, mL) to compare treatment efficacy among patients of different body sizes as V is equal to the patients' total body water. This expression of dialysis dose is analogous to conventional dosing of drugs as mg/kg body weight. The value obtained with this kinetic expression, Kt/V, (see Appendix 1; Equation 9) is unitless and represents the fractional clearance of the urea distribution volume.[27–29,108] Kt/V has become the international reference for dialysis dosing and delivery.[31] This assessment of dialysis dose and intensity is founded on the instantaneous measurement of K$_d$ (see Appendix 1; Equation 4), which may not be constant over the session as well as the imprecise estimation of V from the patients weight and hydration status. It is limited also by simplifying assumptions regarding urea generation, fluid removal, and solute transference during the session, which requires more extensive evaluation.

A more precise understanding and integrated description of solute (ie, urea) dynamics throughout the dialysis session can be derived from kinetic modeling of the intradialytic and interdialytic changes in BUN similar to pharmacokinetic profiles used to describe drug metabolism.[27,109] Urea kinetic modeling is fundamental to understanding the prescription, monitoring, and quality assurance of hemodialysis procedures and must be familiar to all practitioners of this therapeutic modality. It dissects the mutually independent influences of dialysis, residual renal function, nutrition, catabolism, and distribution volume on the intermittent perturbations in urea concentration during and between the dialysis sessions. This kinetic approach to urea metabolism also yields the fractional clearance of urea (Kt/V) as a measure of the integrative dose in addition to G, PCR, and the distribution volume of urea (V) that are interdependent but otherwise beyond clinical assessment.

The simplest kinetic assessment of urea during intermittent hemodialysis is represented by a single-pool (sp), fixed-volume model, in which the entire distribution of urea is contained in a single pool (ie, total body water) that is presumed not to change in volume or urea input during the treatments (see **Fig. 5**).[30,33,105,109] In this simplified model, the only kinetic variable is total urea clearance (K) represented by the sum of residual renal clearance (Kr) and the clearance of the dialyzer (Kd) (see **Fig. 5**, Appendix 1; Equations 5 and 4, respectively).[30] The absolute removal of urea from this system will be reflected by the change in urea concentration at any time during dialysis such that:

$$C_t = C_0 e^{-Kt/V} \tag{1}$$

where C_t is the urea concentration at time = t; C_0 is the predialysis urea concentration at t = 0; K is the total urea clearance; and V is the volume of urea distribution. Rearrangement of Equation 1 provides Equation 2 for sp conditions,

$$_{sp}Kt/V = \ln(C_0/C_t) \tag{2}$$

Equation 2 is the fundamental kinetic expression for the fractional clearance of urea (dialysis dose) during a single dialysis session. In the simplified single-pool model, the kinetic prediction of dialysis dose can derived very simply from the measured predialysis and postdialysis BUN concentrations. It must be emphasized, that this expression represents a gross oversimplification of the events and kinetic variables during therapeutic hemodialysis and should be used only to provide a rough estimate of the integrated dialysis dose.

During a therapeutic dialysis session, the relationships between G, V, and K (illustrated in **Fig. 5**) are more complex, highly interdependent, and cannot be described mathematically by a single simple relationship. Mathematical description of each variable, however, can be defined in terms of the other two with formal urea kinetic modeling (see Appendix 1; Equations 6–9). When one of the variables (G, V, or K) is known, the others can be resolved by simultaneous iterative solution of the equations to yield a unique solution for the unknowns when residual renal clearance (K_r), instantaneous dialyzer clearance (K_d), ultrafiltration volume, and the measured changes in BUN during and after the treatment are known.[30,33,105,109] These computations are performed easily with commercially available software or can be programmed into routine spreadsheet applications.

This simplified single-pool, fixed-volume model loses accuracy if total body water changes during or between treatments, which is typical. The model also loses accuracy during high-intensity treatments of short duration, when urea distribution does not behave as a single homogenous compartment. Delayed diffusion from the intracellular compartment or variations in diffusion among discrete fluid compartments (eg, skin, muscle, gut) with different perfusion and transference characteristics creates a solute disequilibrium between compartments that promotes a postdialysis rebound of urea that is not predicted by immediate postdialysis blood sampling.[30,39,110] Deviations in the assumptions for single-pool, fixed-volume kinetics can be minimized by measurement of the postdialysis urea at 45 to 60 minutes after the end of the dialysis treatment rather than immediately postdialysis. By this time, intercompartmental shifts (or rebound) have reestablished solute equilibrium, and the plasma concentration reflects the equilibrated concentration of urea across all body compartments.[30,111]

Most dialysis treatments also require ultrafiltration, and urea generation proceeds throughout the session, which further deviate the serum urea concentration from single-pool predictions. These collective deviations from single-pool, fixed-volume assumptions can be incorporated into formal urea kinetic analyses by using more mathematically complex double-pool or noncompartmental kinetic modeling methods.[33] The double-pool variable-volume kinetic model accounts for intercompartmental solute diffusion during and after completion of hemodialysis. The $_{dp}Kt/V$ is regarded as the standard for dialysis dose but is not applied routinely because of its complexity. Optionally, correction algorithms that account for these compartmental deviations have been applied to single-pool assessments using additional blood sampling and appropriate software in human patients.[112] These correction formulas minimize many of the limitations of single-pool estimates but have not been validated in animals. More accurate predictions of dialysis dose can also be obtained using single-pool kinetic calculations by incorporating an equilibrated BUN obtained 45 to 60 minutes after cessation of the treatment as the end-dialysis value. Use of the equilibrated BUN yields $_{e}Kt/V$ as a measure of dialysis dose that closely approximates the $_{dp}Kt/V$ and better reflects whole-patient urea clearance. Both the $_{e}Kt/V$ and the $_{dp}Kt/V$ assessments of dialysis dose will be lower than the dose predicted as the $_{sp}Kt/V$.

Ionic Dialysance

Online measurement of these kinetic determinants of dialyzer performance and dialysis dose can be derived for each dialysis treatment as an alternative to blood-based modeling methods with ionic dialysance techniques available on modern delivery systems.[113–116] Dialysance is a measure of solute mass transfer across the dialysis membrane when the solute is present in both the blood and dialysate. The clearance of a solute by the dialyzer is equal to its dialysance when the solute is present only in the blood and is absent in the dialysate. Ionic dialysance is a kinetic assessment of the transfer characteristics of the ionic solutes in the blood and dialysate. The collective concentration of ionic solutes in solution can be measured by the conductivity of the solution to the passage of an electric current. The conductivity of both plasma and the dialysate is influenced primarily by the concentration of sodium and chloride and will change with perturbations of these solutes.[113,115] The collective dialysance of small molecular weight ions (eg, sodium) is considered equivalent to the dialysance of urea, and, consequently, ionic dialysance can be used as a reasonable surrogate for the dialysance of urea. In conventional single-pass hemodialysis circuits in which the dialysate contains no urea, urea dialysance becomes equal to urea clearance, and ionic dialysance becomes an acceptable predictor of the urea clearance of the dialyzer, $K_{d\text{-urea}}$. The ionic dialysance is computed from measurements of dialysate conductivity (concentration of ionic solutes) at the inlet and outlet ports of the dialyzer in response to transient changes in inlet conductivity of the dialysate and the instantaneous dialysate and blood flow rates.[115,117–121]

When ionic dialysance is programmed sequentially during the dialysis treatment, serial updates of the instantaneous clearance ($K_{d\text{-ionic}}$) of the dialyzer can be monitored, and the depurated volume for treatment ($K_{d\text{-ionic}} \times t$) is predicted at the end of the session. The $_{ionic}Kt/V$, as a surrogate for $_{sp}Kt/V$, is provided when the ionic dialysance is indexed to urea distribution volume, V. The availability and simplicity of ionic dialysance to predict dialysis delivery at every treatment should promote a better understanding of the kinetics of dialytic therapy and the efficacy of dialysis prescriptions.

It is also possible to make interim projections of the $_{ionic}Kt/V$ for the session to insure the treatment targets will be met by the end of the scheduled session time. If therapeutic targets will not me met under current circumstances, adjustments to treatment time, blood flow, and dialysate flow, access repositioning, or dialyzer exchange can be initiated to modify the forecast treatment to assure adequacy.[122] Sudden or progressive decreases of $K_{d\text{-ionic}}$ during the treatment can alert to possible clotting in the dialyzer or development of access recirculation that may compromise the adequacy of the treatment (**Fig. 6**).

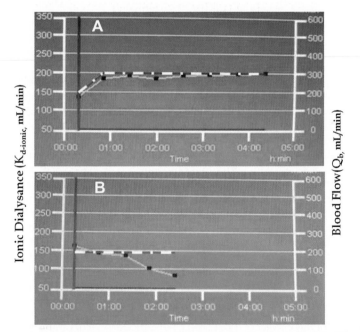

Fig. 6. Screen shots of the ionic dialysance display of the Gambro Phoenix (Gambro USA, Lakewood, CO, USA) illustrating the ionic dialysance (*solid line*, left axis) and blood flow (*dashed line*, right axis) throughout a dialysis session. Panel *A* demonstrates constant dialyzer performance and extraction ratio during the treatment with a $K_{d\text{-ionic}}$ of approximately 195 mL/min at a Q_b of 300 mL/min (extraction ratio, 0.65). Panel *B* illustrates a marked and progressive decrease in $K_{d\text{-ionic}}$ after 1.5 hours of treatment associated with extensive clotting of the dialyzer necessitating termination of the treatment. (*From* Cowgill LD, Francey T. Hemodialysis and extracorporeal therapy. In: DiBartola SP, editor. Fluid therapy in small animal practice. St Louis (MO): Elsevier; 2010, in press; with permission.)

Hemodialysis Schedule

Animal hemodialysis is provided intermittently three times weekly based on human convention. This schedule represents a compromise between clinical benefits, time constraints, and financial burden. However, there are marked theoretical efficiencies and clinical benefits to schedules with increased dialysis frequency.[38,75,76,123–126] For example, six treatments per week at a $_{sp}Kt/V$ of 1.0 per treatment are more efficient and provide better clinical outcomes than three conventional treatments per week with a $_{sp}Kt/V$ of 2.0 per treatment. To reconcile these differences, the concept of standard Kt/V ($_{std}Kt/V$; see Appendix 1; Equation 10) has been proposed to compensate for the differences in efficiency when comparing schedules with different intermittence.[28,103,125,127] Standard Kt/V is a hypothetical continuous urea clearance that would achieve a constant blood urea concentration identical to the average pre-dialysis urea concentration for all intermittent treatments provided during the week. This theoretical concept allows comparisons among dialysis schedules with differing dialysis times and intervals, including the extreme case of continuous therapy.

A dialysis schedule with 3 4-hour treatments per week with a $_{sp}Kt/V$ of 2.0 per treatment is equivalent to a $_{std}Kt/V$ of 2.7. Increasing the schedule to 6 2-hour treatments per week ($_{sp}Kt/V$, 1.0 per treatment) with the same total 12 hours of weekly dialysis substantially increases the amount (efficiency) of dialysis delivered to an equivalent $_{std}Kt/V$ of 3.9 (see Appendix 1, Equation 10). Stated differently, a thrice-weekly, 240-minute treatment schedule ($_{std}Kt/V$, 2.7) requiring 12 hours of treatment could be provided with equivalent efficacy in 70 minutes per session if provided 6 times weekly for a total weekly dialysis time of 7 hours. Although reduction of the individual treatment time is possible according to this analogy (for illustrative purposes), this recommendation would not be clinically prudent.[36,39,125,128] Conversely, decreasing the frequency of dialysis to 2 treatments per week would require extension of each treatment to almost 24 hours to achieve an equivalent $_{std}Kt/V$. These quantitative predictions illustrate the marked benefits to increased frequency of therapy and conversely indicate the difficulty to compensate for decreased frequency of therapy with longer treatment times.[29,30,76]

The intermittent kinetics of hemodialysis can be converted to a continuous equivalent clearance as an alternative to $_{sdt}Kt/V$ for comparing the equivalency of intermittent and continuous therapies, including residual renal function.[29,99,129] This concept is more intuitive for clinicians because the relative contribution of dialysis can be compared directly to residual renal function and to other intermittent or continuous dialytic therapies (see Appendix 1; Equation 11). Total patient clearance (renal clearance, Kr, and dialyzer clearance, EKR) is expressed in the familiar term (milliliter per minute) of clearance, similar to glomerular filtration rate, and the resulting total clearance can be used to predict the expected uremic morbidity, comparable to an earlier stages of kidney disease.

Future Considerations for Outcomes Assessment

A prerequisite for the validity of most urea kinetic modeling algorithms is the presumption of steady-state urea metabolism (ie, constant food intake [quality and quantity]), constant endogenous nitrogen metabolism and catabolism, stable body weight, and a regular dialysis schedule. These conditions rarely exist for most veterinary applications prescribed for acute kidney failure; however, classic double-pool, equilibrated and EKR analyses appear valid under these conditions in human patients if careful attention is paid to the accuracy of all input variables.[130–132]

The rationale to scale dialysis dose to the nebulous index (V) that cannot be readily measured has kinetic justification and historical acceptance. The first-order kinetics of urea removal by dialysis proceeds with an elimination constant equal to K_d/V, which is a measure of the intensity of the treatment. Even though V is not measured directly, it can be derived mathematically to yield the expression, Kt/V, with kinetic modeling. Recently, however, the universality of scaling dialysis dose to the urea distribution volume has been questioned in human patients as the distribution volume varies independently of body size, between genders, and in patients of differing body composition.[133] Consequently, scaling dialysis dose to V may promote undertreatment in some individuals and relative overtreatment in others. The comparative significance of this issue has not been addressed in animals, but it is likely that the diversity of size, species, and breed in addition to gender in animal patients could impose even greater variance in the relative urea distribution volume than seen in humans.

The effect of dose of dialysis on outcome has been demonstrated in humans with end-stage chronic kidney disease in several large-scale clinical studies.[20–23,28,120] The dose of dialysis that is adequate to manage dogs and cats with either acute or chronic kidney failure needs to be established using appropriate tools for treatment quantification. However, until these parameters are established, routine application of UKM extends the therapeutic insights of dialysis delivery far beyond reliance on routine chemistry tests and provides insight into the assessment and clinical management of uremic animals. Kinetic parameters and quantitation of dialysis delivery are important tools for quality assurance of dialytic therapy in animals, but they are not therapeutic goals per se. The provision of a yet-to-be-defined minimal dose of dialysis is only one of the requirements of therapeutic adequacy, and management of uremia necessitates an individually tailored global approach to the animal.

SUMMARY

The establishment of hemodialysis and extracorporeal therapies in animal patients has had a long and sluggish evolution from experimental curiosity to therapeutic mainstream. Currently, hemodialysis stands as a novel and technically complex therapy with narrowly targeted clinical indications and regional availability. Intermittent hemodialysis serves a vital role in the therapeutic stratification of dogs and cats with uremia that remain nonresponsive to conventional medical therapy. Hemodialysis improves survival for animals with AKI beyond what would be expected with conventional management of the same animals. Clinical evidence and experience in human patients suggests a role for earlier intervention with renal replacement to avoid the morbidity of uremia and to promote better metabolic stability and recovery. For a large population of animal patients, it is the advanced standard for the management of acute and chronic uremia, life-threatening poisoning, and fluid overload for which there is no alternative therapy.

APPENDIX 1: MATHEMATICAL EQUATIONS USED FOR DIALYSIS QUANTIFICATION

Equation 1: urea reduction ratio

$$\text{URR}\,(\%) = \frac{_{pre}\text{BUN} - {}_{post}\text{BUN}}{_{pre}\text{BUN}} \times 100$$

or

$$\text{URR}\,(\%) = \left(1 - \frac{_{post}\text{BUN}}{_{pre}\text{BUN}}\right) \times 100$$

Equation 2: creatinine reduction ratio

$$\text{CrRR (\%)} = \frac{_{pre}\text{Crea} - _{post}\text{Crea}}{_{pre}\text{Crea}} \times 100$$

or

$$\text{CrRR (\%)} = \left(1 - \frac{_{post}\text{Crea}}{_{pre}\text{Crea}}\right) \times 100$$

Abbreviations: Crea, creatinine concentration (mg/dl); CrRR, creatinine reduction ratio (%); pre, predialysis; post, postdialysis.

Equation 3: time-averaged urea concentration

$$\text{TAC} = \frac{\text{AUC}}{(t_d + t_i)}$$

Abbreviations: AUC, area under the BUN-Time profile curve (mg/dl x min); TAC, time-averaged urea concentration (mg/dl); t_d, time on dialysis (min); t_i, duration of the interdialytic interval (min).

Equation 4: instantaneous hemodialyzer urea clearance

$$\text{Kd} = Q_b \cdot \frac{\text{BUN}_{in} - \text{BUN}_{out}}{\text{BUN}_{in}}$$

Abbreviations: BUN_{in}, BUN concentration at the dialyzer inlet (mg/dl); BUN_{out}, BUN concentration at the dialyzer outlet (mg/dl); Kd, hemodialyzer urea clearance (ml/min); Qb, blood flow rate through the hemodialyzer (ml/min).

Equation 5: residual renal clearance

$$\text{Kr} = \frac{U_{urea} \cdot V}{\text{BUN}}$$

Abbreviations: Kr, residual renal clearance for urea (ml/min); U_{urea}, urinary urea nitrogen concentration (mg/dl); V, urine flow rate (ml/min).

Equations 6–10: Kinetics of urea using a single-pool fixed-volume model and resulting dose of dialysis: intradialytic and interdialytic BUN concentration (equation 6), urea generation rate (equation 7), and urea distribution volume (equation 8). In equation 6, the interdialytic BUN concentration is obtained by setting Kd as 0. The mathematical solution of equations 7 and 8 requires iterative simultaneous calculations as G is a function of V and reciprocally. The transformation of the dose of dialysis in standard Kt/V (equation 10) allows comparison of different dialysis schedules and modalities.

Equation 6: BUN concentration at time t

$$C_t = C_0 \cdot e^{-(K_r + Kd)t/V} + \frac{G \cdot \left[1 - e^{-(K_r + K_d)t/V}\right]}{K_r + K_d}$$

Equation 7: urea generation rate

$$G = K_r \cdot \left[\frac{C_3 - C_2 \cdot e^{-K_r T_i / V}}{1 - e^{-K_r T_i / V}} \right]$$

Equation 8: volume of distribution of urea

$$V = \frac{(K_r + K_d) \cdot T_d}{\ln \left[\frac{G - C_1 (K_d + K_r)}{G - C_2 (K_d + K_2)} \right]}$$

Equation 9: single-pool Kt/V

$$spKt/V = K_d \cdot T_d / V$$

Equation 10: standard Kt/V

$$stdKt/V = \frac{10080 \cdot (1 - e^{-Kt/V})}{T_d \cdot \left[\frac{(1 - e^{-Kt/V})}{Kt/V} + \frac{10080}{N \cdot T_d} - 1 \right]}$$

Abbreviations: C_t, BUN concentration at time t (mg/ml), where t = 0 at the beginning of the interval analyzed, t = 1 predialysis, t = 2 postdialysis, t = 3 predialysis for the next session; G, urea generation rate (mg/min); Kd, dialyzer urea clearance (ml/min); Kr, residual renal urea clearance (ml/min); $_{sp}$Kt/V, single-pool Kt/V; $_{std}$Kt/V, standard Kt/V; N, number of dialysis treatments per week; T_d, duration of the dialysis session (min); T_i, duration of the interdialytic interval (min); V, urea distribution volume (ml).

Equation 11: continuous equivalent of intermittent clearance

$$EKR = G/TAC$$

Abbreviations: EKR, continuous equivalent of urea clearance (ml/min); G, urea generation rate (mg/min); TAC, time-averaged BUN concentration (mg/ml).

REFERENCES

1. Cowgill LD, Elliott DA. Hemodialysis. In: DiBartola SP, editor. Fluid therapy in small animal practice. Philadelphia: WB Saunders; 2000. p. 528–47.
2. Cowgill LD, Francey T. Acute uremia. In: Ettinger SJ, Feldman EC, editors. Textbook of veterinary internal medicine: diseases of the dog and cat. Philadelphia: WB Saunders; 2004. p. 1731–51.
3. Cowgill LD, Langston CE. Role of hemodialysis in the management of dogs and cats with renal failure. Vet Clin North Am Small Anim Pract 1996;26:1347–78.
4. Langston CE, Cowgill LD, Spano JA. Applications and outcome of hemodialysis in cats: a review of 29 cases. J Vet Intern Med 1997;11:348–55.
5. Cowgill LD, Francey T. Hemodialysis. In: DiBartola SP, editor. Fluid therapy in small animal practice. St Louis (MO): Elsevier; 2006. p. 650–77.
6. ICowgill LD, Langston CE. History of hemodialysis in dogs and companion animals. In: TS Ing, MA Rahman, CM Kjellstrand, editors. Dialysis: history, development and promise. Singapore: World Scientific Publishing Company, in press.
7. Cowgill LD, Francey T. Hemodialysis and extracorporeal blood purification. In: DiBartola SP, editor. Fluid therapy in small animal practice. 4th edition. St Louis (MO): Elsevier, in press.

8. Fischer JR, Pantaleo V, Francey T, et al. Veterinary hemodialysis: advances in management and technology. Vet Clin North Am Small Anim Pract 2004;34: 935–67, vi–vii.

9. Winchester JF. Dialysis and hemoperfusion in poisoning. Adv Ren Replace Ther 2002;9:26–30.

10. Smith JP, Chang IJ. Extracorporeal treatment of poisoning. In: Brenner BM, editor. Brenner and Rector's The Kidney. 8th Edition. Philadelphia: Saunders/ Elsevier; 2008. p. 2081–102.

11. Scott NE, Francey T, Jandrye K. Baclofen intoxication in a dog successfully treated with hemodialysis and hemoperfusion coupled with intensive supportive care. J Vet Emerg Crit Care 2007;17:191–6.

12. Vanholder R, De Smet R, Glorieux G, et al. Review on uremic toxins: classification, concentration, and interindividual variability. Kidney Int 2003;63:1934–43.

13. Vanholder R, Van Laecke S. Glorieux G. The middle-molecule hypothesis 30 years after: lost and rediscovered in the universe of uremic toxicity? J Nephrol 2008;21(2):146–60.

14. Vanholder R, Baurmeister U, Brunet P, et al. European Uremic Toxin Work Group. A bench to bedside view of uremic toxins. J Am Soc Nephrol 2008; 19(5):863–70.

15. Raff AC, Meyer TW, Hostetter TH. New insights into uremic toxicity. Curr Opin Nephrol Hypertens 2008;17(6):560–5.

16. Depner TA. Uremic toxicity: urea and beyond. Semin Dial 2001;14:246–51.

17. Vanholder R, Glorieux G, De Smet R, et al. New insights in uremic toxins. Kidney Int 2003;63:S6–10.

18. Vanholder R, Glorieux G, De Smet R, et al. Low water-soluble uremic toxins. Adv Ren Replace Ther 2003;10:257–69.

19. Vanholder R, Glorieux G, Van Biesen W. Advantages of new hemodialysis membranes and equipment. Nephron Clin Pract 2010;114(3):c165–72.

20. Held PJ, Port FK, Wolfe RA, et al. The dose of hemodialysis and patient mortality. Kidney Int 1996;50:550–6.

21. Lowrie EG, Laird NM, Parker TF, et al. Effect of the hemodialysis prescription of patient morbidity: report from the National Cooperative Dialysis Study. N Engl J Med 1981;305:1176–81.

22. Owen WF Jr, Lew NL, Liu Y, et al. The urea reduction ratio and serum albumin concentration as predictors of mortality in patients undergoing hemodialysis. N Engl J Med 1993;329:1001–6.

23. Parker TF 3rd, Husni L, Huang W, et al. Survival of hemodialysis patients in the United States is improved with a greater quantity of dialysis. Am J Kidney Dis 1994;23:670–80.

24. Henle T, Miyata T. Advanced glycation end products in uremia. Adv Ren Replace Ther 2003;10:321–31.

25. Herget-Rosenthal S, Glorieux G, Jankowski J, et al. Uremic toxins in acute kidney injury. Semin Dial 2009;22(4):445–8.

26. Johnson WJ, Hagge WW, Wagoner RD, et al. Effects of urea loading in patients with far-advanced renal failure. Mayo Clin Proc 1972;47:21–9.

27. Gotch FA. Evolution of the single-pool urea kinetic model. Semin Dial 2001;14: 252–6.

28. Suri RS, Depner T, Lindsay RM. Dialysis prescription and dose monitoring in frequent hemodialysis. Contrib Nephrol 2004;145:75–88.

29. Depner TA, Bhat A. Quantifying daily hemodialysis. Semin Dial 2004;17(2): 79–84.

30. Depner TA. Hemodialysis adequacy: basic essentials and practical points for the nephrologist in training. Hemodial Int 2005;9(3):241–54.
31. Hemodialysis Adequacy 2006 Work Group. Clinical practice guidelines for hemodialysis adequacy, update 2006. Am J Kidney Dis 2006;48(Suppl 1): S2–90.
32. Vanholder RC, Glorieux GL, De Smet RV. Uremic toxins: removal with different therapies. Hemodial Int 2003;7:162–7.
33. Sargent JA, Gotch FA. Principles and biophysics of dialysis. In: Maher JF, editor. Replacement of renal function by dialysis: a textbook of dialysis. Boston: Kluwer Academic Publishers; 1989. p. 87–143.
34. Eknoyan G, Beck GJ, Cheung AK, et al. Effect of dialysis dose and membrane flux in maintenance hemodialysis. N Engl J Med 2002;347:2010–9.
35. Winchester JF, Audia PF. Extracorporeal strategies for the removal of middle molecules. Semin Dial 2006;19(2):110–4.
36. McFarlane PA. More of the same: Improving outcomes through intensive hemo-dialysis. Semin Dial 2009;22(6):598–602.
37. Yeun JY, Depner TA. Complications related to inadequate delivered dose: recognition and management in acute and chronic dialysis. In: Lameire N, Mehta RL, editors. Complications of dialysis. New York: Marcel Dekker, Inc; 2000. p. 89–115.
38. Goldfarb-Rumyantzev AS, Cheung AK, Leypoldt JK. Computer simulation of small-solute and middle-molecule removal during short daily and long thrice-weekly hemodialysis. Am J Kidney Dis 2002;40(6):1211–8.
39. Eloot S, Van Biesen W, Dhondt A, et al. Impact of hemodialysis duration on the removal of uremic retention solutes. Kidney Int 2008;73(6):765–70.
40. Flanigan MJ. Role of sodium in hemodialysis. Kidney Int Suppl 2000;76:S72–8.
41. Stiller S, Bonnie-Schorn E, Grassmann A, et al. A critical review of sodium profiling for hemodialysis. Semin Dial 2001;14:337–47.
42. Brummelhuis WJ, van Geest RJ, van Schelven LJ, et al. Sodium profiling, but not cool dialysate, increases the absolute plasma refill rate during hemodialysis. ASAIO J 2009;55(6):575–80.
43. Phipps LM, Harris DC. Review: modeling the dialysate. Nephrology (Carlton) 2010;15(4):393–8.
44. Al-Hilali N, Al-Humoud HM, Ninan VT, et al. Profiled hemodialysis reduces intra-dialytic symptoms. Transplant Proc 2004;36:1827–8.
45. Coli L, Ursino M, Donati G, et al. Clinical application of sodium profiling in the treatment of intradialytic hypotension. Int J Artif Organs 2003;26:715–22.
46. Sherman RA. Modifying the dialysis prescription to reduce intradialytic hypoten-sion. Am J Kidney Dis 2001;38:S18–25.
47. Song JH, Park GH, Lee SY, et al. Effect of sodium balance and the combination of ultrafiltration profile during sodium profiling hemodialysis on the maintenance of the quality of dialysis and sodium and fluid balances. J Am Soc Nephrol 2005; 16:237–46.
48. Zhou YL, Liu HL, Duan XF, et al. Impact of sodium and ultrafiltration profiling on haemodialysis-related hypotension. Nephrol Dial Transplant 2006;21(11): 3231–7.
49. De Nicola L, Bellizzi V, Minutolo R, et al. Effect of dialysate sodium concentration on interdialytic increase of potassium. J Am Soc Nephrol 2000;11:2337–43.
50. Depner TA, Ing TS. Toxic fluid flux? Am J Kidney Dis 2010;56(1):1–4.
51. Redaelli B, Bonoldi G, Di Filippo G, et al. Behaviour of potassium removal in different dialytic schedules. Nephrol Dial Transplant 1998;13(Suppl 6):35–8.

52. Locatelli F, Covic A, Chazot C, et al. Optimal composition of the dialysate, with emphasis on its influence on blood pressure. Nephrol Dial Transplant 2004;19: 785–96.
53. Redaelli B. Electrolyte modeling in haemodialysis–potassium. Nephrol Dial Transplant 1996;11(Suppl 2):39–41.
54. Karnik JA, Young BS, Lew NL, et al. Cardiac arrest and sudden death in dialysis units. Kidney Int 2001;60(1):350–7.
55. Arieff AI. Dialysis disequilibrium syndrome: current concepts on pathogenesis and prevention. Kidney Int 1994;45:629–35.
56. Arieff AI, Lazarowitz VC, Guisado R. Experimental dialysis disequilibrium syndrome: prevention with glycerol. Kidney Int 1978;14:270–8.
57. Feriani M. Behaviour of acid-base control with different dialysis schedules. Nephrol Dial Transplant 1998;13(Suppl 6):62–5.
58. Polzin DJ. Chronic Kidney Disease. In: Ettinger SJ, Feldman CE, editors. Textbook of Veterinary Internal Medicine. Philadephia: Saunders Elsevier; 2010. p. 1990–2020.
59. Cowgill LD, Langston CE. Acute Kidney Injury. In: Bartges J, Polzin D, editors. Nephrology and Urology of Small Animals. Wiley-Blackwell, in press.
60. Langston CE. Acute Uremia. In: Ettinger SJ, Feldman CE, editors. Textbook of Veterinary Internal Medicine. Philadephia: Saunders Elsevier; 2010. p. 1969–84.
61. Spalding EM, Chamney PW, Farrington K. Phosphate kinetics during hemodialysis: Evidence for biphasic regulation. Kidney Int 2002;61(2):655–67.
62. Messa P, Gropuzzo M, Cleva M, et al. Behaviour of phosphate removal with different dialysis schedules. Nephrol Dial Transplant 1998;13(Suppl 6):43–8.
63. Kuhlmann MK. Phosphate elimination in modalities of hemodialysis and peritoneal dialysis. Blood Purif 2010;29(2):137–44.
64. Chow MT, Di Silvestro VA, Yung CY, et al. Treatment of acute methanol intoxication with hemodialysis using an ethanol-enriched, bicarbonate-based dialysate. Am J Kidney Dis 1997;30:568–70.
65. Noghnogh AA, Reid RW, Nawab ZM, et al. Preparation of ethanol-enriched, bicarbonate-based hemodialysates. Artif Organs 1999;23:208–9.
66. Locatelli F, Buoncristiani U, Canaud B, et al. Haemodialysis with on-line monitoring equipment: tools or toys? Nephrol Dial Transplant 2005;20:22–33.
67. Maggiore Q. Isothermic dialysis for hypotension-prone patients. Semin Dial 2002;15:187–90.
68. Maggiore Q, Pizzarelli F, Santoro A, et al. The effects of control of thermal balance on vascular stability in hemodialysis patients: results of the European randomized clinical trial. Am J Kidney Dis 2002;40:280–90.
69. Selby NM, McIntyre CW. How should dialysis fluid be individualized for the chronic hemodialysis patient? Temperature. Semin Dial 2008;21(3):229–31.
70. Chesterton LJ, Selby NM, Burton JO, et al. Cool dialysate reduces asymptomatic intradialytic hypotension and increases baroreflex variability. Hemodial Int 2009;13(2):189–96.
71. van der Sande FM, Wystrychowski G, Kooman JP, et al. Control of core temperature and blood pressure stability during hemodialysis. Clin J Am Soc Nephrol 2009;4(1):93–8.
72. Rosales LM, Schneditz D, Morris AT, et al. Isothermic hemodialysis and ultrafiltration. Am J Kidney Dis 2000;36:353–61.
73. Pergola PE, Habiba NM, Johnson JM. Body temperature regulation during hemodialysis in long-term patients: is it time to change dialysate temperature prescription? Am J Kidney Dis 2004;44:155–65.

74. Suranyi M, Chow JS. Review: anticoagulation for haemodialysis. Nephrology (Carlton) 2010;15(4):386–92.
75. Depner T. Benefits of more frequent dialysis: lower TAC at the same Kt/V. Nephrol Dial Transplant 1998;13:20–4.
76. Suri R, Depner TA, Blake PG, et al. Adequacy of quotidian hemodialysis. Am J Kidney Dis 2003;42:42–8.
77. Ishibe S, Peixoto AJ. Methods of assessment of volume status and intercompartmental fluid shifts in hemodialysis patients: implications in clinical practice. Semin Dial 2004;17:37–43.
78. Jaeger JQ, Mehta RL. Assessment of dry weight in hemodialysis: an overview. J Am Soc Nephrol 1999;10:392–403.
79. Lambie SH, McIntyre CW. Developments in online monitoring of haemodialysis patients: towards global assessment of dialysis adequacy. Curr Opin Nephrol Hypertens 2003;12:633–8.
80. Schroeder KL, Sallustio JE, Ross EA. Continuous haematocrit monitoring during intradialytic hypotension: precipitous decline in plasma refill rates. Nephrol Dial Transplant 2004;19:652–6.
81. Zhu F, Kuhlmann MK, Sarkar S, et al. Adjustment of dry weight in hemodialysis patients using intradialytic continuous multifrequency bioimpedance of the calf. Int J Artif Organs 2004;27:104–9.
82. Zhu F, Sarkar S, Kaitwatcharachai C, et al. Methods and reproducibility of measurement of resistivity in the calf using regional bioimpedance analysis. Blood Purif 2003;21:131–6.
83. Steuer RR, Bell DA, Barrett LL. Optical measurement of hematocrit and other biological constituents in renal therapy. Adv Ren Replace Ther 1999;6:217–24.
84. Agostoni PG, Marenzi GC. Sustained benefit from ultrafiltration in moderate congestive heart failure. Cardiology 2001;96:183–9.
85. Marenzi G, Lauri G, Grazi M, et al. Circulatory response to fluid overload removal by extracorporeal ultrafiltration in refractory congestive heart failure. J Am Coll Cardiol 2001;38:963–8.
86. Ronco C, Ricci Z, Brendolan A, et al. Ultrafiltration in patients with hypervolemia and congestive heart failure. Blood Purif 2004;22:150–63.
87. Sheppard R, Panyon J, Pohwani AL, et al. Intermittent outpatient ultrafiltration for the treatment of severe refractory congestive heart failure. J Card Fail 2004;10:380–3.
88. Ronco C, Giomarelli P. Current and future role of ultrafiltration in CRS. Heart Fail Rev October 23, 2010 [online].
89. Kazory A, Ross EA, Emerging therapies for heart failure: renal mechanisms and effects. Heart Fail Rev August 31, 2010 [online].
90. Wertman BM, Gura V, Schwarz ER. Ultrafiltration for the management of acute decompensated heart failure. J Card Fail 2008;14(9):754–9.
91. Holubek WJ, Hoffman RS, Goldfarb DS, et al. Use of hemodialysis and hemoperfusion in poisoned patients. Kidney Int 2008;74(10):1327–34.
92. Borkan SC. Extracorporeal therapies for acute intoxications. Crit Care Clin 2002;18(2):393–420.
93. Tyagi PK, Winchester JF, Feinfeld DA. Extracorporeal removal of toxins. Kidney Int 2008;74(10):1231–3.
94. Winchester JF, Harbord NB, Rosen H. Management of poisonings: core curriculum 2010. Am J Kidney Dis 2010;56(4):788–800.
95. Bayliss G. Dialysis in the poisoned patient. Hemodial Int 2010;14(2):158–67.

96. Shalkham AS, Kirrane BM, Hoffman RS, et al. The availability and use of charcoal hemoperfusion in the treatment of poisoned patients. Am J Kidney Dis 2006;48(2):239–41.

97. Chandy T, Sharma CP. Activated charcoal microcapsules and their applications. J Biomater Appl 1998;13(2):128–57.

98. Segev G, Kass PH, Francey T, et al. A novel clinical scoring system for outcome prediction in dogs with acute kidney injury managed by hemodialysis. J Vet Intern Med 2008;22(2):301–8.

99. Waniewski J, Debowska M, Lindholm B. Theoretical and numerical analysis of different adequacy indices for hemodialysis and peritoneal dialysis. Blood Purif 2006;24(4):355–66.

100. Sherman RA, Cody RP, Rogers ME, et al. Accuracy of the urea reduction ratio in predicting dialysis delivery. Kidney Int 1995;47:319–21.

101. Lowrie E, Lew N. The urea reduction ratio (URR): a simple method for evaluating hemodialysis treatment. Contemp Dial Nephrol 1991;12:11–20.

102. Daugirdas JT. The post:pre-dialysis plasma urea nitrogen ratio to estimate K.t/V and NPCR: mathematical modeling. Int J Artif Organs 1989;12:411–9.

103. Gotch FA. Is Kt/V urea a satisfactory measure for dosing the newer dialysis regimens? Semin Dial 2001;14:15–7.

104. Lopot F, Valek A. Time-averaged concentration–time-averaged deviation: a new concept in mathematical assessment of dialysis adequacy. Nephrol Dial Transplant 1988;3:846–8.

105. Sargent JA, Lowrie EG. Which mathematical model to study uremic toxicity? National Cooperative Dialysis Study. Clin Nephrol 1982;17:303–14.

106. Lowrie EG, Teehan BP. Principles of prescribing dialysis therapy: implementing recommendations from the National Cooperative Dialysis Study. Kidney Int Suppl 1983;S113–22.

107. Levine J, Bernard DB. The role of urea kinetic modeling, TACurea, and Kt/V in achieving optimal dialysis: a critical reappraisal. Am J Kidney Dis 1990;15:285–301.

108. Shinaberger JH. Quantitation of dialysis: historical perspective. Semin Dial 2001;14:238–45.

109. Sargent JA, Gotch FA. Mathematic modeling of dialysis therapy. Kidney Int Suppl 1980;10:S2–10 1980.

110. Schneditz D, Daugirdas JT. Compartment effects in hemodialysis. Semin Dial 2001;14:271–7.

111. Smye SW, Tattersall JE, Will EJ. Modeling the postdialysis rebound: the reconciliation of current formulas. ASAIO J 1999;45:562–7.

112. Daugirdas JT. Second generation logarithmic estimates of single-pool variable volume Kt/V: an analysis of error. J Am Soc Nephrol 1993;4(5):1205–13.

113. Mercadal L, Ridel C, Petitclerc T. Ionic dialysance: principle and review of its clinical relevance for quantification of hemodialysis efficiency. Hemodial Int 2005;9(2):111–9.

114. Moret K, Beerenhout CH, van den Wall Bake AW, et al. Ionic dialysance and the assessment of Kt/V: the influence of different estimates of V on method agreement. Nephrol Dial Transplant 2007;22(8):2276–82.

115. Gotch FA, Panlilio FM, Buyaki RA, et al. Mechanisms determining the ratio of conductivity clearance to urea clearance. Kidney Int Suppl 2004;(89):S3–24.

116. Carl DE, Feldman G. Estimating dialysis adequacy using ionic dialysance. Ren Fail 2008;30(5):491–8.

117. Polaschegg HD. Automatic, noninvasive intradialytic clearance measurement. Int J Artif Organs 1993;16:185–91.
118. Petitclerc T. Festschrift for Professor Claude Jacobs. Recent developments in conductivity monitoring of haemodialysis session. Nephrol Dial Transplant 1999;14:2607–13.
119. Kuhlmann U, Goldau R, Samadi N, et al. Accuracy and safety of online clearance monitoring based on conductivity variation. Nephrol Dial Transplant 2001;16:1053–8.
120. Di Filippo S, Manzoni C, Andrulli S, et al. Ionic dialysance allows an adequate estimate of urea distribution volume in hemodialysis patients. Kidney Int 2004; 66:786–91.
121. Di Filippo S, Manzoni C, Andrulli S, et al. How to determine ionic dialysance for the online assessment of delivered dialysis dose. Kidney Int 2001;59:774–82.
122. Chesterton LJ, Priestman WS, Lambie SH, et al. Continuous online monitoring of ionic dialysance allows modification of delivered hemodialysis treatment time. Hemodial Int 2006;10(4):346–50.
123. Heidenheim AP, Muirhead N, Moist L, et al. Patient quality of life on quotidian hemodialysis. Am J Kidney Dis 2003;42:36–41.
124. Lindsay RM, Leitch R, Heidenheim AP, et al. The London Daily/Nocturnal Hemodialysis Study—study design, morbidity, and mortality results. Am J Kidney Dis 2003;42:5–12.
125. Gotch FA, Levin NW. Daily dialysis: the long and the short of it. Blood Purif 2003; 21(4–5):271–81.
126. Toussaint ND. Review: differences in prescription between conventional and alternative haemodialysis. Nephrology (Carlton) 2010;15(4):399–405.
127. Leypoldt JK, Jaber BL, Zimmerman DL. Predicting treatment dose for novel therapies using urea standard Kt/V. Semin Dial 2004;17(2):142–5.
128. Depner TA, Gotch FA, Port FK, et al. How will the results of the HEMO study impact dialysis practice? Semin Dial 2003;16:8–21.
129. Casino FG, Lopez T. The equivalent renal urea clearance: a new parameter to assess dialysis dose. Nephrol Dial Transplant 1996;11:1574–81.
130. Casino FG, Marshall MR. Simple and accurate quantification of dialysis in acute renal failure patients during either urea non-steady state or treatment with irregular or continuous schedules. Nephrol Dial Transplant 2004;19:1454–66.
131. Kanagasundaram NS, Greene T, Larive AB, et al. Prescribing an equilibrated intermittent hemodialysis dose in intensive care unit acute renal failure. Kidney Int 2003;64:2298–310.
132. Debowska M, Lindholm B, Waniewski J. Adequacy indices for dialysis in acute renal failure: kinetic modeling. Artif Organs 2010;34(5):412–9.
133. Daugirdas JT, Levin NW, Kotanko P, et al. Comparison of proposed alternative methods for rescaling dialysis dose: resting energy expenditure, high metabolic rate organ mass, liver size, and body surface area. Semin Dial 2008;21(5): 377–84.

Extracorporeal Removal of Drugs and Toxins

Kelly N. Monaghan, DVM[a], Mark J. Acierno, MBA, DVM[b],*

KEYWORDS

• Drug • Toxin • Dialysis • CRRT • Dosing

This article reviews the principles of drug and toxin removal by extracorporeal circuits and the appropriate management of patients on renal replacement therapy. The principles of drug removal and therapeutic dosing in intermittent and continuous therapies as well as the use of intermittent hemodialysis for the removal of toxic substances are discussed. The considerations involved in the calculation of drug dosages and toxin removal are reviewed; however, there is a paucity of information related to veterinary patients. Therefore, much of this information is extrapolated from human data.

The type of extracorporeal therapy used can greatly affect the extent of drug and toxin removal. The available modalities include intermittent hemodialysis and three types of continuous renal replacement therapies (CRRTs). Intermittent hemodialysis is primarily a diffusive process, whereas CRRT uses a combination of diffusion, convection, and adsorption. The continuous modalities include continuous venovenous hemofiltration (CVVH), a purely convective modality; continuous venovenous hemodialysis (CVVHD), a diffusive modality; and continuous venovenous hemodiafiltration (CVVHDF), which combines the aspects of both convection and diffusion. Convection uses hydrostatic pressure to force fluids and dissolved solutes out of the blood and across the semipermeable membrane of the dialyzer, whereas diffusion uses the tendency of solutes to move from an area of high concentration to that of low concentration to remove substances from the blood. Convective modalities allow for the removal of small- and medium-sized molecules, whereas diffusive modalities are limited to smaller molecules.[1] This difference has significant implications regarding drug removal. The final mechanism of solute clearance is adsorption, which refers to the adherence of solutes to filter membranes, leading to increased removal from plasma. Adsorption is saturable and therefore plays only a minor role in clearance unless the filter is changed more frequently than every 18 to 24 hours.[2]

[a] Department of Small Animal Internal Medicine, Tufts Cummings School of Veterinary Medicine, 200 Westboro Road, North Grafton, MA 01536, USA
[b] Department of Veterinary Clinical Sciences, School of Veterinary Medicine, Louisiana State University, Skip Bertman Drive, Baton Rouge, LA 70810, USA
* Corresponding author.
E-mail address: Dialysis@vetmed.lsu.edu

Vet Clin Small Anim 41 (2011) 227–238
doi:10.1016/j.cvsm.2010.09.005
0195-5616/11/$ – see front matter © 2011 Elsevier Inc. All rights reserved.
vetsmall.theclinics.com

In addition to the type of extracorporeal therapy chosen, there are numerous other variables that play a role in determining the extent of drug removal or clearance during treatment, including the various membrane and solute characteristics.

MEMBRANE AND PRESCRIPTION CHARACTERISTICS

Membrane characteristics affecting drug clearance include the filter material, filter pore size, and filter surface area. In addition, the dialysis prescription, namely the ultrafiltration rate (Q_{uf}), dialysate rate (Q_d), blood flow rate (Q_b), and for convective modalities, the selection of pre- versus post-dialyzer replacement fluids have a considerable effect on the clearance.[3] Higher permeability filters can result in significantly higher drug clearance rates than less permeable membranes, especially for intermediate–molecular weight drugs such as vancomycin.[4] The age of the filter can also affect the clearance because its performance changes over time, particularly in continuous treatment modalities.[5]

DRUG AND TOXIN (SOLUTE) CHARACTERISTICS

The solubility, volume of distribution (V_d), molecular weight, protein binding, charge, and degree of renal and nonrenal eliminations contribute to the clearance of a drug during extracorporeal renal replacement therapies.[3] Antibiotics are arguably the most important group of drugs to consider because they are commonly administered to patients with acute kidney injury undergoing dialysis and their blood levels can be significantly influenced by extracorporeal therapy. This is a critical point because underdosing of antibiotics may result in treatment failure, whereas overdosing may result in unacceptable toxic side effects for the patient.

Several antimicrobial properties influence dialytic clearance. Solubility describes whether a drug is hydrophilic or lipophilic. Hydrophilic drugs, such as β-lactams, glycopeptides, and aminoglycosides, are unable to passively cross the plasma membrane of the cells, and so their distribution is limited to the extracellular fluid. The hydrophilic drugs are usually excreted unchanged by the kidney. Lipophilic drugs, such as macrolides, fluoroquinolones, tetracyclines, and chloramphenicol, may freely cross the plasma membrane of the cells, so they are widely distributed into the intracellular compartment. Lipophilic drugs usually require metabolism through various pathways before elimination.[3]

V_d is another crucial consideration. This term describes the volume in which a drug would need to be dissolved to obtain the observed blood concentration, assuming homogenous mixing in the body. V_d is the primary pharmacokinetic consideration used to determine the initial (loading) dose of an antimicrobial.[6] V_d determines the dose needed to achieve a desired plasma concentration (C_p) for intravenous medications using the following calculation[1]:

$$\text{Dose} = C_p \times V_d \times \text{body weight in kilograms}$$

A large V_d indicates that a drug is highly tissue bound and that only a small proportion of the drug is within the intravascular compartment, available for clearance by extracorporeal therapy.[1] V_d can be increased during critical illness and renal dysfunction but should not be affected by the selected extracorporeal therapy.[6] A large V_d (>1 L/kg) decreases the likelihood of a drug being substantially removed by hemodialysis or CRRT, assuming there is enough time for the drug to distribute. Drugs with a small V_d (≤1 L/kg) are more likely to be cleared by extracorporeal therapies.[5] A drug with a large V_d but high clearance during intermittent hemodialysis is removed from the intravascular space very quickly, but because of its distribution in tissues, only a small amount of the total drug content is removed during any single dialysis session and the plasma concentrations increase between therapies. This phenomenon is termed rebound.[1] In contrast, CRRT has a slow, continuous effect on clearance and does not result in a rapid decline in C_p, with subsequent rebound for drugs with a large V_d because time allows for continuous redistribution of the drug from the tissues to the blood.[1] Overall, drug elimination during CRRT is much slower for drugs with a large V_d than for drugs with a small V_d. Unlike with intermittent hemodialysis, adjustments in drug dosing during CRRT depend more on the relative contribution of the total body clearance rather than on the drug's V_d.[7]

Protein binding of a solute also influences clearance during extracorporeal therapies. A drug that is highly protein bound is less likely to be removed during renal replacement therapy than one that is mostly unbound because an unbound drug can cross the filter membrane, whereas a protein-bound drug cannot.[5] The unbound fraction of the drug can be used to estimate clearance in continuous modalities by multiplying this value by the Q_d or Q_{uf}.[5] However, some studies have shown that clearance in CRRT may be underestimated by this method.[6] In general, drugs that are highly protein bound are poorly cleared by extracorporeal therapies. Disease states such as uremia, hepatic dysfunction, hypoalbuminemia, and nephrotic syndrome have been shown to decrease the protein binding of drugs.[6]

The molecular weight of a solute has a significant effect on its clearance. Most drugs have a molecular weight less than or equal to 500 Dalton (Da), whereas very few have a molecular weight greater than 1500 Da. Low–molecular weight, water-soluble substances can pass easily across a dialysis membrane. However, large, protein-bound or lipid-bound solutes are more difficult to remove.[8] Most hemodialysis membranes favor diffusive clearance of low–molecular weight solutes (<500 Da), whereas membranes used in CRRT have larger pores that allow the removal of solutes via convection, with molecular weights as high as 20,000 to 30,000 Da.[1] Therefore, CRRT membranes generally have no significant filtration barrier to non–protein-bound drugs.

Finally, the ionization of a drug may affect its ability to be cleared by extracorporeal therapies, which is because of the Gibbs-Donnan effect,[1] in which retained anionic proteins on the blood side of the membrane decrease the filtration rate of cationic solutes because of complex formation with a negatively charged membrane.

PATIENT CHARACTERISTICS

In addition to the membrane and solute characteristics that may affect the removal of drugs in extracorporeal therapies, there are also several patient variables that can alter drug handling. Systemic pH levels, body fluid composition, tissue perfusion, residual renal function, and contribution of non-renal routes of elimination can affect clearance.[3] An individual's residual renal function can change continuously because of the dynamic nature of kidney injury and critical illness.[5] It is important to remember that renal disease may affect not only the renal handling of drugs but also the other pharmacokinetic parameters, including bioavailability, V_d, and hepatic metabolism, although these alterations may be difficult to quantify.[3] Drug metabolism in patients with acute kidney injury is also likely to be different from that in patients with chronic kidney disease.

Patient characteristics such as obesity, age, gender, thyroid and renal functions, and cardiac output can affect the V_d of a particular drug.[8] As discussed earlier, the V_d of a drug correlates inversely with its C_p, thus affecting the amount of intravascular drug available for elimination by extracorporeal therapies.

CLEARANCE

Clearance describes the theoretical volume of blood from which a solute is removed per unit time.[9] A patient's native clearance depends on the ability of that solute to pass across the glomerular basement membrane; it may be affected by tubular secretion or reabsorption and is a function of the molecular weight, charge, and urine flow rate.[8] Clearance in extracorporeal therapies is defined by the extraction ratio, which is the product of the Q_b and the percentage of the substance removed from the blood as it passes over the filter membrane.[10] Extracorporeal clearance is determined by the intrinsic clearance of the dialyzer membrane, duration of treatment, Q_b, Q_d, and Q_{uf}.[8] If the renal clearance of a drug is less than 25% to 30% of the total body clearance under normal conditions, impaired renal function is unlikely to have a clinically significant effect on drug elimination.[11] Likewise, CRRT has little influence on the total body clearance of such drugs, so it is not necessary to adjust the dose during renal replacement therapy because the therapy has a small effect on overall clearance.[5] Patients with concurrent liver failure may be an exception to this rule because CRRT may contribute a greater extent to clearance in those patients.[1] In continuous modalities, if the therapy is a significant source of clearance as is the case for drugs that are renally cleared, a loading dose followed by maintenance doses should be given.[5] Drug doses also need to be adjusted when the CRRT dose (ie, Q_b and Q_{uf}) is altered or when the patient's volume status changes because of the change in CRRT clearance.[6]

SOLUTE CLEARANCE AND DOSING RECOMMENDATIONS IN INTERMITTENT HEMODIALYSIS

In general, because of the relatively short course of treatment of intermittent therapies, the authors recommend administering medications as appropriate for patients with reduced renal function after the session is completed, eliminating the role of dialysis in drug clearance.

For drugs that are dosed before the treatment session, redosing may be necessary if they are significantly cleared by extracorporeal therapies. As discussed earlier, drugs that are likely to be significantly cleared are those that normally experience more than 25% to 30% renal clearance, with small V_d, low molecular weight, low protein binding, and no lipid binding. Determining the clearance can be helpful in estimating the doses for administering drugs during the treatment. The gold standard for estimating dialytic clearance is the recovery method.[12]

$$Cl_{dialysis} = (C_d \times V_{dialysate})/(C_p \times T)$$

In this equation Cl is clearance, C_d is the concentration of the drug in the dialysate, $V_{dialysate}$ is the volume of dialysate, C_p is the concentration of the drug in the plasma entering the dialyzer, and T is the time of dialysis. Alternatively, clearance can be estimated by using the arteriovenous difference method.[13]

$$Cl_{dialysate} = Q_b [(C_{arterial} - C_{venous})/C_{arterial}]$$

where $C_{arterial}$ is the drug concentration in the arterial line, and C_{venous} is the drug concentration in the venous line. This approach allows for estimation of dialysis clearance without collecting the dialysate for measurement of drug concentrations but may lead to overestimation of the actual clearance.[14] Estimates of clearance are not generally applicable from one dialyzer to the next because of the large differences in membrane characteristics, pore size, and surface area between dialyzers. Clearance increases as the surface area increases and as the membrane thickness decreases.[15]

These theoretical considerations are valuable but, to date, are not commonly used in clinical veterinary patients.

The concept of rebound is also an important consideration in intermittent hemodialysis solute clearance. Drugs with a large V_d experience a rebound in C_p because the drug is redistributed from tissues.[14] After extracorporeal removal is stopped, any drug removed from the extracellular space can have a concentration gradient that causes drugs to move from their intracellular stores to the extracellular space, leading to an increase in the plasma levels.[16]

SOLUTE CLEARANCE IN CRRT

CRRT is thought to be better tolerated by hemodynamically unstable patients and is as effective in removing solutes during a 24- to 48-hour period as a single session of intermittent hemodialysis.[17] Therefore, CRRT is a useful modality in many patients with acute kidney injury requiring renal support. The principles of solute clearance with regard to membrane, solute, and patient variables are similar in both continuous and intermittent therapies. However, the considerations are far more complex because of the prolonged course, the lack of interdialytic period, and the greater potential variabilities in Q_b, Q_d, Q_{uf}, and delivery of pre- versus post-dilution replacement fluids. There are various reports in the human literature evaluating individual medications in different settings of CRRT. These evaluations cannot be uniformly applied in different modalities, diseases, species, or drugs. It is most useful to consider each of the mechanisms in CRRT and individually assess how solute clearance is affected. However, it must be remembered that these techniques are not precise and are only a starting point for the patients until further research is performed in clinical patients. In addition, it must be kept in mind that critically ill patients with renal dysfunction are at a risk for toxicities associated with standard drug dosing because of accumulation and overdosing. However, underdosing of medications may also be life threatening, as is the case with insufficient antimicrobial treatment resulting in treatment failure or bacterial resistance. Therefore, for nontoxic drugs, doses can safely be increased beyond actual estimates and a 30% increase is recommended by some to ensure adequate dosing in CRRT.[18]

CVVHD Clearance

Solute clearance in CVVHD is primarily determined by the Q_d and the dialysate saturation (S_d). S_d represents the capacity of a drug to diffuse through a dialysis membrane and saturate the dialysate. This value can be calculated as follows[19]:

$$S_d = C_d/C_p$$

S_d can then be used to calculate diffusive clearance with the following equation[19]:

$$Cl_{CVVHD} = Q_d \times S_d$$

The efficiency of S_d and thus, solute clearance in CVVHD, a diffusion-based therapy, is determined by the concentration gradient across the membrane and the molecular weight of the solute as well as the porosity and surface area of the membrane.[19] As a solute's molecular weight increases its diffusive clearance decreases because of the limitations on size in diffusion-based therapies. This effect is greater when using conventional dialysis membranes than when using synthetic CRRT membranes. As a rule, the Q_d is equivalent to the diffusive clearance of small unbound solutes when using this treatment modality.[19]

Alternatively, S_d can be approximated by the unbound fraction of a drug when calculating clearance.[19] Increasing the molecular weight of a solute or the Q_d reduces the S_d and consequently, the clearance of the drug because of the slower rate of solute diffusion and the shortened period available for diffusion.[20]

CVVH Clearance

In CVVH, the primary determinants of solute clearance are the Q_{uf}, which drives convection, and the sieving coefficient (S_c). In convective clearance modalities, S_c is used to describe the capacity of a drug to pass through the membrane.[19] S_c is expressed as follows:

$$S_c = C_{uf}/C_p$$

where C_{uf} is the drug concentration in the ultrafiltrate.[19] For most antimicrobials, the S_c can be estimated by the extent of the unbound fraction ($S_c \approx 1 -$ protein-bound portion) because protein binding is the main determinant of drug sieving.[3] However, this estimate does provide potential for error because S_c is a dynamic value that can be affected by the age of the membrane and the amount of blood flow that is ultra-filtrated (filtration fraction).[19] Solutes that freely cross the membrane, such as urea, have an S_c equal to or close to 1.[3]

Unlike diffusive clearance, convective solute removal, or filtration, is not affected by molecular weight up to the given maximum value of the particular membrane being used.[19] The membranes used in CVVH are highly permeable, with cutoff values as high as 50,000 Da, so the molecular weight of antimicrobials have little to no effect on drug removal or sieving.[19]

Over time, drug sieving coefficients decrease likely because of a growing protein layer that builds up on the membrane surface and/or the increasing number of clotting hollow fibers in the filter.[5] The clearance of small solutes, such as urea and creatinine, is not greatly affected by an aging filter, but those of larger molecular weight solutes are likely affected.[5]

In addition, the location of the replacement solution that is used to drive solute removal, either pre- or post-filter, can influence the efficiency of solute removal.[19] In post-filter dilution, blood is not diluted before entering the filter; therefore the clearance can be determined by the product of Q_{uf} and S_c.[19]

$$Cl_{CVVH} \text{ (post)} = Q_{uf} \times S_c$$

However, if ultrafiltration is performed by pre-filter dilution, the patient's blood is diluted before entering the dialyzer, which decreases the concentration of the solute passing through the filter, thus decreasing clearance. In fact, there is a 15% to 19% reduction in clearance for urea and creatinine when the solution is administered pre-filter as compared with postfilter.[21] A similar effect would be expected for drug clearance. In this case, clearance should be corrected for the presence of pre-filter dilution solution using the following equation[19]:

$$Cl_{CVVH} \text{ (pre)} = Q_{uf} \times S_c \times [Q_b/(Q_b + Q_{uf})]$$

At present, there are no data for the calculation of clearance when a combination of pre- and postfilter dilution is used at varying ratios.

CVVHDF Clearance

CVVHDF provides further challenge in the determination of drug clearance, especially with varied Q_{uf} and Q_d rates. Initially, it might be assumed that this modality would result in an additive effect on clearance because of the use of both diffusion and convection. However, this additive effect is not produced and in fact, the opposite is true. Convection and diffusion may interact in such a way that solute removal is reduced as compared with simply adding the effects together.[19] This reduction in solute removal is because of the presence of convection-derived solute in the dialysate, which works to decrease the concentration gradient. This concentration gradient normally serves as the driving force for diffusion and therefore it lowers the overall, S_d.[19] As a result, the diffusive clearance of a drug in this modality cannot be accurately predicted.

Adsorption of drugs to the filter membranes is the final mechanism of clearance resulting from extracorporeal therapy. As discussed earlier, adsorption likely plays a significant role only if the filter is changed very frequently. However, adsorption can result in increased drug removal, and the capacity for adsorption is filter dependent. Dosing adjustments do not account for adsorption effects.[19]

The rule of thumb for drug clearance estimation at a given Q_d and Q_{uf} is that CVVH has a clearance greater than that of CVVHDF, which is greater than that of CVVHD.[5] There is a relatively small difference for small solutes, but the difference can be marked for larger molecules, such as vancomycin which has a molecular weight of 1485 Da.[4]

DOSING ADJUSTMENTS IN CRRT

Dosing adjustments in the various modalities of CRRT can be estimated by using available drug dosing recommendations extrapolated from human clearance studies, by measuring or estimating clearance, or by therapeutic drug monitoring. Given the countless variables that affect clearance of solutes, including the membrane, drug, and patient characteristics, it is nearly impossible to establish a complete dosing guide for every drug in each patient. Therefore, it is important to understand the different principles discussed earlier that affect the clearance and determine the likelihood and extent of drug clearance. Several references from the human literature provide dosing guidelines for specific drugs based on studies in limited patient pools.[6,17,19,22] An additional reference that reports the dialyzability of drugs is the Web site, http://www.ckdinsights.com, which publishes an annual list of numerous drugs and their likelihood of being cleared by the various extracorporeal therapies.[23]

The loading dose of a drug depends largely on the V_d and need not be adjusted in CRRT.[3] However, V_d may be altered by many factors in critically ill patients including total body water, perfusion, protein binding, lipid solubility, pH levels, and active transport systems and may be larger in critically ill patients.[3] Consequently, dosages may need to be increased in critically ill patients to avoid inadequate dosing.

Drugs that are significantly cleared during CRRT, including amikacin, amoxicillin, ceftazidime, fluconazole, metronidazole, sulfamethoxazole, trimethoprim, and vancomycin, may require maintenance dosage increases compared with standard renal dosing by increasing the amount of each dose or decreasing the interval between doses.[3] For the concentration-dependent antibiotics (aminoglycosides, fluoroquinolones, metronidazole), the rate of microbial kill is closely related to the peak concentration above the minimum inhibitory concentration (MIC), therefore it is better to increase the drug dose while maintaining a fixed interval for drugs that are significantly cleared by CRRT.[19] The rate of kill for time-dependent antibiotics (eg, β-lactams, macrolides, tetracyclines, lincosamides) is related to the length of time for which the concentrations exceed the MIC. Therefore the recommended method of administration during CRRT is to shorten the drug-dosing interval and to maintain a fixed dose.[19] This shortened interval can be estimated by the following equation[19]:

$$IV_{EC} = IV_{anuria} \times [Cl_{NR}/(Cl_{EC} + Cl_{NR})]$$

where Iv_{EC} is the dosing interval during CRRT, Iv_{anuria} is the dosing interval in a patient with anuria, Cl_{EC} is extracorporeal clearance, and Cl_{NR} is the nonrenal clearance.

After establishing the clearance of a drug in a particular modality, a dose can be determined. First, the dosing recommendations in patients with anuria should be addressed, by the following equation:

$$D_{anuria} = D_{normal} \times Cl_{anuria}/Cl_{normal}$$

where D is the dose.[1] Here, dosing adjustments can be performed by reducing the dose in proportion to the reduction in total body clearance. Pharmacokinetic tables can be used to determine the established clearance values and dosing intervals in people with or without anuria. In CRRT, dose can be established using the following basic equation[1]:

$$D = D_{normal} (Cl_{anuria} + Cl_{CRRT})/Cl_{normal}$$

Similarly, this equation can be applied to intermittent hemodialysis, if needed. But making these estimates can be time consuming and expensive and requires known pharmacokinetic data which is often unavailable for veterinary species.

Li and colleagues[22] reviewed the current human literature and summarized the following available methods of estimating the antibacterial dose in patients receiving CRRT:

a. CVVH[24]

$$D = C_{ss} \times UBf \times Q_{uf} \times I$$

b. CVVH[25]

$$D = D_n [Cl_{NR} + (Q_{uf} \times S_c)/Cl_n]$$

c. CVVHDF[1]

$$D = D_n \times [P_x + (1-P_x) \times (Cl_{CRtot}/Cl_{CRn})]$$

d. All modes[25]

$$D = D_{anuria}/[1 - (Cl_{EC}/[Cl_{EC} + Cl_{NR} + Cl_R])]$$

where C_{ss} is the blood concentration at steady state, Cl_{CRn} is the normal creatinine clearance, Cl_{CRtot} is the sum or renal and extracorporeal creatinine clearance, Cl_n is the normal total drug clearance, Cl_R is the renal clearance, I is the dosing interval, P_x is the extrarenal clearance fraction (which is equal to Cl_{anuria}/Cl_n), and UBF is the unbound fraction of the drug.

SPECIFIC THERAPY FOR TOXICITIES OR DRUG OVERDOSES

In addition to their use in acute kidney injury and chronic kidney disease, hemodialysis, CRRT, and charcoal hemoperfusion are the commonly used adjunctive treatments for the management of specific drug overdoses and toxic ingestions when activated charcoal, gastric lavage, available antidotes, and supportive care are ineffective or impossible because of the patient's condition. The principles that guide the removal of a certain toxin are similar to those for the removal of drugs and other solutes. As such, the factors that affect the dialyzability of a toxin include protein binding, V_d, molecular weight, solubility, and charge. These factors have been addressed in greater detail earlier.

Indications for dialysis in the case of toxin ingestion include a strong history or known exposure to a dialyzable toxin, persistence of a significant blood toxin concentration, and lack of an effective medical antidote.[26] Hemodialysis is the method of choice for most toxicities and especially for the removal of low–molecular weight water-soluble molecules, with a small V_d, that are not protein or lipid bound.[8] As mentioned earlier, the intravascular concentrations of drugs/toxins that are lipid soluble and have a high V_d decline very quickly after the first session of hemodialysis but increase again as the serum levels reequilibrate from the extravascular space during the interdialysis period. Sessions may need to be repeated because of this rebound effect.[8] CRRT has a theoretical benefit for patients who have ingested substances that are highly lipid bound and have a large V_d with consequently slow transit times from the extravascular to the intravascular space.[8] In this case, clearance is achieved through prolonged treatment sessions using slower blood flow rates. However, CRRT is uncommonly used in these cases unless the solute displays significant rebound or the patient is unable to tolerate the normally used high flow rates because of hemodynamic instability.[8] Hemoperfusion is another modality that may be used for cases of intoxication. This method uses a charcoal filter, either alone or in circuit with the dialysis filter, to adsorb toxins from the blood by binding to activated charcoal or resin rather than by diffusing out of the blood down a concentration gradient.[8] Hemoperfusion filters are saturable and therefore require an exchange every 2 to 3 hours.[8] The use of these charcoal filters is limited by availability, expense, and their large priming size. In human medicine, hemoperfusion has been largely replaced by high-flux high-efficiency hemodialysis and is limited to select cases (eg, paraquat, theophylline).[27] Peritoneal dialysis has low efficacy in removing toxins and is therefore not recommended.[8]

In general, for removal of dialyzable toxins in a nonazotemic patient that is not at a high risk of dialysis disequilibrium, it is recommended to maximize the size of the dialyzer, Q_b, and duration of the session to achieve maximum clearance.[26] Blood flow rates of 10 to 20 mL/kg/min and treatment times of 4 to 6 hours are selected to ensure complete toxin removal.[26] In patients that are azotemic and/or at a high risk for osmotic shifts, the intensity of the dialysis prescription should be limited and CRRT or multiple sequential treatments may be used instead.

Ethylene glycol intoxication is one of the more common toxin ingestions that benefit from hemodialysis in veterinary medicine. Dialysis is able to remove not only the parent compound but also the toxic metabolites of ethylene glycol. The V_d of ethylene glycol is equal to that of total body water, and it has a low molecular weight (62 Da), therefore it is cleared by hemodialysis. The parent compound is metabolized by alcohol dehydrogenase to the more toxic glycolic acid. Glycolic acid is further metabolized to oxalate, which can then deposit in renal tubules as crystals. Dialytic removal is recommended in patients with severe metabolic acidosis (pH<7.25), acute kidney injury or electrolyte imbalances that do not respond to conventional treatment, a significant level of circulating metabolites, or an alcohol level greater than 50 mg/dL.[28] The patient should be dialyzed until the toxic alcohol level is less than 20 mg/dL or for a minimum of 8 hours, with a second session 12 hours later if levels are not available.[28] The elimination half-life in people with ethylene glycol intoxication treated with dialysis is 155 minutes as compared with 626 minutes without dialysis.[29] If dialysis is performed early, before the metabolism of ethylene glycol or renal injury, the prognosis is excellent. However, if the patient already has acute kidney injury, the prognosis is significantly worse than with other causes of acute kidney injury because of the severity of renal injury caused by this toxin.[30]

Other dialyzable toxins reported in human medicine include aminoglycosides, methanol, salicylates, theophylline, paraquat, acetaminophen, lithium, mushrooms, antiepileptics, sedative hypnotics, and metformin.[8,27] In addition, there have been 2 case reports of baclofen intoxication in dogs that were successfully dialyzed using hemodialysis alone and in combination with hemoperfusion.[31,32] Although there are reported cases of dialysis being used to treat lily intoxication and grape/raisin intoxication in cats and dogs, the toxic principle of these plants is not known and therefore dialysis is primarily used for the treatment of the associated acute kidney injury rather than for the removal of the toxin.[33,34]

SUMMARY

Intermittent hemodialysis and CRRT are becoming increasingly more available to veterinary patients for treatment of acute kidney injury and toxin ingestion. Medications are commonly administered to these patients for comorbidities and treatment of the underlying cause of renal injury, but there are no data in veterinary patients as to the appropriate dosing strategies. At present, recommendations must be extrapolated from the human literature and applied practically based on the information available about a given drug, including its V_d, solubility, protein binding, charge, and molecular weight. When medications with a low therapeutic index are used, it is necessary to use therapeutic drug monitoring to avoid toxicity.

The principles of drug handling can also be applied to drug overdoses and other toxicities to predict the dialyzability of the agent. In addition, the human literature may be useful in determining the likelihood of success with various medications and poisonings.

REFERENCES

1. Bugge JF. Pharmacokinetics and drug dosing adjustments during continuous venovenous hemofiltration or hemodiafiltration in critically ill patients. Acta Anaesthesiol Scand 2001;45:929–34.
2. Tian Q, Gomersall LD, Wong A, et al. Effect of drug concentration on adsorption of levofloxacin by polyacrylonitrile haemofilters. Int J Antimicrob Agents 2006;28: 147–50.
3. Bouman CS. Antimicrobial dosing strategies in critically ill patients with acute kidney injury and high-dose continuous veno-venous hemofiltration. Curr Opin Crit Care 2008;14:654–9.
4. Joy MS, Matzke GR, Frye RF, et al. Determinants of vancomycin clearance by continuous venovenous hemofiltration and continuous venovenous hemodialysis. Am J Kidney Dis 1998;31:1019–27.
5. Churchwell MD, Mueller BA. Drug dosing during continuous renal replacement therapy. Semin Dial 2009;22(2):185–8.
6. Choi G, Gomersall CD, Tian Q, et al. Principles of antibacterial dosing in continuous renal replacement therapy. Crit Care Med 2009;37(7):2268–82.
7. Bohler J, Donauer J, Keller F. Pharmacokinetic principles during continuous renal replacement therapy: drugs and dosage. Kidney Int Suppl 1999;56(72):S24–8.
8. Bayliss G. Dialysis in the poisoned patient. Hemodial Int 2010;14:158–67.
9. Goodman JW, Goldfarb DS. The role of continuous renal replacement therapy in the treatment of poisoning. Semin Dial 2006;19:402–7.
10. Daugirdas JT. Physiologic principles and urea kinetic modeling. In: Daugirdas JT, Blake PG, Ing TS, editors. Handbook of dialysis. 4th edition. Philadelphia: Wolters Kluwer; 2007. p. 25–58.

11. Levy G. Pharmacokinetics in renal disease. Am J Med 1977;62:461–3.
12. Gibson TP. Problems in designing hemodialysis drug studies. Pharmacotherapy 1985;5:23–9.
13. Lee CS, Maybury TC. Drug therapy in patients undergoing haemodialysis. Clin Pharm 1984;9:42–66.
14. Atkinson AJ, Umans JG. Pharmacokinetic studies in hemodialysis patients. Clin Pharmacol Ther 2009;86:548–52.
15. Gibson TP, Matusik E, Nelson ED, et al. Artificial kidneys and clearance calculations. Clin Pharmacol Ther 1976;20:720–6.
16. Tyagi PK, Winchester JF, Feinfeld DA. Extracorporeal removal of toxins. Kidney Int 2008;74:1231–3.
17. Trotman RL, Williamson JC, Shoemaker DM, et al. Antibiotic dosing in critically ill adult patients receiving continuous renal replacement therapy. Clin Infect Dis 2005;41:1159–66.
18. Kroh UF. Drug administration in critically ill patients with acute renal failure. New Horiz 1995;3:748–59.
19. Kuang D, Ronco C. Adjustment of antimicrobial regimen in critically ill patients undergoing continuous renal replacement therapy. Yearbook of Intensive Care and Emergency Medicine 2007;2007(12):592–606.
20. Reetze-Bonorden P, Bohler J, Keller E. Drug dosage in patients during continuous renal replacement therapy: pharmacokinetic and therapeutic considerations. Clin Pharm 1993;24:162–79.
21. Brunet S, Leblanc M, Geadah D, et al. Diffusive and convective solute clearances during continuous renal replacement therapy at various dialysate and ultrafiltrate flow rates. Am J Kidney Dis 1999;34:486–92.
22. Li AM, Gomersall CD, Choi G, et al. A systematic review of antibiotic dosing regimens for septic patients receiving continuous renal replacement therapy: do current studies supply sufficient data? J Antimicrob Chemother 2009;64:929–37.
23. Johnson CA. 2010 Dialysis of drugs. CKD Insights; 2010. p. 1–56.
24. Golper TA, Marx MA. Drug dosing adjustment during continuous renal replacement therapy. Kidney Int Suppl 1998;66:S165–8.
25. Schetz M, Ferdinande P, Van den Berghe G, et al. Pharmacokinetics of continuous renal replacement therapy. Intensive Care Med 1995;21(7):612–20.
26. Cowgill LD, Langston CE. Role of hemodialysis in the management of dogs and cats with renal failure. Vet Clin North Am Small Anim Pract 1996;26(6):1347–78.
27. Holubek WJ, Hoffman RS, Goldfarb DS, et al. Use of hemodialysis and hemoperfusion in poisoned patients. Kidney Int 2008;74:1327–34.
28. Winchester JF, Boldur A, Oleru C, et al. Use of dialysis and hemoperfusion in treatment of poisoning. In: Daugirdas JT, Blake PG, Ing TS, editors. Handbook of dialysis. 4th edition. Philadelphia: Wolters Kluwer; 2007. p. 300–19.
29. Moreau CL, Kern SW, Tomaszewski CA, et al. Glycolate kinetics and hemodialysis clearance in ethylene glycol poisoning. J Toxicol Clin Toxicol 1998;36:659–66.
30. Segev G, Kass PH, Francey T, et al. A novel clinical scoring system for outcome prediction in dogs with acute kidney injury managed by hemodialysis. J Vet Intern Med 2008;22:301–8.
31. Scott NE, Francey T, Jandrey K. Baclofen intoxication in a dog successfully treated with hemodialysis and hemoperfusion coupled with intensive supportive care. J Vet Emerg Crit Care 2007;17:191–6.

32. Torre DM, Labato MA, Rossi T, et al. Treatment of a dog with severe baclofen intoxication using hemodialysis and mechanical ventilation. J Vet Emerg Crit Care 2008;18:312–8.
33. Stanley SW, Langston CE. Hemodialysis in a dog with acute renal failure from currant toxicity. Can Vet J 2008;49:63–6.
34. Langston CE. Acute renal failure caused by lily ingestion in six cats. J Am Vet Med Assoc 2002;220(1):49–52, 36.

Nutritional Considerations for the Dialytic Patient

Denise A. Elliott, BVSc, PhD

KEYWORDS

• Nutrition • Dialysis • Malnutrition • Protein

There are numerous causes of protein energy malnutrition.[1–10] The simplest and most apparent cause is inadequate dietary intake mainly because of anorexia secondary to uremic toxicity and anorexigenic effects of concurrent disease.[4,11] Dietary intake is also compromised by nausea and vomiting, which can often occur at the onset of the dialytic treatment, especially if the flow rates are rapidly increased. Concurrent diseases and endocrine abnormalities, including insulin resistance, hyperglucagonemia, and hyperparathyroidism, can also contribute to a catabolic state.[12,13] The kidney is also an important metabolic organ that synthesizes some amino acids (cysteine, tyrosine, arginine, serine).[14] It is possible that the loss of these activities in kidney failure can also promote wasting.

In addition to the removal of uremic toxins, the dialytic process is also associated with the removal of free amino acids, peptides or bound amino acids, and water-soluble vitamins, each of which can contribute to wasting.[15–18] Total dialysate amino acid losses of 6 to 13 g per hemodialysis session have been reported in human patients (0.09–0.17 g/kg body weight [BW]).[16,18–20] Dialysate total amino acid loss in healthy dogs has been reported to be 0.12 g/kg BW.[21] This loss can be even higher in peritoneal dialytic patients who develop peritonitis. Losses of glucose can also occur if glucose-free dialysate is used.

Sustained blood loss is an unavoidable consequence of advanced renal disease and hemodialysis. Blood loss is associated with frequent blood drawing for laboratory testing, occult gastrointestinal bleeding secondary to the uremic syndrome, and the sequestration of blood in the hemodialyzer and dialytic tubing. Blood is a rich source of protein; hence, these losses can contribute to protein deficiency and muscle wasting. Furthermore, anemia can contribute to apathy, lethargy, and reduced food intake, further compounding the wasting syndrome. Therefore, the veterinary care team should be conscientious and make every attempt to minimize unnecessary or excessive blood withdrawals.

Research and Development, Royal Canin SAS, BP-4 650, Avenue de la petite Camargue, 30470 Aimargues, France
E-mail address: Denise.elliott@royalcanin.us

Vet Clin Small Anim 41 (2011) 239–250
doi:10.1016/j.cvsm.2010.10.001
0195-5616/11/$ – see front matter © 2011 Elsevier Inc. All rights reserved.

vetsmall.theclinics.com

Dialytic patients also have increased catabolism from the chronic inflammatory state of uremia, exposure to the extracorporeal circuit (hemodialyzer membranes, tubing, and catheters), or impure dialysate.[22] Hemodialysis activates the complement cascade, triggering the release of catabolic cytokines and acute-phase proteins.[22–28] Activation of these inflammatory mediators as a consequence of the hemodialysis procedure per se has adverse catabolic effects on protein metabolism. An enhanced release of amino acids from skeletal muscle has been reported with sham hemodialysis (ie; in vivo passage of blood through a hemodialyzer but without circulating dialysate) in normal humans.[23,24] In addition, increased plasma concentrations of 3-methylhistidine in sham hemodialytic normal humans demonstrated the importance of increased protein breakdown in the net catabolic process induced by blood-membrane contact.[24] Inflammation may contribute or cause malnutrition because both tumor necrosis factor alpha and interleukin 6 are anorexigens.[29,30] This muscle breakdown can be further aggravated by acidemia.[31,32]

Protein energy malnutrition and chronic inflammation are significant overlapping factors that influence morbidity and mortality.[22,33] Given the significant association of malnutrition with morbidity and mortality, it is clear that every effort must be made to identify those patients at risk and implement proactive nutritional therapies designed to minimize or reverse these complications.

NUTRITIONAL ASSESSMENT

Repeated frequent assessments of the nutritional status of the patient receiving dialytic therapy are extremely important for the timely recognition of nutritional deficiencies. Early proactive nutritional intervention may be able to prevent or improve malnutrition in these patients. In humans, the protein energy nutritional status at the start of chronic dialysis treatment is a good predictor of longevity. Therefore, there is strong impetus to make every effort to maintain or improve nutritional intake during treatment.

Nutritional assessment uses information contained in the history taking, physical examination, and laboratory data to screen for early indicators of malnutrition. All of this information should be clearly documented in the medical record. Indeed, the problem-oriented approach Subjective, Objective, Assessment, Plan (SOAP) should be used for nutritional support to ensure that all metabolic and nutritional problems of patients are assessed and planned for. Accurate documentation facilitates communication between the various members of the veterinary care team and strengthens the importance of nutrition in the overall care of the patient. The importance of clear documentation is exemplified by the study of 276 critically ill dogs in which a negative energy balance occurred in 73% of the hospitalization days.[34] The negative energy balance was attributed to poorly written orders in 22% of cases.

The dietary record should detail the exact amount of food that the patient is consuming, rather than the amount of food that a patient has been offered. If the patient is not consuming food, then the duration of inappetence or anorexia should be recorded. If the patient is consuming food, the name, manufacturer, type (dry, wet, semimoist), amount fed each day (cans or standard 237-mL cups), frequency of food intake, and method of feeding (ad libitum vs meal feeding) should be recorded. The number and type of snacks or human foods that are offered each day and the potential access to other pets' food should be determined. The history should also be explored to fully understand when the current diet was implemented and any changes in the diet or dietary intake, which have recently occurred. The incidence of vomiting and/or diarrhea should be noted, and any additional factors that can affect the nutritional plan, such as cardiovascular instability; concurrent diseases; fluid, electrolyte, or acid-base imbalance; or metabolic abnormalities, such as hyperglycemia or hypertriglyceridemia, should be recorded.

The BW should be included in the examination of every patient, and for hospitalized patients, it should be recorded daily. BW provides a rough measure of total body energy stores, and changes in BW typically parallel energy and protein balance. In the healthy animal, BW varies little from day to day. However, additional challenges arise in the dialytic patient because BW can be falsely altered by dehydration or fluid accumulation. Therefore, the BW should be interpreted in conjunction with the body condition score (BCS) and muscle cachexia score.

The BCS focuses on the assessment of body fat. The 2 most commonly used scoring systems in small animal practice are a 5-point system in which a BCS of 3 is considered ideal or a 9-point system in which a BCS of 5 is considered ideal. The muscle cachexia score evaluates the loss of metabolically active lean body mass. The initial loss of lean body mass can be subtle and is usually first noted in the epaxial, gluteal, scapular, or temporal muscles. Using a subjective cachexia scoring system facilitates the identification of those patients either with cachexia or at risk of impending cachexia.[35]

Bioelectrical impedance analysis (BIA) is an electrical method of assessing body composition, which has the potential of quantifying total body water, fluid volumes, body cell mass, and fat-free mass. Body cell mass approximates the metabolically active lean body tissue. Hence, BIA may be used to provide instantaneous information of body composition.[36,37]

Biochemical indicators of malnutrition include hypoalbuminemia, decreased blood urea nitrogen, hypocholesterolemia, anemia, and lymphopenia. However, alterations of these common laboratory indicators are not specific for malnutrition and are often indistinguishable from those that can occur with concurrent disease.

The historical data on BW change, dietary intake, gastrointestinal symptoms influencing oral intake/absorption, and physical examination are used collectively to categorize the patient as appropriately nourished, mildly malnourished or suspected of being malnourished, or severely malnourished. Nutritional assessment is not used to determine who should be fed and who should not. Rather it is used to determine how much food and what types of nutrient alterations are required and the most effective way of feeding the patient. If the patient is not voluntarily consuming adequate nutrition, intervention in the form of enteral or parenteral nutrition is required. Regardless of the method of nutritional support selected, it is imperative to reassess the effect of the support, making nutritional assessment a routine and cyclical process.

METHODS OF ADMINISTRATION

The simplest and most obvious way to provide nutrition is to offer food to be consumed orally. However, patients with severe kidney disease often have reduced appetites, have an altered sense of taste or smell, or are anorexic. There are multiple possible causative factors that contribute to anorexia. Dialysis can effectively reduce the blood concentration of some of the uremic toxins that contribute to anorexia, and it is clear that a patient seems to feel better and eats willingly at the cessation of a dialytic session. However, despite effective clearance of many metabolic products of uremia, additional metabolic disorders that can contribute to anorexia (eg, chronic inflammatory conditions, anemia) persist. Furthermore, dialytic patients often require multipharmacologic agents to help manage the consequences of kidney disease. Anorexia is a potentially significant side effect of some of these drugs. All of these factors in combination contribute to reduced caloric intake and refusal of diet.

Practical measures to improve intake include the use of highly odorous foods, warming the food before feeding, and stimulating eating by positive reinforcement with petting and stroking behavior. The total daily caloric intake can be divided into several smaller meals per day. It is important that fresh food should be offered at each meal, and the amount that the pet does not eat should be removed and discarded. Appetite stimulants can be considered but are typically not an effective solution to continually ensure adequate caloric intake. Enteral tube feeding or parenteral nutritional therapy should be implemented for patients reluctant to eat appropriate amounts of food ad libitum.

Enteral feeding, facilitated by the placement of nasoesophageal, esophagostomy, or gastrostomy tube, is recommended in all patients who can tolerate them because enteral feeding helps to maintain the gastrointestinal barrier and prevent the translocation of bacteria and systemic infections.[38] Enteral feeding of caloric veterinary renal diets blended with water or using specifically formulated liquid diets should be used. The amount of water to liquefy the commercial diet together with the volumes used for flushing the enteral feeding device should be closely monitored. Dialytic patients are often fluid intolerant. In cases with extreme fluid intolerance, the amount of water used to liquefy the diet can be replaced with a commercial liquid preparation. This unique situation requires the assistance of a board-certified veterinary nutritionist to ensure that the nutritional requirements of the pet are met by the combination of 2 commercial formulations.

The feeding solution can be administered intermittently in a meal-type pattern or, for hospitalized patients, by continuously using a syringe pump. Several enteral renal formulations have been specifically developed for human use; however, these formulations should be closely evaluated before administration to dogs or cats to ensure that they contain adequate amounts of protein; amino acids, such as taurine and arginine; and arachidonic acid (cats). Enteral feeding via gastrostomy tube has been shown to be an effective way to manage dogs with kidney disease.[39]

Parenteral nutrition is indicated for patients with severe gastrointestinal or neurologic dysfunction that precludes the use of the enteral route to meet the nutrient requirements. In addition, the patient must be able to tolerate the additional fluid load.[40] Parenteral nutrition is largely divided into partial parenteral nutrition (PPN) or total parenteral nutrition (TPN). TPN refers to the provision of the daily caloric requirement and essential nutrients and is typically formulated using 50% dextrose, 8.5% amino acids with electrolytes, and 20% intralipid. Consequently, the solution is hyperosmolar and requires administration into a central vein, such as the cranial vena cava. Historically, a dedicated central catheter has been recommended for parenteral nutrition. Clearly, this recommendation is not a viable option for patients with an indwelling hemodialysis vascular access catheter. One port of the hemodialysis access catheter can be used to administer the TPN solution; however, this option is far from ideal and increases the likelihood of thrombosis or infection of the vascular access, critical complications that minimize the effectiveness of hemodialysis and are life threatening for the patient.

PPN involves the administration of isotonic nutritional solutions through a peripheral vein, thereby avoiding the requirement of a central vein necessary for TPN. However, PPN cannot provide the complete nutritional requirements for a patient because the solution is required to be isotonic to avoid thrombophlebitis. A PPN solution is typically formulated with a combination of 5% dextrose, 8.5% amino acids (without electrolytes), and 20% intralipid to provide approximately 50% of the resting energy requirement (RER). The osmolality of the final solution should be in the range of 300 to 600 mOsm/kg to prevent thrombophlebitis. Therefore, PPN should only be used as an adjunct to supplement oral intake or to supply partial temporary nutritional support in animals that are expected to return to normal oral intake in less than 5 days and that can also tolerate the additional fluid burden of the PPN solution.

PPN products are expensive and require strict aseptic formulation, administration, and special monitoring procedures to avoid sepsis and metabolic complications. Modified amino acid formulations for human patients with acute renal failure are available. These preparations have been formulated on the hypothesis that endogenous urea could be use to synthesize nonessential amino acids. However, it is not clear that these specialized formulations are any more effective than traditional amino acid formulations.

There are 2 additional methods that can be considered to provide partial nutritional support and complement enteral feeding. Amino acids and additional glucose can be added to the dialysate fluid, from where they diffuse into the body during the dialytic procedure.[41] Alternatively, supplemental amino acids, glucose, and/or lipids can be infused during the hemodialysis procedure.[42] With this intradialytic form of nutrition, the nutrient solutions are added to the "venous" side of the extracorporeal circuit as the blood leaves the hemodialyzer. This process may also help to minimize the decrease in the circulating amino acid pool as a result of the dialytic process (see the section Protein). The benefits of intradialytic nutrition in human patients are controversial. Intradialytic parenteral nutrition has been shown to improve markers of nutritional status, such as plasma protein concentrations and anthropometric measurements.[43] However, it is not yet clear if intradialytic parenteral nutrition has a significant effect on morbidity or mortality.[42,44,45] Furthermore, intradialytic nutrition has not been reported in canine or feline patients receiving dialysis.

ENERGY

Monitoring caloric intake is vital because consuming too few calories compromises nitrogen balance and causes loss of lean body mass. Studies in human dialytic patients indicate that dietary energy intakes and body fat are low.[46,47] The energy requirements of canine or feline dialytic patients are unknown. The energy expenditure of an individual patient may be assessed by indirect calorimetry; however, this technique is not widely available in veterinary hospitals.[48] For patients with acute kidney injury, provision of the RER ($70 \times$ [weight in kilogram]$^{0.75}$) is logical. In such critically ill patients, there is little advantage to providing excess calories because energy metabolism can promote hypercapnia, especially if pulmonary function is impaired.

The amount of energy to provide to the patient with CKD who is receiving dialysis should approach the maintenance energy requirements (canine, $132 \times$ [BW in kilogram]$^{0.67}$; feline, $50 \times$ BW in kilogram). However, energy requirements vary widely, and hence the energy intake needs to be adjusted according to individual patient needs based on serial nutritional assessment. Carbohydrate and fat provide the nonprotein sources of energy in the diet. Diets designed for the management of renal failure are usually formulated with a relatively high fat content because fat provides approximately twice the energy per gram than carbohydrate and increases palatability and energy density of the diet, which allows the patient to obtain nutritional requirements from a relatively smaller volume of food. The reduction in feeding volume with high–energy density diets can help minimize nausea and vomiting secondary to gastric distension.

PROTEIN

Adequate amounts of dietary protein must be provided to the dialytic patient to prevent protein malnutrition, and yet, excessive amounts of dietary protein must be avoided because the accumulation of protein metabolites derived from excessive dietary protein exacerbates uremia. Ideally, protein intake should be matched with catabolism to promote a positive nitrogen balance. However, the measurement of total nitrogen output (TNO) to determine nitrogen balance is not practical for clinical use.

The urea nitrogen appearance rate (UNA) can be used to estimate TNO, and an estimation of nitrogen balance can be determined when the nitrogen intake is known.[49,50] The UNA refers to the amount of urea that appears in body fluids and all body outputs, including urine, dialysate, draining tracts, and diarrhea, and is calculated as follows:

UNA (g/d) = urinary urea nitrogen (g/d) + change in body urea nitrogen (g/d) + dialysate urea nitrogen (g/d)

Change in body urea nitrogen (g/d) = (BUN_f − BUN_i g/L/d) × BW_i (kg) × 0.6 L/kg + (BW_f − BW_i kg/d) × BUN_f (g/L) × 1.0 L/kg

where i and f are the initial and final values for the period of measurement; BUN is the blood urea nitrogen; BW is expressed in kilograms; 0.6 is an estimate of the fraction of body water, which is water; and 1.0 is the fractional distribution of urea in the weight that is gained or lost (ie, 100%).

The UNA is highly correlated with the total urinary nitrogen content in hospitalized, critically ill dogs. The relationship between UNA and TNO is described as TNO = (1.3 × UNA) + 1.3.[50] When both the nitrogen intake and the UNA are known, nitrogen balance can be estimated from the difference between the nitrogen intake and TNO calculated from the UNA.[51] Non–urea nitrogen losses can be estimated as 0.031 g of nitrogen/kg/d. Extensive nitrogen losses that may occur with severe diarrhea, exudative lesions, or peritonitis need to be accounted in the calculation of TNO. The UNA provides a simple and an inexpensive and accurate measurement of net protein breakdown and usually correlates closely with TNO. To calculate the dietary protein intake (g/d), the TNO is multiplied by 6.25.

The UNA can also be calculated in patients receiving hemodialysis by urea kinetic modeling. Central to this has been the concept of Kt/V, which describes the dose of dialysis as the hemodialyzer clearance of urea (K) times the duration of dialysis (t) divided by the urea distribution volume (V). Sargent and colleagues[51] described Kt/V as calculated from predialysis and postdialysis BUN and the next predialysis BUN through urea kinetic modeling, a mathematical description of the generation and removal of urea from patients undergoing hemodialysis. This approach has been modified by Daugirdas[52] to a formula, which uses predialysis and postdialysis BUNs, predialysis and postdialysis BWs, and the duration of dialysis to calculate single- or double-pool Kt/V.

Nitrogen balance studies in humans suggest that the average protein intake necessary to maintain nitrogen balance in hemodialytic patients is 1.0 to 1.1 g protein/kg BW/d and 1.05 to 1.20 g protein/kg BW/d in chronic peritoneal dialytic patients.[53] These protein requirements are approximately 30% higher than the recommended daily allowance for healthy adult humans and are designed to compensate for substrate loss during dialytic therapy.[54] Although the optimal dietary protein requirements for cats and dogs undergoing dialysis therapy are not known, it is clear from human medicine that canine and feline patients need more that the minimal protein requirements for healthy pets (the National Research Council [NRC] canine minimal requirement, 2.62 g/kg $BW^{0.67}$; the NRC feline adult minimal requirement, 3.97 g/kg $BW^{0.67}$); 25% to 30% seems a reasonable estimate.[55] This level clearly needs to be adjusted based on consecutive nutritional assessment to minimize excesses in azotemia while simultaneously avoiding protein malnutrition.

High-quality protein sources must be used in the formulation of restricted protein diets to minimize the risks of essential amino acid deficiency. Additional supplementation of taurine should be considered for both canine and feline patients. Although not reported in canine or feline patients, serum and tissue levels of taurine are often low in humans receiving dialysis. Furthermore, studies in healthy adult dogs report significant reductions in plasma taurine concentration during the hemodialysis period, and an average of 47 mg of taurine appeared in the dialysate over a 3-hour treatment period.[21] Although these losses may be insignificant to a healthy adult animal, the potential risk of development of dilated cardiomyopathy secondary to taurine deficiency is a complication that the dialytic patient cannot afford.

VITAMINS, MINERALS, ACID-BASE BALANCE

Virtually all dialytic patients may require restriction of sodium, potassium, and phosphorus. Calcium and magnesium intakes need to be adjusted according to the levels in the dialysate and nutritional intake to maintain the concentrations within the reference range. There is minimal information available on the trace element requirements for the dialytic patient. Clearly, iron supplementation is necessary to complement erythropoietin therapy.

Dietary restriction of phosphate is necessary to control blood phosphate concentrations and the subsequent consequences of hyperphosphatemia and secondary hyperparathyroidism. However, dietary restriction alone is unlikely to adequately maintain blood phosphorus concentrations. Most, if not all, dialytic patients require the addition of phosphate binders to the diet.

The requirements for sodium and water must be managed for each patient individually. Those patients with oliguria/anuria require extreme sodium and water restriction to minimize overhydration and its attendant consequences. Patients receiving peritoneal dialysis can typically tolerate more normal sodium and water intakes because salt and water are removed daily by the hypertonic dialysate. Adequate or mildly increased sodium and water intakes in the patients receiving peritoneal dialysis may facilitate the clearance of small molecules into the dialysate.

The kidney is the major route of excretion of potassium. The patient with renal failure who is receiving dialysis is more likely to develop hyperkalemia as a result of a combination of dietary intake, acidosis, oliguria, hyperaldosteronism secondary to decreased renin secretion by the diseased kidney, and concurrent pharmacologic agents, such as angiotensin-converting enzyme inhibitors. Therefore, the dietary potassium intake needs to be modified for each patient to maintain normokalemia.

Deficiencies of water-soluble vitamins are likely because of the combination of poor food intake and the loss of vitamins during the dialysis treatment. B vitamins are critical for many energy-generating reactions in the body, and vitamin B deficiencies may be a contributing cause of anorexia. Therefore, prevention or replacement of the losses may be beneficial in correcting or preventing anorexia. Commercially available renal failure diets contain additional amounts of water-soluble vitamins, and further supplementation may not be required. If, however, a home-prepared diet is formulated, it may be prudent to additionally provide a B-complex vitamin supplement to ensure adequate daily intake. Supplementation with vitamin A is not recommended because serum retinol–binding protein and vitamin A are increased in CKD.[56]

Metabolic acidosis increases net protein degradation and is associated with the symptoms of lethargy and weakness.[32,57] Protein restriction lessens acidosis by decreasing the endogenous generations of acidic products of protein metabolism. The dialysate is also formulated to assist normalization of acid-base balance predominately by the provision of bicarbonate; however, additional alkali therapy may be needed to maintain a bicarbonate concentration higher than 18 mmol/L.

ADDITIONAL NUTRIENTS OF INTEREST

Dialysis is associated with the production of acute-phase proteins, oxidants, reactive carbonyl compounds, and proinflammatory cytokines that are toxic to the endothelium. These factors can be involved in some of the adverse cardiovascular and cerebral events that can occur in humans on dialysis.[22] Oxidative stress is also particularly significant in patients with acute kidney injury. Decreased plasma concentrations of antioxidant vitamins have been reported in dialytic patients compared with healthy humans, with loss of vitamins A, E, and C into the ultrafiltrate. It seems prudent to provide an antioxidant-enriched diet to maintain normal antioxidant status.[58] Although antioxidant stress has not been evaluated in canine and feline patients receiving dialysis, it is clear that antioxidant status is reduced in cats with CKD, antioxidant supplementation reduces markers of DNA damage in cats with stage II/III CKD, and antioxidant status improves glomerular filtration rate in dogs with surgically induced renal mass reduction.[59–61] Therefore, it is logical that dietary antioxidants can be beneficial to dogs and cats receiving dialysis treatments. The most effective levels and synergistic combinations remain to be determined.

L-Carnitine is a quaternary amine that facilitates the transfer of long-chain fatty acids into the mitochondria for energy generation. Serum-free carnitine concentrations and skeletal carnitine concentrations have been reported to be decreased in human dialytic patients and the concentration of serum acylcarnitines is increased.[62] The reduction in carnitine concentrations is most likely the result of losses into the ultrafiltrate, reduced dietary intake, and perhaps reduced synthesis as a consequence of protein malnutrition (L-carnitine is synthesized from the amino acids lysine and methionine).[63,64] Carnitine supplementation is recommended for humans with clinical symptoms or dialysis complications, including intradialytic arrhythmias and hypotension, low cardiac output, interdialytic and postdialytic symptoms of malaise or asthenia, general weakness or fatigue, skeletal muscle cramps, and decreased exercise capacity or low peak oxygen consumption.[53,65,66] Carnitine supplementation has also been recommended for refractory anemia for which no other apparent cause can be determined.

PHARMACOLOGIC STRATEGIES TO PROMOTE ANABOLISM

It is often difficult to overcome the catabolic state of advanced uremia and achieve positive nitrogen balance with nutritional support alone. Therefore, recent interest has focused on evaluating pharmacologic strategies to promote anabolism in human patients receiving dialysis. Metabolic interventions, including the administration of insulin, anabolic steroids, growth hormone, thyroid hormone, antiglucocorticoids, insulin-like growth factor 1, epidermal growth factor, β hepatocyte growth factor, β2 adrenergic agonists, intracellular proteolytic pathway inhibitors, adenine nucleotides, to facilitate the anabolic process and reduce protein degradation are currently being evaluated as nutritional adjunctives in human medicine.[67,68] Although some of these agents seem promising, improvements in morbidity and mortality in humans have not yet been reported. The efficacy of these interventions in canine and feline patients remains to be seen.

SUMMARY

Although there is a paucity of the literature available on the nutritional requirements of the canine or feline patient receiving dialysis treatments, there is a wealth of information available in human medicine. These studies provide valuable insight, and logical recommendations can be obtained as long as the human data and recommendations are always interpreted in the light of the true, and often unique, nutritional requirements of the dog and cat. It is clear that nutritional intervention must be implemented for patients receiving dialysis. Malnutrition must be prevented. Nutritional therapy must be continually adjusted based on frequent nutritional assessments.

REFERENCES

1. Lowrie EG, Lew NL. Death risk in hemodialysis patients: the predictive value of commonly measured variables and an evaluation of death rate differences between facilities. Am J Kidney Dis 1990;15:458.
2. Cianciaruso B, Brunori G, Kopple JD, et al. Cross-sectional comparison of malnutrition in continuous ambulatory peritoneal dialysis and hemodialysis patients. Am J Kidney Dis 1995;26:475.
3. Palop L, Martinez JA. Cross-sectional assessment of nutritional and immune status in renal patients undergoing continuous ambulatory peritoneal dialysis. Am J Clin Nutr 1997;66:498S.
4. Dwyer JT, Cunniff PJ, Maroni BJ, et al. The hemodialysis pilot study: nutrition program and participant characteristics at baseline. The HEMO Study Group. J Ren Nutr 1998;8:11.
5. Aparicio M, Cano N, Chauveau P, et al. Nutritional status of haemodialysis patients: a French national cooperative study. French Study Group for Nutrition in Dialysis. Nephrol Dial Transplant 1999;14:1679.
6. Williams AJ, McArley A. Body composition, treatment time, and outcome in hemodialysis patients. J Ren Nutr 1999;9:157.
7. Boddy K, King PC, Will G, et al. Iron metabolism with particular reference to chronic renal failure and haemodialysis. Br J Radiol 1970;43:286.
8. Mahajan SK, Prasad AS, Rabbani P, et al. Zinc deficiency: a reversible complication of uremia. Am J Clin Nutr 1982;36:1177.
9. Kopple JD, Mercurio K, Blumenkrantz MJ, et al. Daily requirement for pyridoxine supplements in chronic renal failure. Kidney Int 1981;19:694.
10. Bellinghieri G, Savica V, Mallamace A, et al. Correlation between increased serum and tissue L-carnitine levels and improved muscle symptoms in hemodialyzed patients. Am J Clin Nutr 1983;38:523.
11. Kopple JD, Berg R, Houser H, et al. Nutritional status of patients with different levels of chronic renal insufficiency. Modification of Diet in Renal Disease (MDRD) Study Group. Kidney Int Suppl 1989;27:S184.
12. McCaleb ML, Wish JB, Lockwood DH. Insulin resistance in chronic renal failure. Endocr Res 1985;11:113.
13. Sherwin RS, Bastl C, Finkelstein FO, et al. Influence of uremia and hemodialysis on the turnover and metabolic effects of glucagon. J Clin Invest 1976;57:722.
14. Mitch WE, Chesney RW. Amino acid metabolism by the kidney. Miner Electrolyte Metab 1983;9:190.

15. Blumenkrantz MJ, Gahl GM, Kopple JD, et al. Protein losses during peritoneal dialysis. Kidney Int 1981;19:593.
16. Wolfson M, Jones MR, Kopple JD. Amino acid losses during hemodialysis with infusion of amino acids and glucose. Kidney Int 1982;21:500.
17. Kopple JD, Blumenkrantz MJ, Jones MR, et al. Plasma amino acid levels and amino acid losses during continuous ambulatory peritoneal dialysis. Am J Clin Nutr 1982;36:395.
18. Ikizler TA, Flakoll PJ, Parker RA, et al. Amino acid and albumin losses during hemodialysis. Kidney Int 1994;46:830.
19. Gutierrez A, Bergstrom J, Alvestrand A. Hemodialysis-associated protein catabolism with and without glucose in the dialysis fluid. Kidney Int 1994;46:814.
20. Chazot C, Shahmir E, Matias B, et al. Dialytic nutrition: provision of amino acids in dialysate during hemodialysis. Kidney Int 1997;52:1663.
21. Elliott DA, Marks SL, Cowgill LD, et al. Effect of hemodialysis on plasma amino acid concentrations in healthy dogs. Am J Vet Res 2000;61:869.
22. Kalantar-Zadeh K, Ikizler TA, Block G, et al. Malnutrition-inflammation complex syndrome in dialysis patients: causes and consequences. Am J Kidney Dis 2003;42:864.
23. Gutierrez A, Alvestrand A, Wahren J, et al. Effect of in vivo contact between blood and dialysis membranes on protein catabolism in humans. Kidney Int 1990;38:487.
24. Gutierrez A, Bergstrom J, Alvestrand A. Protein catabolism in sham-hemodialysis: the effect of different membranes. Clin Nephrol 1992;38:20.
25. Pereira BJ, Shapiro L, King AJ, et al. Plasma levels of IL-1 beta, TNF alpha and their specific inhibitors in undialyzed chronic renal failure, CAPD and hemodialysis patients. Kidney Int 1994;45:890.
26. Witko-Sarsat V, Friedlander M, Nguyen Khoa T, et al. Advanced oxidation protein products as novel mediators of inflammation and monocyte activation in chronic renal failure. J Immunol 1998;161:2524.
27. Bologa RM, Levine DM, Parker TS, et al. Interleukin-6 predicts hypoalbuminemia, hypocholesterolemia, and mortality in hemodialysis patients. Am J Kidney Dis 1998;32:107.
28. Mezzano D, Pais EO, Aranda E, et al. Inflammation, not hyperhomocysteinemia, is related to oxidative stress and hemostatic and endothelial dysfunction in uremia. Kidney Int 2001;60:1844.
29. Garcia-Martinez C, Llovera M, Agell N, et al. Ubiquitin gene expression in skeletal muscle is increased by tumour necrosis factor-alpha. Biochem Biophys Res Commun 1994;201:682.
30. Sarraf P, Frederich RC, Turner EM, et al. Multiple cytokines and acute inflammation raise mouse leptin levels: potential role in inflammatory anorexia. J Exp Med 1997;185:171.
31. Mitch WE, May RC, Maroni BJ. Review: mechanisms for abnormal protein metabolism in uremia. J Am Coll Nutr 1989;8:305.
32. Mehrotra R, Kopple JD, Wolfson M. Metabolic acidosis in maintenance dialysis patients: clinical considerations. Kidney Int Suppl 2003;88:S13–25.
33. Zimmermann J, Herrlinger S, Pruy A, et al. Inflammation enhances cardiovascular risk and mortality in hemodialysis patients. Kidney Int 1999;55:648.
34. Remillard RL, Darden DE, Michel KE, et al. An investigation of the relationship between caloric intake and outcome in hospitalized dogs. Vet Ther 2001;2:310.
35. Freeman LM. Nutritional modulation of cardiac disease. WALTHAM Focus Special Edition Advances in Clinical Nutrition 2000;36.

36. Elliott D, Cowgill L. Body composition analysis in uremic dogs: methods and clinical significance. In: American College of Veterinary Internal Medicine Veterinary Medical Forum. San Diego (CA): The American College of Veterinary Internal Medicine; 1998. p. 661.
37. Elliott DA. Evaluation of multifrequency bioelectrical impedance analysis of the assessment of extracellular and total body water in healthy cats and dogs [PhD thesis]. Davis (CA): University of California - Davis; 2001.
38. Deitch EA, Bridges RM. Effect of stress and trauma on bacterial translocation from the gut. J Surg Res 1987;42:536.
39. Elliott DA, Riel DL, Rogers QR. Complications and outcomes associated with use of gastrostomy tubes for nutritional management of dogs with renal failure: 56 cases (1994–1999). J Am Vet Med Assoc 2000;217:1337.
40. Druml W, Kierdorf HP, Working group for developing the guidelines for parenteral nutrition of the German Association for Nutritional Medicine. Parenteral nutrition in patients with renal failure—guidelines on parenteral nutrition, chapter 17. Ger Med Sci 2009;18:1.
41. Kopple JD, Bernard D, Messana J, et al. Treatment of malnourished CAPD patients with an amino acid based dialysate. Kidney Int 1995;47:1148.
42. Dukkipati R, Kalantar-Zadeh K, Kopple JD. Is there a role for intradialytic parenteral nutrition? A review of the evidence. Am J Kidney Dis 2010;55:352.
43. Smolle KH, Kaufmann P, Holzer H, et al. Intradialytic parenteral nutrition in malnourished patients on chronic hemodialysis therapy. Nephrol Dial Transplant 1995;10:1411.
44. Chertow GM, Ling J, Lew NL, et al. The association of intradialytic parenteral nutrition administration with survival in hemodialysis patients. Am J Kidney Dis 1994;24:912.
45. Cano NJ, Fouque D, Roth H, et al. Intradialytic parenteral nutrition does not improve survival in malnourished hemodialysis patients: a 2-year multicenter, prospective, randomized study. J AM Soc Nephrol 2007;18:2583.
46. Wolfson M, Strong CJ, Minturn D, et al. Nutritional status and lymphocyte function in maintenance hemodialysis patients. Am J Clin Nutr 1984;39:547.
47. Blumenkrantz MJ, Kopple JD, Gutman RA, et al. Methods for assessing nutritional status of patients with renal failure. Am J Clin Nutr 1980;33:1567.
48. O'Toole E, McDonell WN, Wilson BA, et al. Evaluation of accuracy and reliability of indirect calorimetry for the measurement of resting energy expenditure in healthy dogs. Am J Vet Res 2001;62:1761.
49. Maroni BJ, Steinman TI, Mitch WE. A method for estimating nitrogen intake of patients with chronic renal failure. Kidney Int 1985;27:58.
50. Michel KE, King LG, Ostro E. Measurement of urinary urea nitrogen content as an estimate of the amount of total urinary nitrogen loss in dogs in intensive care units. J Am Vet Med Assoc 1997;210:356.
51. Sargent J, Gotch F, Borah M, et al. Urea kinetics: a guide to nutritional management of renal failure. Am J Clin Nutr 1978;31:1696.
52. Daugirdas JT. Simplified equations for monitoring Kt/V, PCRn, eKtV, and ePCRn. Adv Ren Replace Ther 1995;2:295.
53. Fouque D, Vennegoor M, ter Wee P, et al. EBPG guideline on nutrition. Nephrol Dial Transplant 2007;22(Suppl 2):ii45.
54. Rand WM, Pellett PL, Young VR. Meta-analysis of nitrogen balance studies for estimating protein requirements in healthy adults. Am J Clin Nutr 2003;77:109.
55. National Research Council of the National Academies N. Nutrient requirements of dogs and cats. Washington, DC: National Academies Press; 2006.

56. Raila J, Forterre S, Kohn B, et al. Effects of chronic renal disease on the transport of vitamin A in plasma and urine of dogs. Am J Vet Res 2003;64:874.

57. May RC, Hara Y, Kelly RA, et al. Branched-chain amino acid metabolism in rat muscle: abnormal regulation in acidosis. Am J Physiol 1987;252:E712.

58. Morena M. Rationale for antioxidant supplementation in hemodialysis patients. Saudi J Kidney Dis Transpl 2001;12:312.

59. Yu S, Paetau-Robinson I. Dietary supplements of vitamins E and C and beta-carotene reduce oxidative stress in cats with renal insufficiency. Vet Res Commun 2006;30:403.

60. Brown SA. Oxidative stress and chronic kidney disease. Vet Clin North Am Small Anim Pract 2008;38:157.

61. Keegan RF, Webb CB. Oxidative stress and neutrophil function in cats with chronic renal failure. J Vet Intern Med 2010;24:514.

62. Hiatt WR, Koziol BJ, Shapiro JI, et al. Carnitine metabolism during exercise in patients on chronic hemodialysis. Kidney Int 1992;41:1613.

63. Guarnieri G, Toigo G, Crapesi L, et al. Carnitine metabolism in chronic renal failure. Kidney Int Suppl 1987;22:S116.

64. Wanner C, Forstner-Wanner S, Rossle C, et al. Carnitine metabolism in patients with chronic renal failure: effect of L-carnitine supplementation. Kidney Int Suppl 1987;22:S132.

65. Ahmad S, Robertson HT, Golper TA, et al. Multicenter trial of L-carnitine in maintenance hemodialysis patients. II. Clinical and biochemical effects. Kidney Int 1990;38:912.

66. Golper TA, Wolfson M, Ahmad S, et al. Multicenter trial of L-carnitine in maintenance hemodialysis patients. I. Carnitine concentrations and lipid effects. Kidney Int 1990;38:904.

67. Kopple JD. Uses and limitations of growth factors in renal failure. Perit Dial Int 1997;17(Suppl 3):S63.

68. Dong J, Ikizler TA. New insights into the role of anabolic interventions in dialysis patients with protein energy wasting. Curr Opin Nephrol Hypertens 2009;18:469.

Index

Note: Page numbers of article titles are in **boldface** type.

A